# Hall Jackson and
the Purple Foxglove

J. Worth Estes

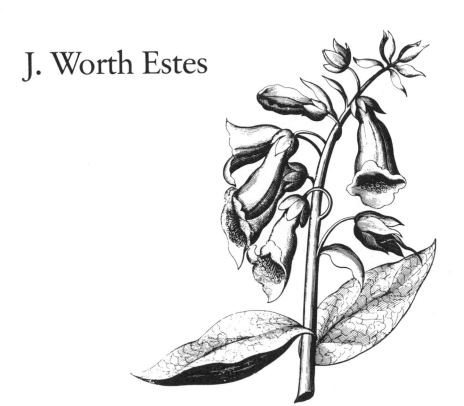

# Hall Jackson and the Purple Foxglove

## MEDICAL PRACTICE AND RESEARCH IN

## REVOLUTIONARY AMERICA 1760-1820

Published by the University Press of New England

Hanover, New Hampshire 1979

Copyright © 1979 by Trustees of Dartmouth College
All Rights Reserved
Library of Congress Catalogue Card Number 79-63083
International Standard Book Number 0-87451-173-9
Printed in the United States of America

Library of Congress Cataloging in Publication data
will be found on the last printed page of this book.


**The University Press of New England**

Brandeis University
Clark University
Dartmouth College
University of New Hampshire
University of Rhode Island
University of Vermont

For my wife, Cynthia,
and in memory of
Joseph A. Estes and
Paul Dudley White
because all of them have
contributed to the making
of the author of this book

# Acknowledgments

I AM ENTHUSIASTICALLY INDEBTED to the many people who have directed me to sources I should probably never have discovered on my own. Some of these people who have so generously shared their knowledge, and their collections, with me, in the spirit of the characters in this book, are acknowledged in citations to their specific contributions, for which I am most grateful. I would like to stress my very special thanks to Mrs. Henry B. Shepard, who, as the result of our chance meeting described on page 271, below, provided the necessary stimulus to the development of this study.

Richard J. Wolfe, Curator of Rare Books and Manuscripts and Garland Librarian at the Boston Medical Library in the Francis A. Countway Library of Medicine, was my continually indispensable guide to the standard as well as the unconventional medical historical literature. Edward W. Pelikan, M.D., of the Department of Pharmacology and Experimental Therapeutics at the Boston University School of Medicine, made important calculations for me, directed me to the first importations of the foxglove, tried to teach me the limits of what can legitimately be inferred from even the most appropriate statistical analyses, and generally encouraged this study in a way that probably makes him unique among department chairmen. Philip Cash, Ph.D., of Emmanuel College, Boston, guided my understanding of the relationships among medicine, war, and politics in the Revolutionary War period.

Among other scholars and librarians who furnished valuable clues and assistance are Harriett Lacey and Frank C. Mevers, Ph.D., of the New Hampshire Historical Society, in Concord, and Dorothy M. Vaughan of the Portsmouth Public Library. Lloyd E. Hawes, M.D., now at the University of Massachusetts Medical Center, in Worcester; Diana Long Hall, Ph.D., of Boston University; Lester S. King, M.D., at the *Journal of the American Medical Association*; and John J. Byrne, M.D., at the Boston City Hospital and Boston University School of Medicine all made helpful comments on early versions of the manuscript, as did Dr. Cash.

Jenifer Woodworth and, before her, Joyce Greene, cheerfully typed—and retyped—the evolving manuscript.

My wife Cynthia followed Hall Jackson's footsteps with me all over New England during the eight years since I began this study, and our good friends William and Amey Wieting of York Harbor, Maine, provided us hospitality and good cheer of the kind that one likes to associate with the eighteenth century while we explored Jackson's New Hampshire and local archives. Dr. Wieting arranged my first opportunity for displaying Hall Jackson's work in public, at a meeting, appropriately, of the Portsmouth Medical Society. Irene Buonapane generously contributed an original drawing.

Small portions of this work have appeared in the following, although more recently discovered data have permitted me to modify or amplify some of my earlier conclusions: *Bulletin of the History of Medicine*, 47 (1973): 394–408; ibid., 50 (1976): 536–552; *Harvard Medical Alumni Bulletin*, 49 no. 4 (March/April 1975): 16–21; ibid., 50 no. 4 (March/April 1976): 31–39; *Boston University Medical Centerscope*, 7, no. 3 (Summer 1975): 22–29; *Bulletin of the New York Academy of Medicine*, 52 (1976): 617–626; and *Journal of the History of Medicine and Allied Sciences*, 31 (1976): 271–291.

Throughout I have used exact transcripts of both original spellings and grammatical constructions, unless noted otherwise, and I have clarified only the most confusing punctuation. I note this here to avoid the repetitious use of the often distracting convention of *sic*.

*Boston, Massachusetts*                                                    J.W.E.
*November 1978*

# Contents

# Tables

# Figures

# Illustrations

# Preface

IN 1785 Dr. William Withering of Birmingham, one of England's most distinguished scientists, published the first large-scale study of any drug in which sound principles of scientific investigation were employed. Within six months his *Account of the Foxglove*, in which he clearly demonstrated that digitalis can relieve the symptoms of dropsy, now called congestive heart failure, had reached Portsmouth, New Hampshire. That town's leading physician, Dr. Hall Jackson, recognized the value of the new drug for his own practice; and since foxglove did not grow in America, he immediately wrote to Withering to ask for a supply of seeds.

The immediate stimulus of this book was my discovery of Withering's original letter of reply, with which he sent Jackson seeds for growing the new wonder drug. My investigations were designed to explore several questions that the letter raised:

1. What was Hall Jackson's professional life like? What kinds of medical and surgical skills did he have, how had he acquired them, and how did he use them? To what extent did they contribute to the well-being of his patients?

2. What was the state of the health of the population of eighteenth-century New Hampshire? How did it compare with that of the rest of America, and of Europe, at the same time? That is to say, what was the medical milieu in which Hall Jackson, William Withering, and their colleagues, worked?

3. How did these physicians think of the origins and symptoms of dropsy? How did they come to understand the way in which digitalis benefited their patients? What kinds of data helped them to reach these conclusions?

4. What difference did it make, after all, that Jackson was the first to introduce digitalis to American medicine, and what were the immediate consequences of his having done so?

5. Finally, how was medical research carried out in the Age of Enlightenment? What was its extent, what were its methods, and how were its results communicated? What difference did medical research make in the care of patients two hundred years ago?

In the course of answering these questions, insofar as they are answerable, I will use the introduction of the foxglove into therapeutics as a case history of medical practice in the eighteenth century. Because foxglove is still the source of our most helpful drug for treating heart failure, its history will help us to view the written roots of medicine in the perspective of their authors' own times and places and ideas, and, in turn, to place today's medical knowledge and practice into their longer perspectives.

I have found it expedient and necessary to answer my questions in chapters that tell two interconnected but sometimes separable stories. The first concerns Dr. Jackson and his medical practice in the context of health and disease in eighteenth-century America. The second describes the introduction of digitalis into the medicine of eighteenth-century America and of England, then the source of most American medical knowledge. Because neither story can be completely subsidiary to the other, the book consists of two interwoven narratives. On the one hand, conditions of health and disease converged with Jackson's professional skills, such as post-mortem examinations, the special needs of military surgery, and techniques for preventing smallpox, all of which had been important since long before Jackson began his practice. On the other hand, the equally ancient clinical problem of dropsy converged, on a date which can be precisely determined, with digitalis, the first drug to promise predictable relief from the disease.

The evidence for these convergences comes largely from communications between and among the physicians and natural philosophers of America and England. In fact, my two major stories will intersect most clearly in Withering's letter to Jackson. The apparent digressions in those stories are designed to illuminate that intersection in particular, and to bring the aggregate of my explorations within a common framework.

The world was to me a secret which I desired to divine. Curiosity, earnest research to learn the hidden laws of nature, gladness akin to rapture, as they were unfolded to me, are among the earliest sensations I can remember ...None but those who have experienced them can conceive of the enticements of science. In other studies you go as far as others have gone before you, and there is nothing more to know; but in a scientific pursuit there is continual food for discovery and wonder.
> —*Victor Frankenstein, in Mary Shelley,*
> Frankenstein, *1816*

There is no general dogma [of medicine] other than this: disease is to be treated by anything that is proved to cure it.
> —*Oliver Wendell Holmes, 1869.*

CHAPTER ONE

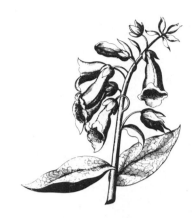

# 'The Grand Phiz for Enockalation'

## A COLONIAL PHYSICIAN

## AT WORK

THE STORY OF the introduction of the purple foxglove into general medical use, from Leonhard Fuchs's naming of the plant in 1542, through Dr. William Withering's careful ten-year evaluation of the drug and establishment of its therapeutic standards, to its present place in the treatment of the failing heart, has been told in several different settings.[1] The story of the foxglove in newly independent America, however, has not been told in terms of medical practice. Withering's study appeared at the end of the Enlightenment, the period in which reason, human understanding, and, most of all, science began to gain on authority, despotism, and tradition. It inaugurated what might be called the birth of pharmacology, even though pharmacology as a distinct discipline did not appear for another seventy years.

Dr. Hall Jackson, the man responsible for the systematic introduction of digitalis into America, was well known in the New England colonies and states as both physician and patriot. Like Withering, he was a man of many talents and interests; Boorstin has commented, "The man who could not be a little bit of everything was not qualified to be an American...Versatility was no longer merely a virtue; it was a necessity."[2] Withering and Jackson together exemplified Henry May's definition of the Enlightenment as consisting "of all those who believe two proposi-

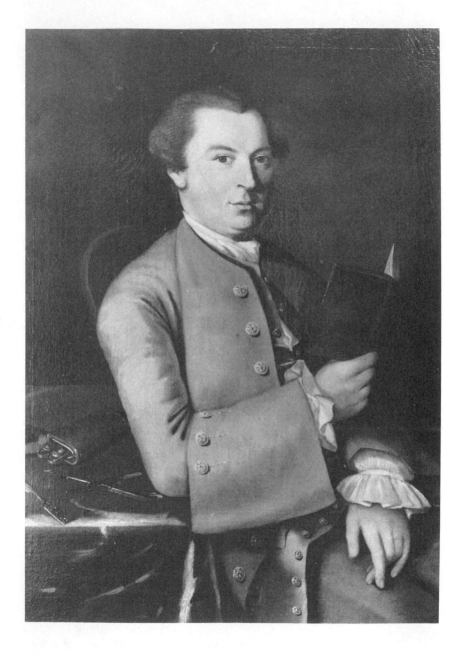

1. *Dr. Hall Jackson. Portrait attributed to John Singleton Copley. (Mead Art Museum, bequest of Herbert L. Pratt)*

tions: first, that the present age is more enlightened than the past; and second, that we understand nature and man best through the use of our natural faculties." When Benjamin Franklin made a proposal for promoting useful knowledge among the British plantations in America in 1743, among the topics he suggested for correspondence among the members of what became the American Philosophical Society were "new methods of curing or preventing diseases...and all philosophical experiments that let light into the nature of things, tend to increase the power of man over matter, and multiply the conveniences or pleasures of life." Jackson's professional career was entirely consistent with Franklin's goals for his new Society's members, and the physician's tempestuous foray into the Revolutionary War will illustrate, in a special way, May's generalization that "liberty...was associated above all with rationality." [3]

At the time Withering's book appeared, Dr. Hall Jackson (1739–1797) was a prominent New Hampshire physician. Born in Hampton, he had studied medicine with his father, Dr. Clement Jackson, after the family moved to nearby Portsmouth. It has been reported that Hall attended lectures and teaching rounds at the Middlesex Hospital in London for three years, and that when he returned to Portsmouth he opened an apothecary shop, while continuing his medical studies with his uncle, Dr. Anthony Emery, in Hampton. Conflicting but definitive evidence from Jackson's own pen, showing that he spent only the year 1762 abroad, will be presented later. He does seem to have received some form of recognition in London for "an ingenious invention by which a ball was extracted from a gun shot wound, which had baffled the skill of all the Surgeons." [4]

Before the Revolution, Jackson and three other physicians, including his brother-in-law, Dr. Stephen Little, were practicing in Portsmouth. Thus the overall ratio of about one physician to one thousand population throughout the colonies also held for Portsmouth in Hall Jackson's day, although it ranged as high as about seven per thousand in Williamsburg. Recalculation of Eric Christianson's data shows that the number of medical practitioners in eighteenth-century Massachusetts doubled more rapidly (every 27 years) than did the general population (every 37 years), as the doctor-to-population ratio increased from 1.0 per thousand in 1700 to 2.4 in 1780, although Boston doctors contributed less to the increased ratio than they do today. In the late twentieth century, estimates of the ratio of actively practicing physicians to the American population range from about 0.65 to 1.8 per thousand, although even these estimates vary widely with population density. At present, no substantive increments in medical manpower needs are being solicited; perhaps the two-hundred-year-old traditional ratio is the optimum. Nonetheless, Whitfield Bell's assessment of the colonists' medical needs is familiar today: "The people called for more medical care while the physicians complained that they could not make a living." [5]

Of the approximately 3500 practitioners of medicine in America at the outbreak of the Revolution, only 5 percent had university degrees in

Table 1.
M. D. Degrees Earned by
Americans at the University of
Edinburgh to 1820

| Years | Number of M.D.'s Awarded to Americans |
|-------|---------------------------------------|
| 1740–1750 | 1 |
| 1751–1760 | 5 |
| 1761–1770 | 25 |
| 1771–1780 | 22 |
| 1781–1790 | 23 |
| 1791–1800 | 42 |
| 1801–1810 | 30 |
| 1811–1820 | 11 |
| TOTAL | 159 |

The first M.D. degree was awarded to
John Moultrie of Charleston, South
Carolina, in 1749.
SOURCE: Samuel Lewis, "List of the
American Graduates in Medicine in
the University of Edinburgh from
1705 to 1866, with Their Theses,"
*New England Historical and Genea-
logical Register*, 42 (1888), 159–165.

medicine. Few Americans could afford to attend English or European
schools, and few English medical graduates were likely to emigrate to a
relatively undeveloped area like colonial America. For instance, 159
Americans earned degrees at the leading eighteenth-century medical
school, Edinburgh, from 1749 through 1820, although some attended
other European schools, chiefly in Leyden and Germany, and some
studied with individual teachers, such as the renowned Hunter brothers
in London, or on hospital wards.[6]

Table 1 shows that the Revolutionary War between England and her
colonies did not diminish the number of Americans who sought the best
medical education obtainable abroad. The postwar years saw an increase
over what might have been expected on the basis of the increasing population of immigrants to America. The decline in the numbers of Americans at Edinburgh after the first decade of the nineteenth century may
be attributable to the growing sense of independence, and of nation-

alism, after the War of 1812, as well as to the growing number of medical schools at home.

Most colonial American doctors, in fact, received no academic training at all. They learned their profession, in what they were now coming to think of as their native country, under any of several alternative systems. The prospective doctor might, for instance, be indentured, or he might pay a fee of as much as a hundred pounds for up to seven years of on-the-job training as an apprentice.[7]

The quality of instruction for medical apprentices varied widely, because standardization of the curriculum was not possible. Some must have learned by imitating their preceptors, without understanding much of what they were doing. Formal curricula in the Edinburgh tradition were evolving at the two American medical schools founded before the Revolution, Pennsylvania and King's College (renamed Columbia in 1792), but neither was yet having any marked influence on the national medical scene. Not until three more had been established, at Harvard, Philadelphia, and Dartmouth, by the end of the century, could America even begin to meet its own medical manpower needs.[8]

Colonial laws designed to ensure uniform standards of training as a prerequisite to professional licensing were few. The only state medical society chartered before the War was that of New Jersey, formed in 1766 as much to protect qualified physicians against unfair competition from quacks as to upgrade professional standards.[9]

We can conclude, from what we can learn of Hall Jackson's own career, that his training with his father and his uncle was not only adequate but, at least, stimulating. He also participated in the training of future physicians himself, with certain limits: a friend wrote that Jackson "was remarkable for his friendship, his readiness to advise, instruct, & patronize all young physicians within the sphere of his acquaintance, whom he considered worthy of being countenanced."[10]

In 1765 he married Mary Dalling, widow of Royal Navy Lieutenant Daniel Wentworth, a member of the prominent family that provided New Hampshire's last two Royal governors. The Jacksons had three children, but both sons died young, as did their daughter's only daughter, Hall Jackson's only grandchild. It has been reported that at the time of his marriage he gave up his apothecary shop to devote himself exclusively to the practice of medicine. According to a newspaper advertisement, however, his shop was in operation as late as 1774.[11]

Eighteenth-century medical books and articles often were written for the lay public as much as for the profession. In fact, newspaper accounts provide some of the most detailed accounts of Dr. Jackson's professional accomplishments, while recording kinds of medical problems that occurred more frequently in colonial New Hampshire than now. For instance, in February 1768 the *New Hampshire Gazette* reported:

> About three weeks ago a young lad of 17 Years of Age, belonging to Hampton, in crossing Winnipisaukee Pond, froze both his legs to

that Degree, there was a Necessity of cutting them both off last Week; which was perform'd by Dr. Jackson of this Town.[12]

A week later the paper printed a follow-up on this case, and added an even more bizarre medical story:

> We hear from Hampton, that the Lad mentioned in our last, who had his Legs cut off, is in a fine Way of Recovery. The Servant Boy of Mr. Gibbs of this Town, who had his Leg taken off the next Day, after the above, is also in a good Way: This Boy ran away from his Master, and secreted himself on board a Vessel in the Harbour in order to go off, but she not sailing so soon as expected, he lay on board three Days & Nights, the Weather being extremly cold, he froze in such a manner that he lost Part of both Feet immediately; about a Week after he was seiz'd with those terrible Symptoms the Lock'd Jaw, and convulsive Cramp, he lay near three Weeks stiff and immoveable, no Force that could be apply'd would bend one Joint of his Body, nor could the Edge of the Knife be forced between his Teeth: the Nerves and Tendons of the remaining Parts of one foot being bare, with violent and almost constant Spasms in the same Leg, it was tho't adviseable to take it off, which gave him immediate Relief; his bad Symptoms are gone off, and he is so far recovered as to astonish every one who has seen him.—We hear this Lad took in eighteen days one Ounce two Drams of solid Opium, besides a large Quantity of Musk, notwithstanding which, he did not sleep one Hour in twenty-four during the whole time. Doctor HALL JACKSON has had the Care of this Lad as well as the former.[13]

Even if the boy could not have had the benefit of general anesthesia during the amputation, his immediate postoperative feeling must have been one of great relief.

It is probable that even the more potent narcotic painkillers of today would not have helped him to sleep any more than he did, considering the extent of his injuries. The possibility of major surgery without anesthesia is frightening today, but eighteenth-century surgeons could accomplish it because, as one pointed out with pride, "almost the whole of the sufferings of the patient may be comprized within the space of two minutes."[14] In Jackson's own journals he listed only three amputations which he performed, of "crockett's Arm" (April 1780), "Dan.l Littlefields Arm" (September 1794), and an unidentified man's thigh (June 1786). The latter patient died less than twenty-four hours later.[15]

In 1791 Jackson treated a Captain Smith for a "broken" plantaris tendon in the ankle. That the injury was actually a sprain is suggested by the treatment, which consisted of an "anodyne" or pain-killing ointment composed of nightshade, tobacco, henbane, Jimson weed, and turpentine. Not even Jackson could have supposed it would be helpful to a physical separation in the tendon.[16]

Another aspect of Jackson's surgical reputation was based on his skill in performing cataract operations. He properly refused to operate on persons who had any sight remaining in either eye, "but when wholly blind nothing can be feared. The inflammation that sometimes happens after the operation in a diseased eye, might so effect the one not diseased as to deprive it of sight."[17] This condition is now known as sympathetic uveitis.

The cataract operation that Jackson performed was called couching. Used by the Romans and described as early as the first century A.D. by Celsus (born 25 B.C.), couching involved dislocating the pathologically opacified lens of the eye with an instrument introduced through the cornea.[18] Preparation for eye surgery in the eighteenth century was as trying for the surgeon as for the patient:

> An assistant stands behind the patient, who puts his right hand under the patient's chin, after having covered the right eye, supposing it to be the left which is to be operated upon; the assistant then places the back part of the patient's head on his breast, at the same time directing the face upwards, to prevent the discharge of the vitreous humor. He afterwards lifts up the superior eyelid with two or more of his fingers, taking care not to press upon the globe of the eye above; the operator at the same time depresses the inferior part of the globe of the eye till the incision is made. The patient must look straightforwards, and a little upwards. The operator now fixes his right elbow upon his right knee, after having put his right foot firmly on the patient's seat for this purpose. He then suddenly and resolutely introduces the point of his knife through the external part of the cornea.[19]

Celsus himself described the details of the intraocular part of the operation in sufficient detail for the instruction of a surgeon today, two millennia later:

> In order also that the eye to be treated may be held more still, wool is put over the opposite eye and bandaged on: further the left eye should be operated upon with the right hand, and the right eye with the left hand. Thereupon a needle is to be taken pointed enough to penetrate, yet not too fine: and this is to be inserted straight through the two outer tunics at a spot intermediate between the pupil of the eye and the angle adjacent to the temple, away from the middle of the cataract, in such a way that no vein is wounded. The needle should not be, however, entered timidly, for it passes into the empty space; and when this is reached even a man of moderate experience cannot be mistaken, for there is then no resistance to pressure. When the spot is reached, the needle is to be sloped against the suffusion itself and should gently rotate there and little by little guide it below the region of the pupil; when the cataract has passed below the pupil it is pressed upon more firmly in order that it may settle below. If it sticks there the cure is accomplished; if it returns to some extent, it is to be cut up with the same needle, and separated into several pieces which can be the more easily stowed away singly, and form

smaller obstacles to vision. After this the needle is drawn straight out; and soft wool soaked in white of egg is to be put on, above this something to check inflammation; and then bandages. Subsequently the patient must have rest, abstinence, and inunction with soothing medicaments.[20]

The modern operation for complete extraction of a diseased lens was first described in 1748 by Jacques Daviel (1696–1762), who developed the technique to avoid the complications that often occurred when a dislocated lens was left in the anterior chamber of the eye. Daviel's innovation seems not to have been employed widely until the nineteenth century, and Hall Jackson and his contemporaries continued to couch for cataract.[21] His friend William Plumer thought that Jackson was the first to introduce couching to New Hampshire, or, perhaps, to America.[22] This claim of priority is somewhat doubtful because we do not know just which technique Jackson himself used. However, lens extraction was being performed by other Portsmouth surgeons within at least nine years of his death, so it may be that Jackson did introduce the newer technique to his own colleagues.[23]

Two hundred years ago it was not thought unethical if unsolicited testimonials to a physician's skill or character appeared in the local newspapers. The satisfied owner of a slave who had been couched by Jackson wrote to the *New Hampshire Gazette:*

> As there is without Doubt, many persons in this Country who labour under that inexpressable Misfortune, the loss of SIGHT, and from such Causes as might be removed by the Hands of an ingenious and skilful Surgeon or Operator, did they know where to apply, I thought myself in Duty bound, not only to those unhappy Persons, but also in Justice and Gratitude to the Merit and Generosity of Doctor HALL JACKSON of Portsmouth, to publish the following remarkable case.
>
> I have a Negro Man of near sixty Years of Age, who for many Years late past, has been *totally Blind*, not able to discern any object whatever, or scarce distinguish Day from Night: In this unhappy situation I suppose he would have ended his Days, not having the least Thoughts that it was possible for any Person to relieve him, until Doctor HALL JACKSON, in his Way to the Eastward, accidentally call'd at my House, and seeing the Negro, he humourously upbraided me with keeping such an Incumbrance in my Family, when he could be so easily cured, and at the same Time generously offered to perform the Cure the next Time he came this Way; a few Days after he called at my House again, and according to his Promise perform'd some kind of Operation on one of the Fellow's Eyes, which instantaneously restored him to Sight, so that he has been capable all this Season of working in the Fields, and takeing Care of Cattle: About two Months ago he called again, and perform'd the same Operation on the other Eye, which has compleated his Cure,

his Sight being now good; he is capable of doing as much business as can be expected from a Man of his Years.

Samuel Clarke

York, September 24th, 1770

N.B. Doctor JACKSON has repeatedly performed the Operation on other blind Persons, with the like good success.[24]

A further case report seems almost to have been written by a modern neurologist, or at least by someone skilled in describing a patient's ophthalmological history:

About five Weeks ago, was brought to Dr. Hall Jackson of this Town, one Fletcher, of Winter Harbour, he is now in the thirty-ninth Year of his age: when he was six months old, he lost his sight, and remained perfectly blind ever since; the next Day after his Arrival here, he had his left Eye couched, but besides the Disease that attended this Eye, from his Infancy, he had received a Blow from the End of a Mop Staff, which had rendered the Disorder so complicated, as to afford little or no Prospect of success, notwithstanding it so far succeeded, as to make him capable of distinguishing some Objects, tho' not with any great Degree of exactness; he in some Measure, though not wholly, lost the little Benefit that he received by a violent Inflammation that succeeded the Operation, and this retarded it's being performed on the other Eye, until last Thursday week, when it was done with all the success that could be expected or desired: No sooner was the instrument out of his Eye, when he was able clearly and distinctly to see the many Persons and Objects that surrounded him, in all of which he immediately perceived a Difference, but how or in what this Difference consisted, he could give no account, as he had no Idea of Form, Colour, Magnitude, distance, or such a Plurality of Things but what he had formed in his Mind, from the Sense of Hearing and Feeling; which plainly demonstrates that were we deprived of the Use of our sensory Organs we could have no Ideas of Things whatever.

All objects and Colors seem'd equally agreeable to this Person except Red and green, the former of which, he could not look upon with any Degree of Satisfaction, but with the latter he appeared to be very much pleased.

The Joy expressed by this Person in being restored to so valuable a Sence, did by no means appear so great as in those that have been before sensible of the enjoyment of it.

About ten Days ago a Negro Man belonging to Mr. Nathaniel M[illegible] of Durham, who had been blind for some Years, had both his Eyes Couched by Doctor Hall Jackson, and perfectly restored to sight.[25]

One wonders why Jackson did not include any cataract operations among his few journal notes on patients he treated from 1774 to 1795,[26] unless it was because he thought the operation deserved no particular mention, or because he was more interested in other uses of his records (a subject to be explored in Chapter 3).

Plumer credits Hall Jackson with another "first," the introduction of "the method of healing wounds by the first intention, & if it was after the practise had been tried in Europe, with him it was entirely original, & the result of experiment and observation." Whether a wound heals by first intention is, of course, not the result of a "method"; it is the expected outcome when the wound is clean. The concept of healing by second intention—the idea that the formation of pus in a wound was a desirable occurrence ("laudable pus")—had been established by the early Middle Ages. In contrast, when a wound heals by first intention, no pus forms. It is not difficult to understand that doctors who were accustomed to the presence of pus in wounds might be reluctant to accept its absence as a desirable goal. Not until the nineteenth century, in fact, when bacteria and specific means of combatting them were first brought to the notice of the profession, could healing by first intention be universally accepted. John Hunter's book on inflammation, in which he advocated healing by first intention, was published in 1794 and first reprinted in America in 1796, a year before Jackson died. Again, it is difficult to be sure, on the basis of Plumer's evidence alone, whether Jackson was the first to introduce the newer concept to America.[27]

A trip to the doctor's office in Jackson's Portsmouth had more inconveniences than lack of anesthesia and antiseptic measures. One of Jackson's patients inserted this notice in the *New Hampshire Gazette* in 1775: "The person who took a gun out of Dr. Hall Jackson's entry-[way] is requested to return the same to George Dame [the town tax collector], or he will be prosecuted as a Thief."[28]

In general, Jackson regarded Portsmouth as a healthy place in which to live. In 1789 he wrote:

> Portsmouth is without exception as healthy a Place as any in America, or perhaps on the Globe; there has not been a continued fever, or any acute Disorder of consequence, (the Influenza excepted), the last twelve months in this large Town. No person was ever known to have regular intermittent, or what is commonly called the fever of ague, in the Town of Portsmouth, unless contracted in some other climate or place.[29]

Jackson saw at least three cases of endemic goiter in the late 1780's. Two of them were sisters from inland New Hampshire. Appreciating the value of salt water fish in this condition, although ignorant that it was their iodine content that was responsible, he sent the girls to live near coastal salt water marshes. Their goiters disappeared, leaving only a little sagging skin below their necks. One sister later returned home, whereupon her goiter reappeared.[30]

As a physician in a seaport town, Jackson might have been likely to encounter at least a few cases of intermittent fevers, or agues, now called malaria, among the many visiting seamen. One of the first specific drugs for the treatment of any disease, quinine, then known as Peruvian bark after its chief source, or as Jesuit's bark after its chief suppliers, had been used successfully for 150 years to treat ague. (Unfortunately, the bark's specificity for the fever of ague was extrapolated to include its supposed specificity for any fever, regardless of its origin.[31] We will examine the supposed homogeneity of fevers in Chapter 4.)

Jackson employed at least one other treatment for ague. In 1789 he wrote: "The common American *Willow*...is certainly possessed with virtues similar to those of the Peruvian bark; I have recommended it in...a considerable number of cases of low continued fevers, when there has been evident marks of putridity, and I think with good success."[32] He may have come across, although perhaps only at second hand, a discovery by the Reverend Edward Stone of Chipping Norton in Oxfordshire, who had read a paper entitled "An Account of the Success of the Bark of the Willow in the Cure of Agues" to the Royal Society of London in 1763. Stone reasoned that because the willow bark, like the Peruvian bark, tastes bitter and grows in marshy places, where malaria is often endemic, it, too, should be able to cure the same diseases as those for which the Bark was specific therapy. It was only much later that willow (*Salix alba*) bark was indeed found to contain a salicylate that is much like aspirin and which can reduce moderate fevers, as does aspirin. Although willow bark cannot cure malaria or "fevers [with] marks of putridity," Jackson probably used it in his practice because at least it could alleviate some common pains and fevers. Alternatively, some of his patients may well have recovered regardless of treatment.[33]

Jackson did not find Portsmouth to be completely healthy at all times. In the same letter in which he praised the town's general health, he testified:

> I am perswaded Consumptions [i.e., tuberculosis] are more frequent than formerly: Nothing is more evident than consumptive Parents leaving hereditary dispositions, to the Disorder, to their Children; as population increases the disease must become more frequent, besides, I have been convinced from my own observations that Consumptions are contagious.

The latter observation is, of course, correct, but it could not be confirmed until the late nineteenth century. For treating consumption, Jackson favored a "pectoral decoction" which included zinc sulfate, columbo root, quassia wood, and orange peel, a mixture designed to strengthen all the body's working fibers.[34]

In 1786 in a twenty-eight page book entitled *Observations and Remarks on the Putrid Malignant Sore-Throat* he described an epidemic of diphtheria associated with scarlet fever which had been plaguing New Hampshire for two years. The monograph was published anonymously, "By a Gentleman of the Faculty." Jackson's authorship is attested by the inscription on one of the few existing copies: "From the Benevolent Author Dr. Hall Jackson to Jeremy Belknap June, 1787." Jackson's non-medical friends mentioned the book, so it must have been known to others, but his reasons for preferring that his name not appear on the title page are not known.[35]

The word "faculty" in the by-line refers not to a medical school—there has never been one in Portsmouth—but, following common usage of the day, to the local medical profession in general, who did have an instructional function within the profession, long hallowed by the Hippocratic Oath. In 1793 Dr. David Morril wrote to Dr. Levi Bartlett that he had consulted with Jackson, in the latter's capacity as "censor," about medical texts that Morril should study. Morril expected to pay a "premium" for Jackson's instructional services. In the late eighteenth century, "censor" and "premium" had academic connotations they have now lost, but which are implicit in their contexts here. Two years earlier, in 1791, only five years after the publication of the book on diphtheria, Jackson was the official censor for the eastern region of the newly formed New Hampshire Medical Society, in which capacity he administered examinations and certified to the candidates' abilities.[36]

Jackson wrote his small book for the guidance of patients and their parents perhaps more than for other physicians. He also intended the book to help reduce the incidence of the most severe consequences of the disease, by preparing its victims before they contracted it:

> [These remarks] were thrown together at a late hour, after the fatigues of a busy day, as well as for the author's own satisfaction, as the purpose of adopting some concise and regular method of treating a disease that is so rapidly spreading, and in all probability will become general, amongst us.[37]

Diphtheritic sore throat had been known as a distinct disease since 1748. Jackson described its spread through New Hampshire and Massachusetts since the autumn of 1784. It was not then new to that area; it had first appeared in Massachusetts in 1659, although it was not recognized as a clinically distinct syndrome.[38] Jackson could not blame adverse climactic conditions, as was often done, nor generalized debility among the populations affected: "more general health never prevailed through the country, excepting in the summer of 1784; when puerperal fevers were remarkably common through the country in general."[39] He thought that the sore throat was a contagious disease, but:

> Whatever then may be the remote or predisposing cause of the present disease, must remain one of those mysteries that baffle human researches. Blindly to puzzle for peccant causes, is oftentimes as futile and absurd, as prescriptions founded on prejudice and conjecture are unjustifiable.[40]

In other words, a physician must bring the same kinds of skills and reasoning to bear on diagnosis as on drug therapy.

> From a consideration of these foregoing symptoms we are led to conclude, that the present disorder, is a disease of a highly putrid nature, and that the indications of cure are to be sought for, only,

in such remedies as may obviate the tendency to putrefaction, quiet the septic ferment in the habit, and support the system: How irrational then, must be the practice of those, that urge the cooling regimen, antiphlogistic remedies, antimonials, mercurial purges, and other evacuants: by these a debility is induced; the vital energy impaired, and the spreading putrefaction greatly encouraged: Has not the great mortality that has attended this disease in many parts of the country been in some measure owing to the too frequent use of these remedies? [41]

Jackson reasoned that "The tonic as well as the antiseptic powers of the Bark must render it a medicine not only proper, but highly necessary in this disorder," in the absence of antibiotics or antitoxin for his diphtheria patients. He could not have known that quinine has no effect on diphtheria bacteria, because he could not have known of bacteria. Jackson was so convinced of the bark's merits that he resorted to seemingly heroic measures to ensure that his patients received an adequate dose of it into their bodies:

> ...there are many cases where...it cannot be got down, or the stomach will not retain it;...to obviate this difficulty, we have now a method of conveying into the habit, a sufficient quantity of this noble medicine by the means of a pediluvium...It is found that the hand, after being well chafed, will imbibe in an hours time near an ounce and a half of warm water, and allowing that the surface of the hand is to that of the whole body as one to sixty, the absorption of the whole in the same space of time would amount to upward of seven pounds. [42]

Jackson's usual treatment for diphtheria, when the patient could not take the bark by mouth—and he usually could not—was to have him soak his feet and legs (because the foot has about the same surface area as the hand) in a "decoction" (that is, extracted in boiling water) of bark, Virginia snakeroot, and camomile flowers. Presumably a portion of the bark might be absorbed through the skin, but it would have had to be well abraded in order for appreciable amounts of drug to have gained entry into the blood. Furthermore, quinine is a local irritant, and its effects on exposed skin capillaries would have tended to inhibit its absorption into the rest of the body. Because quinine is now known not to affect the course of diphtheria under any circumstances, it was most likely fortuitous that any of Jackson's patients recovered after undergoing this treatment.

In his own journals he does not attribute to putrid malignant sore throat one single death among all his patients who died from 1774 to 1795, even in the years during which he thought the epidemic was at its peak, 1784–86. Moreover, during those three years he lost no more of his patients from all causes than in any other years. [43] His book may well have been devoted to rhetorical exaggeration of a phenomenon that was otherwise routine in his practice.

Jackson seems to have been a regional expert on purulent diseases. In 1788 Dr. Levi Bartlett of Kingston sent him a patient with a serious ear infection. Jackson replied that the infection would disappear eventually if kept clean, and that he had seen this occur even if mastoiditis supervened.[44]

In the same letter, apparently in reply to another question from Bartlett, Jackson gives some evidence of his knowledge of the current medical literature. He writes about *Cicuta maculata*—water hemlock, or cowbane—a potent poison that produces death by convulsions:

> I have never seen one instance where I could perceive the Cicuta answer any valuable purpose; and a late publication in G. Britain declares it pernicious in all cases, useful or salutary in none. It proves Doctor Storck [Anton Stoerck, who did perform a number of appropriate experiments with poisonous plants] an impostor[;] he [the author of the English article] has been at Vienna, and other parts of Germany and could find not one cure of consequence performed by Dr. Storck, or any other person with the Cicuta, and challenges all Great Britain to produce one.[45]

The most frightening disease in eighteenth-century America was smallpox. The Reverend Cotton Mather (1662–1728), pastor of the Second Church in Boston, described it in 1724 as "A Distemper so well known, and so much Felt, that there needs no Description to be given of it." He went on to postulate that some biological agent was involved: "It begins now to be Vehemently Suspected That the Small-Pox may be more of an Animalculated Business, than we have been generally aware of. The Millions of [illegible] which the Microscopes discover in the Pustules, have Confirmed the Suspicion."[46]

When Hall Jackson participated in the colonists' sporadic wars against smallpox forty years later, which first established his professional reputation throughout New England, Mather's "animalcules" remained unknown to medicine. Puritan Mather, unable to differentiate between microbiological and theological causes of disease, had attributed the ultimate cause of the disease to just retribution from a vengeful God:

> Glorious God, Such a Sharp, and indeed such a New Rebuke [Mather knew that small pox was unknown to classical civilizations, and thought that it had followed the Moors in their conquest of Europe] of thine upon us, Correcting us for our Iniquity, and Consuming our Beauty as a Moth, (yea, as a Lion,) Why, Why must it come upon us?... The Answer which Heaven thunders down upon us, is: Ah, Sinful Generation, a People Laden with Iniquity, a Seed of Evildoers, Children that are Corrupters; They have forsaken the Lord! ...Tis because ye Revolt more and more![47]

Man's only course was to prepare himself for the dread disease by completely accepting and adhering to the teachings of the New Testament; there was no likelihood of escape in Mather's Presbyterian theology, founded squarely on Original Sin. Once afflicted, the patient could achieve at least an easier departure from this world through piety and confession.

Mather's great contribution to medicine arose from his confusion of theology and biology in his observation that "It has hardly ever been seen, that any after having Suffered [smallpox] Once, comes to Suffer it a Second time...It is to be hoped, O Man, That this observation will be verified in thy Moral Experience; and that the Grosser Sins, which thou hast once Repented of, thou wilt Never again fall into them." His long pages of reputed remedies, which even he could realize were not likely to be of much help to the smallpox victim, give way finally to his description of inoculation as a safe and effective measure for smallpox prevention.[48]

When a smallpox epidemic broke out in Boston in May 1721, Mather suggested that the town's doctors try the inoculation method newly described in letters to London from Constantinople. The only Boston physician who would venture to try the experiment was Zabdiel Boylston (1679–1766). Together they must have worked out the details of the technique much as Hall Jackson would employ it later. Mather's was the more succinct description of it:

> We make usually a Couple of Incisions in the Arms...Into these we putt Bitts of Lint...which has been dipt in some of the Variolous Matter, taken in a Vial, from the Pustule of one...that has the Small Pox of the more Laudable sort now turning upon him; And so we cover them with a Plaister...Yett we find the Variolous Matter fetched from those that have the Inoculated Small Pox, as Agreeable and Effectual as any other...In four and twenty Hours, we throw away the Lint; and the Sores are dressed once or twice, Every four and twenty Hours, with Warmed Cabbage-Leaves...About the Seventh Day, the Patient feels the Usual Symptoms of the Small-Pox coming upon him; and he is now managed as in an Ordinary Putrid Fever. If he can't hold up, he goes to Bed...If he be very Qualmish at the Stomach, we give him a gentle Vomit, yea, We commonly do these things almost of Course...whether we find the Patient want them or no. And if the Fever be too high...we Bleed a Little...Upon or About the Third Day...the Eruption begins ...The Eruption is made without their suffering one Minute of any Sensible Sickness for it...The Eruption being made, all Illness Vanishes; There's an End on't.[49]

Mather and Boylston also tried the crucial experiment to confirm the efficacy of their new method, with success: "The Transplantation has been tried on such as have gone through the Small-Pox formerly in the Common way; and has had no Effect upon them." [50]

Boylston's description of the procedure is more detailed; its chief historical value lies in his presentation of the numerical results of the first great therapeutic experiment, the first statistical epidemiological study, in America.[51] His data and those of other Boston epidemics and some elsewhere are summarized in Table 2 and discussed below.

Not until 1798 did Edward Jenner develop the method still used today, vaccination, in which immunity is induced not with smallpox virus but with cowpox virus, which is so closely related that it also induces immunity to smallpox, while producing even fewer and much less severe symptoms than inoculated smallpox. Cowpox had never been known to be fatal to man. Before 1800 it required considerable courage to undergo inoculation and risk death with the artificially induced smallpox, although the risk was known even then to be much less than with the naturally acquired disease, as Table 2 shows.

Early in its history, inoculation was opposed by some clergy who thought it was sinful, by others because it prevented their parishioners from attending church, and by still others because preventive medicine "tends to anticipate and banish Providence out of this world." Outbreaks of smallpox during the Revolutionary War did much to popularize inoculation and to make it acceptable to both military and non-military populations.[52]

Nathaniel Adams of Portsmouth wrote of the smallpox epidemic that visited Boston in 1764:

> The small-pox was very prevalent in Boston, and from the continual intercourse, which was kept up between that place and this, both by land and water, there was great danger of its being brought here, and communicated to the inhabitants. To prevent which, the selectmen [of Portsmouth] had a fence built across the road at Great Swamp, and a small house erected, to smoke all persons and baggage, coming from Boston by land. After they were thoroughly cleansed by the guard set there for the purpose, they received certificates, and were permitted to pass. The same caution was used in relation to all vessels from Boston, which were required to perform quarantine, and every prudent method was adopted to destroy the infection.
>
> Dr. Hall Jackson resided in Boston for two or three months, and carried several classes safely through the disorder by inoculation; a large number went there from this town, to put themselves under his care.[53]

A "class" was a group of persons who were inoculated at the same time and who lived together until the smallpox induced by inoculation had run its course, in about three weeks, and there was no danger of transmitting it to others.

Although the prophylactic value of large-scale public inoculation had been proved statistically at its first introduction to the Western world in Boston in 1721, forty years later it was still an emotional issue in relatively isolated colonial communities that understood the contagious nature of smallpox all too well. The 1764 epidemic began in Boston after the brigantine *Nancy* docked on December 21, 1763. Not until the following March 13 did town meeting finally vote to permit the selectmen, as the public health authority, to establish inoculation hospitals at Point

Shirley and Castle William in the harbor, and to permit the establishment of private inoculation hospitals in privately owned homes. Those insular accommodations in Boston harbor were the first hospitals specifically designated for inoculation. To accommodate the large number of persons who came to Castle William to be inoculated, forty-eight of the fort's barracks rooms were renovated and each furnished for ten patients. Among those who took advantage of the inoculation at this time, although in a private home, was John Adams, who was treated by Dr. Nathaniel Perkins. When the epidemic began to abate, all the Boston smallpox hospitals were closed by the selectmen, as of April 20, and those in Charlestown on May 12, less than two months after their opening.[54]

Earlier, when the disease had threatened to spread faster than the citizens could be inoculated, the selectmen of Boston had solicited the assistance of experts in inoculation from other New England towns. On March 29 Hall Jackson and Dr. Isaac Foster advertised the availability of lodgings for inoculation in Charlestown, and urged that prospective patients come before the inoculation permit expired. The houses in which Jackson and Foster inoculated were marked with red flags, as warnings. Jackson was paid 48 shillings for each inoculation he administered in Boston at the time, but it is not known whether he inoculated at the official hospitals as well as privately. Neither do we know precisely why Jackson chose to help quash this latest in Boston's recurring smallpox outbreaks. His work there did help to establish his reputation, and led to specific requests for his participation in later mass inoculations.[55]

The success of the Boston program, as shown in Table 2, was clear by June 30. Of 699 Bostonians who contracted smallpox naturally, almost 18 percent died; but of the 4977 (including about 400 from other towns, like Portsmouth) who had the mild form of the disease induced artificially, fewer than one percent died. Approximately one third of Boston's 15,700 inhabitants were inoculated during the program, many of the others having been immunized from earlier inoculations or infections; the last epidemic had occurred only twelve years before. The inoculations in 1764 were the first to affect markedly the long-range death rate attributable to smallpox in Boston, because the poor, who usually could not afford the necessary costs but were the most likely to contract the disease, were treated free of charge for the first time.[56]

Table 2 shows the data pertaining to the safety and efficacy of inoculation which were available by 1764, and some Boston data that were collected afterward. We cannot be sure that Jackson had seen any of these data, but he surely understood their implications. That so few people contracted smallpox in Boston in 1764 (4.5 percent) is attributable to the short interval since both widespread infection and inoculation had last increased the proportion of immune persons in the town. The 1721 epidemic alone had left relatively few people susceptible to the virus when it next struck nine years later; only a handful had been inoculated that first time. But the long interval of twenty-two years between the

Table 2.
Results of Smallpox Inoculation Programs in Boston and Charleston,
1721–1792

| | Persons with Naturally Acquired Smallpox | | | | Died |
|---|---|---|---|---|---|
| | Died | | | Number | |
| Location | Number | Fraction | % | Survived | Number |
| *Boston, 1721–22* | | | | | |
| | 844 | 1/7 | 14.7 | 4915 | 6 |
| *Boston, 1730* | | | | | |
| | 500 | 1/8 | 12.5 | 3500 | 11 |
| *Boston, 1752* | | | | | |
| Total | 514 | 1/10 | 10.2 | 5030 | 30 |
| Whites | 452 | 1/11 | 8.9 | 4607 | 23 |
| Blacks | 62 | 1/8 | 12.8 | 423 | 7 |
| *Boston, 1764* | | | | | |
| | 124 | 1/6 | 17.7 | 575 | 46 |
| *Cambridge, 1764* | | | | | |
| | 4 | 1/10 | 10.5 | 34 | 2 |
| *Boston, 1776* | | | | | 28 |
| *Boston, 1778* | | | | | 19 |
| *Boston, 1792* | | | | | 165 |
| *Charleston, S.C., 1738* | | | | | |
| Total | 480 | 1/5 | 21.9 | 1710 | 7 |
| Whites | 180 | 1/4 | 25.7 | 520 | 4 |
| Blacks | 300 | 1/5 | 20.8 | 1190 | 3 |

* The population of Boston was about 11,000 in 1721, and about 16,000 in 1764; the population of Charleston was about 5,000 in 1738.

The absolute numbers of patients, and the fractional numbers, were the only data published in the original sources. When the numbers of persons dying are compared with the numbers of persons surviving following naturally acquired and inoculated smallpox, values of chi-square are sufficiently large to permit the inference that death was less likely to follow inoculation at $P < 0.025$ in all instances for which data are available.

SOURCES: Zabdiel Boylston, *An Historical Account of the Small-Pox Inoculated in New England* (London, S. Chandler, 1726), p. 40. John B. Blake, *Public Health in the Town of Boston 1630–1822* (Cambridge, Mass., Harvard University Press, 1959), pp. 243–249. John Duffy, *Epidemics in Colonial America*, 1953 (rep. Baton Rouge, Louisiana State University, 1971) p. 36. Francis R. Packard, *History of Medicine in the United States*, 2 vols. (New York, Paul B. Hoeber, 1931), Vol. 1, pp. 72–94.

| Persons Inoculated with Smallpox | | | Per Cent of City's Population* | | | |
|---|---|---|---|---|---|---|
| Died | | Number | Died of all | Infected with | Inoculated with | Died of Natural or Inoculated |
| Fraction | % | Survived | Causes | Smallpox | Smallpox | Smallpox |
| 1/47 | 2.1 | 274 | 12.9 | 54.5 | 2.8 | 7.9 |
| 1/46 | 2.2 | 500 | 6.7 | 28.6 | | 3.6 |
| 1/69 | 1.4 | 2083 | 6.4 | 35.4 | 14.1 | 3.6 |
| 1/83 | 1.2 | 1951 | | | | |
| 1/20 | 5.0 | 132 | | | | |
| 1/108 | 0.9 | 4931 | 3.5 | 4.5 | 32.1 | 1.1 |
| 1/323 | 0.3 | 647 | | | | |
| 1/178 | 0.6 | 4960 | | | | |
| 1/112 | 0.9 | 2102 | | | | |
| 1/55 | 1.8 | 8987 | | | | |
| 1/120 | 0.8 | 843 | | 43.8 | 17.0 | 9.7 |
| 1/112 | 0.9 | 446 | | | | |
| 1/133 | 0.8 | 397 | | | | |

1730 and the 1752 epidemics left many more Bostonians susceptible to the disease because the average life expectancy at the time was only about thirty years (see Chapter 3).

Zabdiel Boylston and other eighteenth-century physicians published or examined data presented as fractions of the population at risk who died, using a common numerator of one. The idea of presenting similar data more efficiently with a common denominator of 100 did not develop until the 1780's, when Jeremy Bentham began to use percentages to express rates or proportions percent, although they had been used for calculating interest on principal since at least 1568. The nineteenth century would be half over before percentages came into common usage by scientists to express the relative proportions of parts in the whole.[57]

Table 2 shows why Jackson did not need to know modern statistical techniques to compare the numbers of people dying after inoculation or naturally acquired smallpox with the numbers of survivors, in order to assess the safety of the preventive technique. For populations for which appropriate data for chi-square analyses are available, the relative safety of inoculation is demonstrable in all cases at a high probability level (less than 0.025), even for blacks in Boston in 1752. The halving of the death rate following inoculation over the years is probably attributable to measures taken to protect classes of patients undergoing inoculation from other diseases. Boylston concluded that at least four of his six patients who died following inoculation had actually died from other causes.[58]

In 1764 smallpox virus commonly was inoculated into a small incision made in the patient's skin with a piece of lint soaked in pus from another patient's pocks. Dried thread was bound around the wound, to permit sufficient irritation and inflammation to occur, so that the hypothetical causative agent of the disease could readily drain from the sore. The patient was subjected to a series of emetics and purges, chiefly drugs containing mercury or antimony, to further facilitate the escape of the disease from the body. In Chapter 4 we will explore this escape theme, which will recur throughout this book.

The inoculation procedure was well organized, and measures long in common use for controlling the spread of the disease from inoculated patients in 1764 were codified in Massachusetts law in 1777. The physician in charge had to provide a "cleansing-house" and guards. After a patient recovered from the artificially induced disease, but no sooner than three weeks after he had been inoculated, he had to report to a "shifting room" where, supervised by a "cleanser," he would undress, wash in rum or vinegar, and be fumigated. After dressing in fresh clothes in another room, the patient could then be discharged. At no time during a class could a patient or staff member go outside certain official limits without the physician's permission. To facilitate enforcement of this restriction, many inoculation hospitals were built on islands. In addition, patients were required to post a bond of ten pounds, and physicians five hundred pounds, to assure that they would obey the regulations.[59]

Twelve-year old Peter Thacher described his experience with inoculation in Boston in 1764:

Boston, Saturday, April 14, 1764, I was inoculated at the George Tavern by Doct. Joseph Gardiner. . . . Att. Night we took Each of us a Pill.

Sunday, April 15, we took a Powder in the Morning w[hich] worked me Nine Times. Felt very Sick in the Morning but better in the After Noon. Att Night took one Pill which work'd me once. . . .

Tuesday, April 17. . . . Took a Powder w[hich] work'd me ten times.

Wednesday, April 18, took two Pills which did not work me at all. At Night took a Pill.

Thursday, April 19. Took a Powder which worked me 5 times up & once down. Felt very sick in the Morning but did not in the afternoon.

Friday, April 20. . . . Felt very poorly all Day. . . .

Saturday, April 21. Took a Powder which worked me 4 Times down and once up. Felt very sick in the Morning & did not get up till 10 o'clock. I have some Pock come out to Day.

Sunday, April 22. Felt charmingly all Day. I had more Pock come out to Day. At Night took Brimstone in Milk for a sore Mouth.

Monday, April 23. Felt very well. The Pock still continue coming out. Took Brimstone.

Tuesday, April 24. Pretty well in the Morning but towards Night I had a Sore Throat. . .

Wednesday, April 25. Felt very Dull & heavy by reason of a sore Throat which afflicts me much. Took Brimstone & Molasses. . .

Friday, April 27. Better. My Throat is sore yet. My Pocks are turned & turning. . .

Sunday, April 29. Took Physic to dry away my Pock & to cleanse my Blood from its Small Pox. Felt very poorly in the Morning but better in the Afternoon. My Physic worked me 7 times.

Monday, April 30. Went down Stairs. Dined below & in the Afternoon I went to see Stephen Whiting. . .

Wednesday, May 2. . . I was very well at Day but Dull at Night.

Thus, through the Mercy of God, I have been preserved through the Distemper of the Small Pox which form[erly] was so fatal to many Thousands. The Distemper is very mortal the natural Way. I should have a thankful Heart for so great a Favor. I confess I was undeserving of it. Many and heinous have been my Sins but I hope they will be washed away.[60]

Hall Jackson's record in Boston prompted some of his neighbors in Portsmouth to urge him to establish an inoculation program there. In

April of 1766 the Portsmouth selectmen agreed to let him use the Town Pest House on Shapley's Island in the harbor for administering the inoculations. Twelve years later Jackson and two of his Portsmouth colleagues ran still another inoculation hospital there. In that year, 1778, two of Jackson's patients died of smallpox.[61] Nathaniel Adams, who was there, described the organization and rules designed to prevent uncontrollable outbreaks of the disease in the town:

> A committee was appointed to apply to the committee of safety for leave to inoculate, which was granted. The Pest, Henzell's, and Salter's Islands, were fixed upon, as suitable places for the hospital. Regulations were established for the government of it, and the whole was put under the care of a committee, who were to give permission to the surgeons, or physicians, to inoculate. No person was allowed to visit the hospital without leave from the committee, nor to be inoculated without a written license from them; and previous to obtaining a license, he was obliged to deposit in the hands of the committee a sum sufficient to defray all the expense. No person was allowed to leave the hospital in less than twenty-one days after inoculation, nor until he had procured a certificate from his physician that he was free from infection, and was thoroughly cleansed by a person, appointed for that purpose by the committee. The physicians were allowed eight dollars for each patient under their care, excepting every tenth person, who was a pauper sent by the committee, and who was inoculated and attended through the disorder gratis. There were two classes carried through this disorder, containing about four hundred and twelve persons in all, at the expense of sixteen dollars each.[62]

This was clearly a publicly regulated public health program, as it had been in Boston, although it can hardly be regarded as an early form of socialized medicine. The town took half of the fees, for furnishing room and board for the three weeks' stay in the public pest house, while half was allotted to the professional men who administered the inoculations and looked after the patients with smallpox.

Four years later still, in 1782 (a year in which Jackson lost three patients in an epidemic), he superintended an inoculation hospital which he and three colleagues established on Henzell's Island in Portsmouth Harbor. The town was not involved officially in this hospital.[63]

We have Jackson's detailed notes on the 365 patients from southeastern New Hampshire inoculated on Henzell's Island from March 2 to June 15, 1782. The patients ranged in age from infancy to 51 years; half of them were 12 or less, and 75 percent were under 20. They were not inoculated in classes, as they had been in Boston and elsewhere, but daily; Jackson inoculated from one to thirty-one patients daily during the life of the Henzell's Island hospital. They were given from one to four doses of a cathartic pill, with smaller doses administered to children than to adults. The accounts in the back of Jackson's notebook show that the most frequently used cathartics were calomel (mercurous chloride), rhubarb, Glauber's salts (hydrated sodium sulfate), and a prepackaged cathartic powder—although tartar emetic (antimony and potassium tartrate), paregoric, and laudanum were also prescribed when necessary. All the patients stayed for the usual period of three weeks, during which they developed the expected pocks; 14 percent developed one sore, 64 percent developed two, 21 percent developed three, and one percent developed four or more (one patient developed as many as 30 sores). The outcomes were favorable in all instances; although one patient did develop an abscess at the site of his inoculation, it seems to have disappeared by the time he was discharged from the hospital.[64]

Jabez Dow (1776–1839) of Dover, New Hampshire, studied medicine with Hall Jackson for a year or two just before Jackson died. Dow, who spent much of his professional career making notes for books he never published, has left us a marvellously detailed account of inoculated smallpox as he saw it at Jackson's smallpox hospital on Shapley's Island, Portsmouth, in 1796. Dow's observations are quoted at length so that they can be compared with the more gastrointestinally oriented notes of patients like Peter Thacher and John Adams:

The small pox by inoculation requires some attention, to be certain that the Contagion has taken effect, which may be always ascertained by the third day. On the sixth or seventh Day from inoculation, there are flushes of heat, succeeded by cold shiverings, the patient continually complaining of pain in his back, loins, darting thro' the shoulders, & almost every part of the Body, a constant pain in the head, with febrile heat, high coloured urine &c. These are what are called, the symptoms of Small pox.

Some have [illegible] symptoms, others mild, & some exceeding distressing.

On the ninth Day, the symptoms, in common Cases disappear totally or partially. But in one Case in 160 patients, the symptoms continued till the incrustation. About this time (on the 9th [day]) the pustules begin to appear; which are of two kinds; viz. the Confluent (Variola confluens) & the distinct (Variola discreta) The former sometimes fatal, & the latter generally salutary. In the confluent small pox, the inflammatory pustules, come out thick, less prominent, & are one continued surface, the pock communicating with each other at their Base; leaving no intermediate surface unpustulated. The distinct come out in prominent, circumscribed, & less inflammatory pustules.

Many have but few pustules, & those of the distinct kind; some have none,[2] [Dow's note 2: "It has been observed to me...by H. Jackson...that if a patient is inoculated, & the inoculation takes, & the patient stays three weeks in an infectious hospital, among infectious patients, there is no kind of danger of taking the small pox ever after if they have had neither symptoms, pock, nor any kind of illness."], others but two or three; & in a very few instances, those who have the symptoms bad, will have no pock, & in several, but few.

On the twelfth Day there appear Vesicles on the Apices of the pustules, containing white variolous matter, each succeeding Day (to the fifteenth) enlarging & inclining to a well digested pus; at which time the patient complains of being very sore, unable to stir, & generally refractory.

After the pustules have matured, & the Vesicles full, there appears a dark livid spot on the apex of each; this is the commencement of incrustation, which takes place first on the Crown of the head, inclining downwards. In the confluent small pox, the surface is so loaded with Matter & the patient being much debilitated, that in some cases, at the beginning of incrustation when the vesicles are full of matter, it takes a retrograde motion into the System, the pock flatten, & immediate Death the consequence.

From the twelfth to the fifteenth [days], the head swells in the confluent species & frequently Blindness [is] the consequence, lasting sometimes many Days.

On the eighteenth Day the incrustation is compleat, & the scabs begin to fall off in the order before mentioned of the incrustation; This is the last stage of the small pox, & is compleated on the 21st Day, when the patient is free from Contagion, altho' a desquamation succeeds the falling off [of] the pustular incrustation, leaving a Cicatrice for each pustule; these cicatrices are called pock-pitts, which remain sometimes only a few weeks or months, but often times they are permanent, & are said to increase in mediocrity [size] thro' life.

This is a Description of the mild small pox; but these & the following observations are accurately made with the whole appearances of 160 patients, out of which not one died.

REGIMEN. A vegetable Diet is all that is necessary or allowable. The Farinacea possessing a sufficiency of Nutriment & being least subject to fermentation, compose the principal regimen in the small pox. The fermentative and putrefactive tendency of this disease sufficiently inculcates the entire prohibition of animal food. Milk deprived of its butyraceous parts [butter fat] from its innocency may be used without hesitation. The use of vegetable acids is eminently advisable.

ADMINISTRATION. By way of antidote Calomel combined with Tartar [of Antimony] was prescribed to check the violence of the disease & continued from inoculation till the eruption, unless prohibited by the intervention of loose teeth or tumefied [swollen, because of the mercury in calomel] gums.

Thirty grains to a robust, 25 gr. to a middling & 20 gr. to slender constitution, of Pulv. Jalap [powdered jalap, a potent cathartic] was given every third morning[4] [Dow's note 4: "Some think Doses of Glauber's Salts sufficient in all common cases."] from the inoculation to the eruption, the dose however to be varied as their operation may indicate. If the stomach loathe this medicine in substance, the Tinct[ure] Jalap is a good substitute.

For delicate constitutions the acrimony of the virus, produces such irritations, as to threaten disagreeable nervous affections, in which cases opium may be prescribed with freedom. Instances of full confluent pock, with constipated habits, urges early attention to relieve & prevent constipation, for this hurries putrefaction.

REMARKS. If the patient takes his food or drink more than blood-warm he will have his mouth & throat full of pock which will be exceeding distressfull. Also all wounds & inflammations will have the same consequences; sometimes they advance to sphacelation [ulcers].

The sooner the symptoms & eruption appear, the less violent ye Disease; the Virus having less time to accumulate, & the habit better adapted to visit the violence of its operation. And this may be the reason why more patients in the natural small pox have the confluent kind.[5] [Dow's note 5: "Two patients had the symptoms not till the tenth & the eruption not till the fifteenth."]

The kind of contagion does not determine the pustules to be confluent or distinct. Take the Contagion from confluent pock & inoculate, it is as likely to produce good distinct pustules[7] as otherwise, & vice versa; so it appears that the violence of this Disorder depends more on the temperament and predisposition of the Constitution, than the quality of the contagious Matter introduced by incision [Dow's note 7: "Five patients were inoculated at the same time with the same kind of Matter, & by the same person; one had very confluent, two less confluent, & the other two very distinct pock"].

Cleanliness is of the greatest importance to patients, not only of their persons, but of their apartments, especially to ventilate & [illegible] or besprinkle their apartments with vinegar or limewater every day, more particularly on the Days of incrustation.

It has been a prevalent opinion that ye contagion may be kept months or even years, & then be capable of producing the Disease, upon which an eminent practitioner[10] informed me that he had discovered the contrary to be true, by actual experiments.[11] [Dow's notes: "10. Dr. Hall Jackson. 11. He has kept the contagious Matter in a phyal; in sponge in like manner, in open air, both in thread & sponge, & in open air without anything containing it, & at the expiration of six weeks, was totally incapable of producing the Small pox."]

The invaluable benefits resulting from the inoculated small pox[12] [Dow's note 12: "It is observed that the natural small pox is fatal to patients, baffling to Physicians, & terrifying to bystanders; out of seven patients, three will die, ruin the constitution of two, & two only perfectly recover."] which saves every one from the awful effects in the natural way; (as no one was ever known to have it twice) is known to most people, yet there are superstitious few, who think attempts to evade the Dispensations of heaven unavailing. But if a person, after once having this Disease, is inoculated a second time, it will take & inflame in a considerable Degree, & have a similar appearance to the first inoculation; And those who give constant attendance to infected persons, will frequently have spurious pox, which shows the habit is susceptible of this Contagion a second time, tho' the Constitution possesses an unknown power in every instance, to which the operation of the Contagion is incompatible.[65]

Only six months before he died in 1797 Jackson and Dr. William Cutter received permission from the Portsmouth selectmen to open a smallpox hospital on Shapley's Island.[66] The era of inoculation was, however, about to end when Jenner's demonstration of the equal effectiveness and lesser risk of vaccination was brought to Boston by Dr. Benjamin Waterhouse three years later.

Following the outbreak of smallpox in Marblehead in the summer of 1773, four leaders of the patriot party in that Massachusetts fishing port —Elbridge Gerry, Azor Orne, and the brothers John and Jonathan Glover—obtained permission from the town to build a hospital for smallpox inoculation on Cat (or Catta) Island in Marblehead Harbor. Ashley Bowen, a sometime sail rigger and frequent indefatigable observer of Marblehead life, dated the onset of the epidemic from the arrival, on June 1, of a ship whose crew had been exposed to smallpox while boarding a French ship.[67]

Many Marbleheaders objected to the building of the Essex Hospital, as it was called, because they feared that the presence of smallpox in the neighborhood would lead to its further spread in the community. They also said it would frighten off the shipping on which the town depended for its livelihood and supplies. In general the proponents of the hospital were patriots, while the local Tories made up the opposition.

Some opponents vilified the hospital as a get-rich-quick scheme on the part of the four proprietors. The fee had been fixed at five pounds fifteen shillings for inoculation, room, board, and nursing care for each patient, although the proprietors agreed to inoculate one needy person free of charge for every ten paying guests. Unlike the later hospitals in Portsmouth Harbor, this one was privately owned, all the profits after expenses for room, board, and professional services going to Messrs. Gerry, Orne, and Glover. They hired Dr. Hall Jackson as superintendent of the hospital. He was assisted by Dr. Ananias Randall of Long Island for the first month, and then by "Doctoress Hawes from Boston." [68]

The new hospital consisted of two buildings. The smaller, of one story only, had one room for "shifting" and another for storing clean clothes for the patients when they left the island. The hospital building itself had three stories. Each of its ten rooms for patients contained four beds, although over 100 patients were inoculated in each class. A kitchen and staff quarters completed the facility. [69]

Bowen's voluminous notebooks testify to the importance of smallpox in Marblehead. In October 1773, on "Thirdsday ye 14," it astonished Bowen that "Nobody brok out with Small Pox. Grate Preporation of ye Ospet on Catt Island for Enockalation." A week later the dockside gossip recorded that "this day the Chief of our Time is Spent about ye Enockalation Hospitall." Among those who took a dim view of the Essex Hospital, Bowen devoted one whole diary to it. In his notes he ridiculed the whole business as a play military operation:

> [October 15, 1773] this day Came to Town Gener Hall Jackson Grand Phiz for Enockalation on Catt Island With a number of Vollanteers with him...
> [October 19, 1773] [They] Layed Seague to the Castle of Pox, General Jackson Commander in Chief[,] Genl Randall Leftent General of Castol Pox...Tis supposed this Seague will Last Thirty Days— by an Expres from Castle Pox Generill Jackson had a Smart Engagement and Wounded [near] a 100...of Colonel Ornes Body of Wollonteers...[70]

Despite his sarcasm the conservative Ashley Bowen was frightened of smallpox. Jackson had been in Marblehead three months before and had diagnosed it in Bowen's wife and young son, both of whom recovered. Not long afterward, Bowen wrote a poem in which Cotton Mather's avenging God plays the key role:

> A sore distemper is crept in
> It seized on all both bold and young
> But by what means I cannot tell
> And very fatal proves to some.
>
> In Scripture we may plainly see
> And read such words as these
> Can evil in the city be
> Except the Lord be pleased.

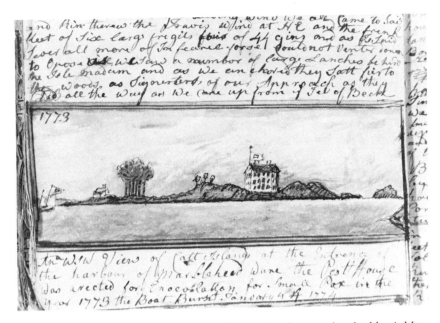

11. *The Essex Hospital, Cat Island, Marblehead Harbor, as sketched by Ashley Bowen in 1773. (Courtesy of the Marblehead Historical Society)*

Short-sighted creatures as we are
Could not our danger see
Tho often-times distressed with fear
What this disease should be.

Surely the hand of Providence
Over us did bear a sway
Tho we so much distressed with fear
Must fall an easy prey.

The 24 day of July
We were all fenced around
Before the 17 of August came
Eight bodies are lain in the ground

How do you think dear friends
What we must feel within
To see so many carried out
That had our neighbors been.

Not only neighbors until some
But their dear friends likewise
Which makes our very hearts relent
And draws tears from our eyes.

Let's not impute it all to chance
Nor merely second cause

> But let us view the hand of God
> As what we do deserve.[71]

The usual precautions against spread of the disease were taken. They were emphasized, to allay the public's fears, in an advertisement for the hospital's services in the *Essex Gazette* for the week in which the hospital opened, 19–26 October 1773:

> The Proprietors of the Essex Hospital beg Leave to inform the Public, that any Person, who has a near Relation in the first Class, may, within ten Days from Tuesday last, have permit to go to the Hospital, and there tarry until the Class comes out; after that Time none can be admitted, unless their Friends should have unfavourable Symptoms, or be in Difficulties from some other Disease.—No letters can come from the Patients; but Memorandums are taken by the Boatmen, and may be known by applying to the Stores of the Subscribers, where Letters and Packages may be lodged, and daily conveyed to the Patients.
>
> We would further inform the Public, that the Hospital Book will be opened for the second Class on Thursday next, and Patients may enter their Names by applying to the Stores mentioned from that Day until the Class is full.[72]

Jackson himself, on at least one occasion, broke the restriction on outgoing mail during an inoculation class, but he assured the Selectmen of Portsmouth, to whom he wrote, that the letter was not contaminated.[73] The day before the official opening, the proprietors may have had an unscheduled difficulty. According to Ashley Bowen, "It seems that the first Cow that they had on the Isle was so DisContented that She took her Calf on her Back and Swam for ye Neck and was Discovered and Carried Back."[74]

Otherwise, the hospital opened on schedule, and the Marbleheaders were given a chance to reassure themselves about the safety measures taken at an open house. According to the *Gazette*,

> On Tuesday last the first Class of Patients went down to the Essex Hospital. As a Number of respectable Persons, of both Sexes, went in it, and the Hospital was clear of infection, many Gentlemen of the Town accompanied it to the Island, and the Hospital was thronged in every Quarter. In the Afternoon the House was cleared, and Doctor Jackson proceeded to inoculate the Patients, being One Hundred and Three in Number [even if there were only forty beds] ... The Patients are daily displaying their Signal of Health [a flag] from the Middle of the Island, and are all in high Spirits.[75]

As the first class entered the Essex Hospital, an advertisement for the "Suttonian Inoculation for the Smallpox" appeared in the *Essex Gazette*. This alternative method was extolled by Mr. Latham, Surgeon to the King's Regiment of Foot stationed near Albany, as superior to any other.[76] Disputes about the efficacy of therapeutic regimens were not then debated in the pages of scholarly journals or research meetings as often as in the public press. Such public debates were designed not for professional consumption but to persuade potential customers.

The front page of the next week's issue of the *Gazette* was devoted to arguments for each of the two methods, presented by two anonymous contributors. The first included a lengthy extract from a home medical manual, pointing out that inoculation with material from smallpox sores succeeds in preventing the severe consequences of the naturally acquired disease, no matter how it is done. The author follows the Suttonian line, however, by suggesting that laymen can perform the treatment as well as physicians; he decries the mystery that usually surrounds doctors, as do irregular healers and medical quacks even today. He also agrees with the Suttonian aversion to preparing patients for inoculation with anything more than a mild purgative. That Suttonian inoculators often prepared their patients by isolating them for two weeks (during which they required room and board) before the inoculation was administered may also have increased their profits.

The equally unknown second author—perhaps one of the proprietors of the Essex Hospital, or even Jackson—accuses the practitioners of Sutton's method of gaining more money and publicity than increased protection for their patients from their efforts. Jackson and his colleagues, following current teaching, believed that mercurial drugs would lessen the severity of the disease brought on by inoculation—hence Jackson's reliance on calomel at Henzell's and Shapley's Islands.[77]

The anonymous discussers of the Suttonian method had, in fact, merely stooped to irrelevant name-calling. Robert and Daniel Sutton's method, which had gained preeminence in England in the 1760's and for which they were granted a patent in 1766 (although the Suttons themselves did not publish their method until 1796, others had described it as early as 1767), was primarily a dietary regimen, in which milk, gruel, and plant foods were the chief ingredients. These foods were selected because they were thought to be "cooling" foods, as opposed to "heating" foods, like meat, other animal products, liquor, and spices. The Hippocratic concept of hot and cold aspects of diseases and their therapies can still be found in the United States even today.[78]

Another difference was that the Suttonians administered the smallpox virus in a very small dose, with a lancet recently dipped into a fresh pock. Although they could not have known it, this method was preferable to using pus from older pustules in which bacteria and white blood cells (Mather's "animalcules") were likely to be swarming. The patient was kept in the open air as much as possible, and not restricted to a small room or house, as was otherwise usual. Only mild doses of emetics and purgatives were administered. In fact, the Suttons' method had the distinct advantage of being less unpleasant and less likely to be fatal than the traditional method, although data for making conventional statistical comparisons are lacking. The newer method finally gained general acceptance when Dr. John Morgan of Philadelphia endorsed it enthusiastically in 1776.[79]

In the local news section of the same issue of the *Gazette*, the latest bulletin from Cat Island was encouraging:

> It is with Pleasure that we can inform the Publick, that the hundred and three Patients, first entered at the Essex Hospital, are well recovered of the Small Pox. Six others were inoculated on Tuesday last, and among them were two Gentlemen from Salem, who a Day or two before had been with infectious Persons. The last mentioned patients have been daily out since they went to the Hospital, and we hope will have no Occasion to be confined any more than the first. We must however expect that some [illegible] News mongers will be much concerned for them this Week, as they despaired of most of the Class the past Week, and in their Grief readily reported that some of them were dead.[80]

Another story going around the county, very likely spread by pro-Suttonians, prompted the Essex Hospital proprietors to insert yet another notice in the *Gazette*, this one over Jackson's signature:

> Whereas a Report has been industriously propagated, that the Dysentery prevails at the Essex Hospital; and also, that a great Number of Patients have been thrown into a Salivation by the too profuse Use of Mercurials: This may certify that there is not the least Complaint or Disorder in the Hospital excepting the Small-Pox; and that out of One Hundred and Eleven Persons inoculated, not five have made any Complaints from the Use of Mercurials; nor has one Patient been affected by the Small-Pox, or otherwise, so far as to oblige him to confine himself to the House one Day since his first Arrival on the Island. Not one third of the Mercurials recommended and used by some popular Practitioners, are made Use of at the Essex Hospital, and those of a much milder and less dangerous nature.[81]

In spite of all the rumors, or even honest confusion, three weeks after admission the first class was reported to have graduated with distinction and promise:

> The second Class of Patients have gone down to the Essex Hospital, and many of the Gentlemen and Ladies, who were earliest, have their Pox out. We hope to see them come off in as high Spirits as the former Class, than which it can hardly be expected that a hundred and odd Persons can be more favourably dealt with by such a grievous Distemper. Few of the recovered Patients have any Recipe [trace] of the Disorder in their Countenance; and those who had fullest are very little pitted. Those who were somewhat delicate in their Constitutions can give convincing Proofs that the preparative Medicines have proved no Ways prejudicial; for certain it is, that some slender Patients have come out of the Hospital much healthier than they went into it.[82]

The inoculation procedure, however, did not put everyone into either high spirits or more flesh, even long after the novelty had worn off in New England and the procedure's worth had been proven over and over again. A patient just discharged from an inoculation hospital at Beverly, north of Boston, in 1794 committed his feelings to verse that is not completely devoid of humor:

> Pinch'd with the Symptoms, chill'd for want of fuel,
> Made lean by Jallop [a cathartic], [Glauber's] Salts,
>     & Water Gruel
> For full three weeks with Patience we have borne
> To be from roast meat, toast and coffee torn.
> With Job's few comforts, but with all his grief,
> At length we find arrived the wish'd relief!
> Hail! BACON, BUTTER, EGGS! Before our Eyes
> We see hot puddings, beef & gravy rise!
> We bid our fellow sufferers all Adieu,
> And, be assured, we wish good Luck to You![83]

It would seem that this anonymous poet had been subject to both current evacuant therapy and the Suttons' diet.

Two months later the third class was discharged, completely recovered and in spite of possible unfavorable circumstances, such as dysentery, pregnancy, and old age among the patients. The only untoward incident involved a particularly bloody accident, for which all of Hall Jackson's surgical skill was needed and, apparently, used. According to the account in the *Gazette*:

> Among others, who left the Essex Hospital, is Capt. Lowell of
> Newbury-Port whom we some time ago mentioned to have been
> wounded by the discharge of a cannon. The cure of this person does
> great honour to the Physician who has the care of the Hospital. He
> [Capt. Lowell] had been inoculated but twelve days, and the Small-
> Pox was just making its appearance, when the accident happened,
> by which his left arm was blown off and never found, and the re-
> maining part was amputated within four inches of his shoulder: The
> right hand and part of the arm were torn to pieces; and this arm was
> amputated just below the elbow: The large vessels of the neck, the
> windpipe and the lower jaw-bone from the chin to the ear, laid quite
> bare; and three of the upper fore teeth broken off with a piece of
> the jaw: The coats of the right eye pierced and its humours
> discharged, and the bone between the eye and nose broken through:
> The other eye greatly hurt; the whole skin of the face and breast
> much burnt, and several shivers of bones driven into his cheeks in
> different places: besides this, he also had a wound four inches long
> in the inside of his thigh, which was so filled with powder that it
> was not discovered 'till several days after the accident. Notwith-
> standing, in the short space of thirty-seven days he is so far re-
> covered as to need no further care of a Surgeon.[84]

This man's cure would have been a remarkable feat in our own time; for the eighteenth century it is remarkable testimony to Hall Jackson's surgical abilities.

Notwithstanding the precautions taken by Jackson and his employers and the undoubted good results among the classes of patients inoculated, the hospital on Cat Island was closed by the local authorities, largely because of rising political pressures brought by the Tories. Following an attempt by some patients returning from the Hospital to land at an unauthorized place, mobs of Marbleheaders created disturbances in the town, unsuccessfully trying to force closure of the hospital.[85]

The next incident was more successful. Ashley Bowen probably knew the men who tried to stir up the town's fear of the spread of smallpox by taking advantage of the regulations requiring the patients' clothes be thoroughly cleaned before they could be returned to the mainland. He tells the story very tersely in his diary: "[Wednesday, January 19, 1774] this Evening John Granday [,] [J?] Broaden [,] James Delap [,] J. Cleark and a servant of Grandays all went to Catt Island in aldor to Steel Close that was Left out a Cleaning and they wear Detected by Colo Orne..."[86] The next day the Marbleheaders expressed their fear of what Granday and his friends might have brought about: "this day the Inhabteant[s] Tarid and feathered the 4 men that Went to Catt Island and Carried them to Sailem and back again."[87]

The *Essex Gazette* for February 1, 1774, had this to say about the end of the Essex Hospital:

> "On Monday, last week a Meeting was called at Marblehead, to put a Stop to the Disorders which for several Days before had happened in the Place. As the Dispute respected the Essex Hospital, it was agreed by the Proprietors to shut it up; at their Desire a Committee was chosen to inspect the cleaning of Furniture, Apparel, &c. On Tuesday the Committee went to the Hospital, and attended their Business until Wednesday Night, when they awaked with the Rest of the Family, being eleven in Number, surrounded with Flames. The Ruffians, who perpetrated this Act, went from the Town prepared with Tar Tubs, &c. and proceeded setting fire to all Parts of the House without any Attempt to awake the People. So infernal were the Villains that they struck down one Man who in Amazement had jumped from his Bed, and was running from the Flames... And others were turned out, cold as it was, with scarcely any Thing to cover them.—The Perpetrators are not yet apprehended.—The Town is in such Confusion that a military Watch is nightly kept, as it's thought Lives and Properties are not safe without it."
>
> The above Account we received from a Correspondent; in Addition to which, we hear, that the Number of People who went over to Cat Island, to burn the Hospital, was about 20; Part of them, in Disguise, went up from where they landed, and set Fire to the Building, which contained 70 beds, with Bedding, and all the other Furniture belonging to the Hospital, the whole of which was consumed,

together with a Barn.—The Loss to the Proprietors (four in Number) is estimated at Two Thousand Pounds.[88]

Of the fire, Ashley Bowen noted only that "this Night the Hospitol Took fier and was Consumed with Barn [,] Litt[le] House [for cleansing] and all."[89]

A month later he recorded the proprietors' attempt to bring the arsonists to justice:

> [February 25, 1774]...the Properaiters of Esex Hospitol took two men up on Suspision of there being Concerned in Burning the Hospitol at Catt Island and carried them to Salem and put them in Prisone but our fishermen all Rise in a body and Went to Salem and brougth home again...[90]

The proprietors finally gave up trying to prosecute the men when, according to Bowen: "We hear the Propriaters of Esex Hospitol have with drown the Write against Burning the Hosp."[91]

So Hall Jackson's model hospital went up in flames, partly in political flames, at the instigation of or with the tacit consent of the local Tories, as Billias has shown. Unfortunately, Jackson's own thoughts on the subject have not been passed on to us, and the episode may well have been but another in the long series of riots on what now seem like flimsy excuses that characterized the decade before the Revolution.[92]

Three years later Jackson was recalled to Marblehead for the same purpose. By that time the town had not only come to realize the safety and usefulness of inoculation, it had also, since the start of the Revolution, ceased to believe all that the Tories said. This time Jackson's invitation came not from private entrepreneurs, but from the town meeting, under the new regulatory statute. Consequently, he could offer his patients a peaceful course of treatment. Yet when he left Marblehead for the second time, it was with a bitterness that would become increasingly familiar to him after the Revolution (see Chapter 2).

The town of Marblehead gained more by Jackson's second stay than he ever did. In 1787, ten years later, he wrote to Robert Hooper, Jr. (1741–1814) who, at the specific request of the board of selectmen, had first asked Jackson to superintend the town-funded inoculation program. Jackson asked Hooper to persuade the selectmen to pay him what they owed him for his services in 1777. At that time the town fathers had panicked because small pox was flourishing in towns all around Marblehead. Under the terms of the agreement between Jackson and the selectmen, the town was to pay for the inoculation procedure, Jackson's fees, and any other medicines he might use. Unfortunately for Jackson, there was no written contract to cover the agreement.[93]

Jackson arrived in Marblehead on April 22, 1777. During the five months he remained there, he cared for 1519 patients, of whom he inoculated 448, including four of Ashley Bowen's children. The rest were treated for other conditions, such as dysentery, which was spreading through the town at the same time. The local Small Pox Committee, however, did not have its heart in the program—it actually encouraged those whom Jackson inoculated to pay no more than fifteen shillings for the treatment, whereas in Boston he had been paid 48 shillings per patient in 1764, 20 shillings at the Essex Hospital in 1773, and 30 shillings in Portsmouth in 1787. Because he had purchased a stock of medicines out of his own pocket before going to Marblehead the second time, on the understanding that he would be reimbursed, he ruefully informed the Marblehead selectmen in 1787 that medicines that had cost him fifteen pounds before the war cost him 316 pounds in 1777, a remarkable degree of inflation. He assured Hooper that he asked only for an opportunity to negotiate with the selectmen, if they would give him a definite appointment to meet with them.[94]

Jackson's attempts to be compensated continued for another six years, but to no avail. In November 1793 the Marblehead selectmen informed him that: "They do not hold themselves accountable, nor can they make acknowledgement for the same." Thus ended only one of Hall Jackson's attempts to be reimbursed for professional services by a government agency.[95] After the Revolutionary War he found it just as difficult to convince the Continental Congress to make good its financial responsibilities to him.

Although Jackson tried in vain to obtain back wages from the State of New Hampshire and the United States Government, as well as the town of Marblehead, it is hard to assess his actual need for money. It seems to have been relatively small, in spite of his protests. He himself wrote that his prewar income was 350 pounds a year, which would have enabled him to live comfortably.[96] It is likely that his pleas for compensation are now magnified by the preponderance of his letters on the subject that have survived, largely because they were addressed to public officers, who would have kept complete correspondence files.

The Portsmouth tax rolls show that during his entire life in Portsmouth Jackson paid at least as much in taxes as, if not more than, most heads of household in that town on the assessed value of his possessions. And over the thirty years following 1766 he received about 100 to 150 pounds annually from the town for smallpox prevention and care, as well as expenses for medicines used.[97]

In 1774 Jackson billed the Province of New Hampshire for £5/2/6 for services performed during twenty-three professional calls on men garrisoned at Fort William and Mary in Portsmouth harbor. He charged 1/6 for extracting a tooth or for bleeding, four or five shillings for various medicines, five shillings for dressing wounds, four shillings for night calls, and ten shillings for reducing a dislocated hip. These fees are like those charged by his brother-in-law, Stephen Little, also in Portsmouth, but they are greater than the fees charged by other New Hampshire physicians, such as Josiah Bartlett and Benjamin Rowe, Jr., both of whom practiced in small towns near Portsmouth. Because Boston physicians commanded fees similar to Jackson's, it seems that fees were generally higher in the larger towns than in the smaller villages.[98]

A more extensive idea of Hall Jackson's fees can be inferred from extracts of the fee bill established by the physicians and surgeons of Portsmouth only nine years after his death. The fees are almost identical with those established twenty-five years earlier in Boston. Some 1806 fees in Portsmouth were:

| | |
|---|---:|
| Visit in ordinary cases with advice, recipie or one dose of medicine, or common application . . . . | $0.75 |
| Visit by night in ordinary cases . . . . . | 1.50 |
| Visits, two necessary, one the same day, with advice, recipie or one dose of medicine, each time . . . | 1.50 |
| Visit and bleeding at the patient's house . . . . | 1.00 |
| Visit and extracting a tooth at patient's house . . . | 1.00 |
| Visit, opening a small abscess and dressing it . . . | 1.00 |
| Visit and reducing a simple hernia . . . . . | 2.00 |
| Visit and reducing compound fractures of the large bones . . . . . . . . . | 6.00 |
| Visit and reducing simple fractures of the large bones . . . . . . . . . | 3.00 |
| Visit and amputating toes & fingers & extirpating small tumours . . . . . . . . | 2.00 |
| Visit and performing paracentesis & for hydrocele . . | 5.00 |
| Visit and introducing Catheter, first time . . . . | 3.00 |
| Visit and dressing recent wound with one stitch . . | 1.00 |
| Cases of midwifery, easy or common . . . . | 6.00 |
| Cases of midwifery, laborious, exceeding 24 hours . . | 8.00 |
| Amputating, trepanning, hernia, couching or extracting a cataract, and amputating cancerous breast . . | 30.00 |
| Using glyster syringe [enema], in 24 hours, visit not included . . . . . . . . | 0.50 |
| Cases of Lues Venerea, simple and soon cured . . . | 5.00 |
| Cases of Lues Venerea of long continuance . . . | 10.00 |
| Inoculating individuals with cowpox . . . . | 3.00 |
| Inoculating families with cowpox, each person . . | 2.00 |
| Almshouse, each year for continuing coverage . . . | 100.00 |
| For each and every dose of medicine, or every half dozen of powders, pills or boluses, after the first, twenty cents, or double the apothecary's price . . . . | 0.20 |

The fee bill allowed for increased charges if the physician had to travel beyond the limits of Portsmouth to see the patient, except when major surgery or a delivery was involved, and for lower charges when the patient was treated in the physician's own office. Physicians were obliged always to render an itemized bill for every professional service performed, but they were also permitted to remit all or a portion of the charges if the patient could not afford the entire bill.[99]

The operations listed above are like those being performed at the same time in the teaching hospitals of Europe, although the variety may have been less in Portsmouth. Of the eight most frequently performed operations today, only cataract surgery and closed reduction of fractures were performed by Hall Jackson and his contemporaries. (Amputations are rarely necessary today.) They were unable to do the intra-abdominal operations, like cholecystectomies and hysterectomies, that are common today, and they did not understand the necessity for tonsillectomies and adenoidectomies, which together account for the most frequent operative procedure in the late twentieth century.[100]

On the average, costs to patients have increased about tenfold in current money over the last two centuries, if this fee bill is compared with the current fees for a practice in a small town in twentieth-century New Hampshire for comparable procedures. As the complexity of the procedure increases, the cost increment is greater, but part of this escalation seems unrelated to modern technological advances, or to mere inflation. For instance, that it now costs a minimum of about $200 for complete pre- and post-natal care in rural New Hampshire, a thirtyfold increase, reflects increasing emphasis on complete care for the prospective mother; in Hall Jackson's day the doctor was not likely to be consulted much before the expected day of delivery.[101]

(Although it is not possible to translate eighteenth-century colonial currencies into modern dollars by any simple formula, Jackson's fees and incomes may be compared with selected annual incomes, in pounds sterling, of contemporary Revolutionary Bostonians in various walks of life: carpenters, 45−90; common laborers, 15−25; artisans, 50; artisan shopkeepers, 500; urban shopkeepers, 250; merchants, 1500; teachers and Harvard professors, 100−180; Superior Court judges, 800; ministers, 150 plus as much as 400 in emoluments; physicians trained at Edinburgh, 700; and lawyers, 1500−3000. A family of seven living in the city needed an income of £50 a year. A brick house sold for £500, and slaves for 35 to 40 each.[102] Modern readers need not envy their ancestor-patients of two centuries ago.)

Because the physicians who signed the Portsmouth general fee bill agreed to charge twice what the apothecaries charged for medicines, it may be inferred that the doctors were attempting to protect the druggists, and, perhaps, that the physicians did not want to become mere apothecaries themselves. As we have seen in Jackson's own case, however, it was not uncommon for a doctor to have had an apothecary shop not many years earlier.

A few years after the Portsmouth physicians and surgeons established their uniform rate schedule, the problem of easy accessibility of over-the-counter drug products was taken under advisement by the state medical society. In order to protect the reputation of the profession, as well as to protect the health of the people, the society took steps that might be appropriate again today. Its members met and:

> RESOLVED, That the practice of depositing medicines in stores, taverns, and grog-shops, with directions to the common people for

their use, is not only pernicious to the health and morals of society, but derogatory to the character and reputation of physicians.
RESOLVED, That we disapprove the encouragement held out to the public through the medium of pompous advertisements, that the daily use of bitters is not conducive to health; and we consider the facility with which Stoughton's Elix[ir,] Spec., bitters etc. may be secured at country stores, one of the most direct means of inducing habits of intemperance (the bane of society) of any within our knowledge.[103]

Stoughton's Elixir, a patent medicine originally licensed in 1712, contained a substantial amount of alcohol, which was thought to be responsible for much disease.[104] This reasoning, however, was probably based more on morality than on pathology.

Jackson left his wife a substantial estate, valued at $19,212.35, of which almost half was in real estate. The detailed inventory of his estate reflects the worldly goods of an active and prominent practitioner. Over the next few years his executors collected an additional $8000 in debts owed Jackson for his professional services and on personal loans. Considering that the average New England laborer earned between $125 and $250 yearly in 1812, Mrs. Jackson inherited a comfortable establishment and income.[105]

It is unfortunate that the inventory does not list the contents of Jackson's surgical kit, or his library. We know, however, that he kept up with the latest medical literature, and that he altered his practice when he was convinced, by new data, that his patients would benefit.

The only extant volume known to have belonged to him was Thomas Johnson's 1633 edition of John Gerarde's *The Herball or General Historie of Plants*.[106] This book would have been about the nearest thing to a textbook of pharmacology available to him. Because it was already over 150 years old when he died, it may have passed on to him from his father or uncle, both of whom were physicians.

The drug plants available to Jackson among those native to New Hampshire were listed, with a hint of pride, by the Reverend Jeremy Belknap in his history of the state. Jackson had contributed to the compilation of Belknap's list of "Native vegetables for medicinal purposes":

Prickly ash, for "chronic rheumatism"
Poke, or Indian tobacco, for its "strong narcotic quality"
Witch hazel (*Hamamelis*) for "inflammation"
*Lobelia*, "a strong emetic"
*Lobelia cardinalis*, "employed in the cure of a disease with the name of which I will not stain my page" [syphilis]
Skunk cabbage (*Arum*), because it is "very efficacious in asthmatic complaints"

For other plants, Belknap does not list their special therapeutic uses because he says they are too well known for their many different effects:

Black elder (*Sambucus nigra*)
Red elder (*Viburnum opulus*)
Maidenhair fern (*Adianthus pedatuus*)
Sarsaparilla (*Aralia*)
Snake root (*Polygala senega*)
Ginseng (*Panax trifolium*)

Belknap recognized still others that are poisons but may have therapeutic properties in special circumstances. For "spasmodic affections" appropriate treatments included doses of:

[Water] hemlock (*Cicuta maculata*)
Thorn apple (*Datura stramonium*)
Henbane (*Hyoscyamus niger*)
Nightshade (*Solanum nigrum*)

Finally, he is not sure whether a second group of poisonous plants has any medicinal value:

Ivy (*Hedera helix*)
Creeping Ivy, or Mercury (*Rhus radicans*)
Swamp sumach (*Rhus toxicodendron*) [Poison Ivy]
Water Elder (*Viburnum opulus*)
Herb Christopher (*Actea spicata*)
Stinking Snakeweed (*Cliffortia trifoliata*)
White Hellebore (*Veratrum album*)

Altogether, this might be considered to be a rather conservative group of drugs; many of them do have proven pharmacological activities (especially water hemlock, thorn apple, henbane, nightshade, and white hellebore, all of which contain potent poisons that are not in general medical use). The entire group probably represented, to Belknap, potential American independence from the mother country for medical supplies, because the putative range of their curative properties is wide, especially when we recall that they were used to treat symptoms rather than specific nosological entities.[107]

Some idea of the medical books in use in Portsmouth at the time, perhaps even by Jackson, may be gained from the list of 120 volumes given by his contemporary and colleague Joshua Brackett (1733–1802) to the New Hampshire Medical Society in 1792. Brackett's donation contained 7 works on anatomy, 6 on general surgery, 5 on midwifery, 33 on general medicine, 4 on fevers, 2 on infectious diseases, 2 on philosophical principles in medicine, 5 pharmacopoeias or dispensatories, volumes of 3 medical journals, and 2 medical dictionaries.[108] Single volumes each were devoted to subjects as diverse and wide-ranging as gout, ulcers, venereal disease, nursing, mercury, lead, chemistry, dentistry, bile, trephining, hydrocoele, consumption, nerves, and lime-water. Among the still familiar authors represented were Bartholin, Bell, Culpeper, Cheyne, Cornaro, Cullen, Currie, Duncan, Fothergill, Galen, Glauber, Huxham, Morgan, Percival, Pott, Paré, Radcliff, Rush, Salmon, Sydenham, Van

Swieten—and Withering, on the foxglove. The list corresponds closely with at least one other, compiled in 1810, of medical books in general use at the time of the Revolution.[109]

Hall Jackson probably was familiar with many of these and perhaps other standard medical books. He was once asked to comment on a similar bibliography as an examiner for the state medical society.[110] We will see later that he read Withering's important new book almost as soon as it came off the press.

Perhaps the best way to explore the range of a man's reading is to examine his writings. The final chapters will confirm that this is true for Dr. Jackson. His professional records, summarized in Chapter 3, are equally informative. They will permit an assessment of the extent to which his professional judgments reflect contemporary thinking among his colleagues, both in his own milieu and in the academic centers from which the English-speaking world drew its medical concepts. Also, Jackson's records, meager as they are, show the extent to which his professional activities were determined by biological forces within his community—forces that, for the most part, Jackson could not manipulate himself.

Before examining these forces, we will consider the political crisis that required Jackson's special skills in the outskirts of Boston in 1775, both on his military patients and on the entire American medical scene. His letters, and those of his superiors, reveal a sad story of medical politics and treason, alongside a surprising estimate of the achievements of American military surgeons during the Revolutionary War.

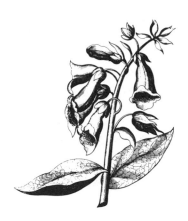

# CHAPTER TWO

# 'A Disagreeable and Dangerous Employment'

## A SURGEON AT THE SIEGE OF BOSTON

NATHANIEL ADAMS described Portsmouth's first reaction to the outbreak of war in neighboring Massachusetts:

> The British troops commenced hostilities, by firing on the people,
> collected at Lexington, in Massachusetts, the 19th of April. The
> news of this attack spread rapidly through the country. This town
> met on the 20th to consider what measures are most expedient to
> be taken at this alarming crisis. They recommended every man to
> furnish himself with a good firelock, bayonet, powder, and balls,
> and every other requisite for defence; that they form themselves into
> companies, and obtain what instruction they can in the military art;
> that one hundred men be enlisted, and properly equipped to march
> at a minute's warning; that they divide themselves into two com-
> panies of fifty men each, choose their own officers, and enter into
> such agreements, so that the strictest subordination and discipline
> be preserved among them. They then chose a committee to consult
> with the provincial committee, and adopt such measures as they
> shall judge necessary.[1]

The alarming—but not unexpected—news prompted Hall Jackson to
lend his professional skills to the cause he already favored. By then his
politics were as well known throughout Portsmouth as his professional
abilities. The royal governor, John Wentworth (1737–1827, governor

1766–1775), was irritated at having to call in a well known patriot in order to obtain the best possible obstetrical care at the birth of his son Charles Mary. The aristocratic governor wrote to a friend, on February 8, 1775:

> There is no doubt S[ullivan] has his spies, and none can be more ready for the office than H. J———n; neither can there be one more deceptive or less to be relied on. He skilfully attended the perilous hour lately in this house, but does not visit here. Even at that time, when retir'd from his professional call, he prefer'd the jolly, laughing servants' hall to the master's parlour, in which I quietly acquiesced. Here his *unmeaning* intention was triumphantly exercised. Obstetric anecdotes, surgery, military instruction, and political phantoms by turns entertained the circle; and the next day his own storys he retail'd on the parade as news from the Province House. The evacuation of this mental dysentery the Major [Sullivan] can have no profit in.[2]

This story of the contagious dangers of republicanism was widely retold at the time. Nathaniel Adams may have had it in mind when he wrote of Jackson that "In the obstetric art he acquired high reputation, & was frequently applied to for advice & assistance in difficult cases, by persons who did not usually employ him."[3]

Like many other Americans in late 1773, Jackson had been caustic in his opinion of Parliament's retention of the Townshend tax on tea imported by the colonies. A week before the Boston Tea Party he wrote, in the third person, from the Essex Hospital to the Portsmouth Selectmen:

> He hopes that the Valiant and Patriotic General Gains will not slacken his endeavours to keep out that pernicious, banefull, and poisonous Herb which the wicked East India Company are endeavouring to cram down (in such abundance) into the Gullets of a free…People; hopes his endeavours will be as successful in this respect, as they were conducive towards the repeal of the *Stamp-Act and Honour of Great Pitt*; he humbly conceives the manner of imposing this noxious weed on us, is unconstitutional, so far as it will tend to prejudice the Healths and Constitutions of those that make use of it.[4]

This was certainly not the last time that toxicology and politics were to be utterly confused by American physicians and politicians.

Jackson seems not to have been an excessively passionate patriot, however. A few years before the war, he signed a petition seeking a peaceful settlement of the colonists' grievances with England. As the war approached its end, he signed another petition requesting that the new state of New Hampshire explore legal ways of dealing with the royalists' property, without having to resort to outright confiscation; in this case, he may have had his sister's interests in mind, because her Tory husband had fled to England. Jackson's own undoubted loyalty to the cause of independence had been recognized in his appointment to the Portsmouth

Committee of Forty-Five which functioned as a Committee of Safety, in May 1775, and to a town committee charged to draw up instructions for its delegates to the Provincial Congress at Exeter seven months later.[5]

He must not have waited for the Portsmouth town meeting on April 20, 1775; he had arrived in Cambridge by that evening so that he could help the wounded.[6] Probably because the wounded numbered less than forty, Jackson was back in Portsmouth four days later, when he wrote to Colonel Jeremiah Lee (1721–1775) of Marblehead, congratulating him on his recent close escape from the British on April 18th, along with Azor Orne and future American Vice-President Elbridge Gerry, after a meeting with John Hancock and Samuel Adams at Menotomy (now Arlington). He went on to describe his anxiety to join in the fight:

> Could it be thought advisable for us to leave the seaports, I should long before this have been with you at the head of a company as good as ever twanged a bow. Inferior in military discipline to none, they are anxious and eager to be with you.
>
> You will know how the art military has been my hobby horse for a long time past. I have vanity enough to think that the recommendation of an immediate perusal of the enclosed volume to the officers in the United army will not be thought impertinent at this time, considering the nature of our country; considering the natural genius of our men, no piece could be better adapted to our circumstances...
>
> I have published some pieces in our papers but the *New Hampshire Gazette* can hardly be called a proper channel to convey one's ideas to the Publick. Might not some of the principal parts of the Partisan be given in manuscript to some of our officers?... As I apprehend there is not many books in the country, you will make what use of this you think proper, so that I may have it again hereafter.[7]

It is not known what book Jackson might have sent to Colonel Lee. Jackson is known to have "occasionally indulged himself in writing small scraps of poetry," but none appears to have been published.[8] He had not yet written his book on diphtheria; besides, diphtheria is not a disease of soldiers. Although no other more military manual attributed to Jackson has surfaced, "the Partisan" might have been a manual of arms, written for the use of the troops under Jackson's own command at Portsmouth. In the eighteenth century a partisan was also a double-edged form of pike. Such a weapon might have been used by New Hampshire militia, who also "twanged a bow."

Although the letter leads us to conclude that Jackson had expressed his thoughts on Britain's treatment of her North American colonies in the local press, his name is not signed to any political pieces in the *New Hampshire Gazette* in the months preceding the outbreak of the war, and there is none signed "Partisan." He may have been one of those who wrote political tracts and calls to arms under a variety of pseudonyms,[9] since "partisan" was often used in the sense of "patriot."

After returning from Cambridge, Jackson spent much of his time drilling troops raised by the town meeting, as well as studying his military specialty, artillery:

> ...After returning Portsmo' the military spirit running high, I went on as usual instructing two Company's. I carried to Portsmo' a plan of Paddock's Field Pieces, Carriages, and mounted the three Brass pieces found in Jno. Warner's Store, belonging to Col. Mason. I headed the Company which you exercised with when at home augmented by Twenty men from each Town near Portsmo' and brought up 4 24-pounders and 4 32-pounders from Henry Point...While at Cambridge I acquired the art of exercising the Field Pieces.[10]

Less than two months later Portsmouth learned of the battle of Bunker's Hill on the Charlestown peninsula. The next day, June 19, Jackson packed up his medical and surgical equipment and made the thirteen-hour ride to Cambridge once again, at the special request of the Portsmouth Committee of Safety. At least 271 Americans, and about three times as many British, had been wounded in the action. Jackson found their situation deplorable:

> ...to describe the pittiful and miserable condition of our unfortunate wound[ed] Brethren would be impossible, many tho' 48 hours was elapsed, had never had the least application apply'd, many lay bleeding & not a person to assist them. [Of the surgeons who were there], not one of these were possessed of even a needle, or any other proper Instruments, had they been ever so well equipped, the matter would not have been much mended. I amputated several limbs and extracted many balls the first night, the next day I was hurried to all quarters   Dr. Church having got notice of my being at Mistick, [and he] the best Surgeon on the Continent being obliged to supply poor [General Joseph] Warren's place [because of his death at Bunker Hill] at the Congress forced the principle [part] of the wounded on me, I went on with this fatigue 15 days, when a violent inflammation in my eyes forced me to return to Portsmo'. I lost only two of my patients one Col. Gardiner, of Cambridge wounded in his groin, the other one Hutchinson a man from Amhurst whose thigh I amputated close to his body. He survived 7 days, and would have finally recovered had not the fates took exception to his name [which was that of the unpopular prewar governor of Massachusetts].[11]

Colonel Thomas Gardner's wound was elevated into heroic verse a year later by "a Gentleman of Maryland," who, in a dramatic epic version of the battle, has Gardner say:

> A musket ball, death-winged, has pierced my groin,
> And widely op'd the swift curr'nt of my veins.
> Bear me, then, soldiers to that hollow space,
> A little hence, just in the hill's decline.
> A surgeon there may stop the gushing wound,

And gain a short respite to life, that yet
I may return, and fight one half hour more.
Then shall I die in peace, and to my God
Surrender up the spirit which he gave.[12]

If Hall Jackson ever saw this poem, he probably regretted that the anonymous poet did not know the name of the surgeon who vainly tried to save the fatally injured colonel.

Perhaps Jackson used the ball extractor he had invented in London that first night at the New Hampshire camp near Charlestown Neck. Most wounds were inflicted by the smooth bore muskets that were in common use or by artillery shot. Rifles, with spiral grooving, were issued to specialized companies only, because they were then considered to be more difficult to use. The guns of the day delivered all sizes and shapes of shot, from 3 to 24 pounds, as round shot, grape shot, K-shot, bombs, and cannisters, at rates of up to 100 rounds a day for the lighter guns and up to 40 a day for the heavier weapons. Officers and noncommissioned officers employed straight swords and one or two pistols for their personal defense, but bayonets were in wide usage on muskets and rifles.[13]

Most wounds were attributable to burns or to projectiles, which might pierce any part of the body. The first victim at Bunker's Hill, Private Asa Pollard, was beheaded by a cannon shot, and the most illustrious patriot to die there, Dr. Joseph Warren, was felled by a musket shot to the head. Among parts of the body listed as having suffered nonfatal wounds during the battles at Lexington and Charlestown were the foot, leg, knee, thigh, groin, breast, arm, hand, throat, and cheek. One American was wounded by a ball that pierced his right shoulder and emerged through his back; he survived the wound by eleven years, but was crippled by it. Jackson's successful treatment of the captain who was nearly blown up by a cannon at Marblehead two years before (see Chapter 1) was probably the most dramatic surgical service he ever rendered.[14]

Some years ago Duncan estimated that nine times as many Continental soldiers died of disease as of battle wounds, and that the same ratio among the British was only five. Peckham's exhaustive recent compilation shows, however, that of the 200,000 American men in military service at some time during the Revolution, 3.6 percent died in battle and 5.0 percent in their camps, presumably of disease (another 4.3 percent died as prisoners of war in British hands). Others have estimated that a Continental soldier had a 98 percent chance of surviving the battlefield, but only a 75 percent chance of surviving a Continental hospital.[15] Although the newer data lay to rest the popular specter of disease as a remarkably greater killer of men than battle during the war, disease was the more feared, because its victims were less prepared for it and it was the less predictable cause of death.

Recomputations show that the Americans lost about 7200 men during the war; of these, approximately 35 percent were killed and the rest listed only as wounded. The British lost more, about 10,200 men, of whom

27 percent were killed.[16] (Comparable assessments for the Americans' French allies, and the Germans hired by the British, cannot be made.) Thus the two sides seem to have come out about even in terms of actual numbers of casualties sustained in battle.

Jackson went home again to Portsmouth about the first of July, but he was back in Cambridge for a third time two weeks later. He wrote of his latest efforts, probably to John Langdon (1714–1819), a Portsmouth merchant and politician who later became governor of his state and a United States senator. He and Jackson were close friends for many years, although Langdon had courted Mary Dalling Wentworth before she married the surgeon. Because Langdon was representing New Hampshire at Philadelphia, Jackson hoped his friend could obtain a secure military appointment for him:

> About ten days after my leaving the Army I received a formal request from the Field Officers of the following Regiments requesting my return to the Army at their expense should not the Continental Congress grant an appointment to me...tho' I act in capacity of Surgeon General to Sullivan's Brigade more particularly, I am hurried thro' the whole Army. Every other day I attend [Doctor] Church to Waltham to dress Coll's. Brewer and Buckminster, who are still languishing with the wounds they received at Bunker's Hill.
>
> Once in a while a person backs out with a small Pox and are removed. Not a Surgeon in Sullivan's Brigade has had the Disease [and therefore all were likely to come down with it].
>
> I receive my authority to act from the General, but when or how much my pay will be, I know not. It will be hard to expect it from the Army whose pay is not more than adequate to their services. The Gentlemen of the Massachusetts Committee inform me that they have apply'd to the Continental Congress for an appointment for Dr. Church and myself, if so, I doubt not of your favorable interposition in my favor. You know the business I have left for the disagreeable and dangerous employment of a Sickly Camp Hospital the disorders of which are generally of the Contageous kind, you know how difficult it will be for me to regain my business when the campaign is up; should you think me worthy your notice I doubt not but you will consider me in the capacity you think proper to establish me in, from the Battle of Charlestown [Bunker Hill].[17]

In the event, Hall Jackson would receive neither position nor pay from the Continental Congress for any of his wartime services, and he would soon fall out with Dr. Benjamin Church, one of Massachusetts' most vocal patriots. In the meantime, he stayed on with Sullivan's brigade.

Brigadier General John Sullivan (1740–1795) was one of the New Hampshire commanders at the siege of Boston. A lawyer without battle experience, his military career was controversial at best—he never won a major engagement. After the war he became a congressman and then governor of New Hampshire. On September 4, 1775, Sullivan wrote from his camp at Winter Hill (in modern Somerville) to the New Hampshire representatives at Philadelphia, John Langdon and Dr. Josiah Bartlett (1729–1795). Bartlett would later be one of the five physicians to sign the Declaration of Independence, the first president of the New Hampshire Medical Society, and, like Langdon and Sullivan, a governor of his state. In his letter Sullivan was most concerned with the medical care provided his troops:

> There is yet a matter of much greater Importance which I must entreat the Congress to take under their Consideration, which is the Regulation of our Hospital, which if continued under the present Regulation [i.e., Church's] I greatly fear will if it does not Ruin the present Army prevent another being arised in America—when I first came here I found our Army very Sickly, the Sick but ill provided with necessaries, I with great trouble got the Hospital for my Brigade well Regulated. Soon after Dr. Church's appointment he ordered all the Sick to be removed to the Hospital at Cambridge with every article I had provided for them.[18]

The Continental Congress had taken over responsibility for providing medical support to the patriot troops in New England from the Massachusetts Provincial Congress in June 1775, and the new relationship was activated when George Washington took command of the army in Cambridge on July 2. At that time the army had only just begun life as a national organization, but for most of the war the soldiers would continue to think of themselves as belonging to their respective states' own regiments.

Before the creation of the Continental Army, the backbone of the medical care provided to the rebel soldiers in the field had been the individual regimental hospital system, although the hospitals were seldom if ever discrete structures, and the system was often organized only loosely on an ad hoc basis. In theory at least each regiment could provide appropriate care for the ten companies of about forty men each which comprised a regiment, following classical British army tradition.

Dr. Benjamin Church (1734–1778?) of Boston was unanimously elected Director General of the Hospital Department of the Continental Army by the Congress. As soon as he assumed his command he began to reshape his department by establishing a General Hospital headquartered in Cambridge. The General Hospital seems to have been envisioned as a more flexible facility in terms of the actual numbers of men for whom medical care could be provided; it would have to be capable of caring for up to 2200 cases of illness during the month of August. In the Hospital Bill passed on July 27, 1775, Congress authorized the posts of one director general and chief physician at $4.00 per day, four surgeons and one apothecary at $1.33 per day, up to twenty surgeon's mates (i.e., assistant surgeons) at $0.66 per day, and one nurse to every ten patients at $2.00 per month, as well as ancillary support personnel. Similar tables of organization had long been used by the British as alternatives to regimental hospitals, under appropriate conditions. When Church took command in early August, he began to commandeer additional buildings to supplement those in which medical services were already being provided. All together, at least ten homes in Cambridge, Menotomy, Roxbury, and Watertown were utilized by the General Hospital, while at least four more were used as smallpox hospitals. Some of them were expropriated after their loyalist owners had fled to the protection of General Gage's troops who were bottled up on the Boston peninsula.[19]

James Tilton (1745–1822), who became Surgeon General of the Army during the War of 1812, confirmed other contemporary and retrospective accounts of the health of the American troops during the Revolution when he wrote, with very little hindsight necessary: "It would be shocking to humanity to relate the history of our general hospital, in the years 1777 and 1778, when it swallowed up at least one half our army, owing to a fatal tendency to throw all the sick of the army into the general hospital." Tilton regarded the mobile field units, then called flying hospitals, as, indeed, a luxury that the country could ill afford if they were to be totally independent of any central control, and suggested that they should be only temporary services provided by the general hospital facility.[20]

In the end, general hospitals continued to be the chief centers of military medicine throughout the war, and, in fact, ever since. But regimental surgeons and hospitals also remained to a limited extent, because they provided the men in the front lines with emergency treatment. When Church's successor as Director General of the Continental Army, Dr. John Morgan of Philadelphia, drew up regulations for regimental surgeons, he was only formalizing procedures already being followed by Hall Jackson and his colleagues:

> It being the duty of the regimental surgeon and mates, in case of action in the field, to attend the corps to which they belong, in order to dress the wounded in battle; they are to take post in rear of the troops engaged in action, at the distance of three, four or five hundred yards, behind some convenient hill, if at hand, there to dress the wounded who required to be dressed, on or near the field of battle...
>
> The amputation of a limb, or performance of any capital operation, cannot well take place in the heat of a brisk action. It is seldom possible or requisite. What the surgeon has chiefly to attend to, in cases of persons being much wounded in the field of battle, is to stop any flow of blood, either by tourniquet, ligature, lint and compress, or a suitable bandage, as the case may require; to remove any extraneous body from the wound; to reduce fractured bones; to apply proper dressings to wounds; take care on the one hand not to bind up the parts too tightly, so as to injure the blood circulation, increase inflammation, and excite a fever; or, so loosely as to endanger the wounds bleeding afresh, or to allow broken bones, after they are properly set, to be again displaced. The wounded being thus dressed

by the regimental surgeons, are next to be removed to the nearest hospital belonging to the brigade, or to the general hospital, as may be most convenient.[21]

That there was need for regulation of the regimental hospitals was evident from Morgan's own observations at one near New York in 1778:

> On looking into the rooms, they were found to be filled with Sick, and the surgeons who had their care, panting for breath, in the midst of them. It was admidst the sultry heat of summer. In vain I represented to [the regimental surgeon] the danger of engendering a putrid, malignant fever, from crowding so many sick in the house. I forbade him then, as I had uniformly prohibited every regimental surgeon, from taking charge of more than thirty or forty sick. I recommended to him to send at least one half of his men into the barn. He disregarded my advice, a putride fever prevailed, he caught the infection and paid forfeit of his rashness with his life.[22]

Tilton must have seen similar tragedies. Thirty-five years later he wrote that "More surgeons died, in the American service, in proportion to their number, than officers of the line! a strong evidence this that infection is more dangerous, in military life, than the weapons of war."[23]

An occasional observation in the field might prove to be of future therapeutic use, but most Revolutionary War surgeons were too busy for even the most informal and unorganized research efforts. Dr. Charles Gilman of Woodbridge, New Jersey, made one discovery, for himself at least, which illustrates the value of healing by first intention over healing by second intention:

> At the battle of 'Haarlem' Heights, I received a crease wound to the back of the hand. Painful, it would not heal and exuded laudable pus. In camp at Newburgh, I spilled—quite accidentally—for I had had too much rum, some upon the member. I covered it, and in two days I noticed no odor. I removed the cover and the wound was healing. Thereafter, all wounds were soaked in rum clothes before covering.[24]

In 1789 Benjamin Rush (1745–1813) first published his thoughts and observations on the fevers which had plagued the armies of both sides, accounting for the discouraging numbers of fatalities in the garrison. In all likelihood it was not one infectious disease, but a number of dysenteries produced by different Gram-negative bacteria:

> The army when in tents was always more sickly than when in the open air. It was likewise more healthy when it was kept in motion, than when it lay in encampment... Young men under twenty years of age were subject to the greatest number of camp diseases... Those officers who wore flannel shirts or waistcoats next their skins, in general, escaped fevers and diseases of all kinds... The principal diseases in the hospitals were the typhus gravior and mitior of Doc-

tor Cullen. Men who came into the hospitals with pleurisies or rheumatisms soon lost the types of their original diseases, and suffered, or died, by the abovementioned states of fever... The typhus mitior always prevailed most, and with the worst symptoms, in winter. A free air, which could only be obtained in summer, always prevented or mitigated it... In all those cases where the contagion was received, cold seldom failed to render it active. Whenever an hospital was removed in winter, one half of the patients generally sickened on the way, or soon after they arrived at the place to which they were sent... There were many instances of patients in this fever, who suddenly fell down dead, upon being moved, without any previous symptoms of approaching dissolution. This was more especially the case, when they arose to go to stool... The contagion of this fever was frequently conveyed from the hospital to the camp, by means of blankets and clothes... The remedies which appeared to do most service in this disease were vomits of tartar emetic, gentle dozes of laxative salts, bark, wine, volatile salts, opium, and blisters ... An emetic seldom failed of checking this fever, if exhibited while it was in a *forming* state, and before the patient was confined to bed... Those soldiers who were billeted in private houses generally escaped the hospital fever, and recovered soonest from all their diseases.[25]

Rush also noted that typhus did not become prevalent in the Continental Army until it had been supplemented by the addition of men from other regions of the country. In this respect, the ratio of battle casualties, few as they were, to infectious disease patients, must have been much higher during Hall Jackson's attendance at the New Hampshire camp at Winter Hill in the summer of 1775 than the ratio other army surgeons would see for the rest of the war:

It is very remarkable that, while the American army at Cambridge, in the year 1775, consisted only of New Englandmen (whose habits and manners were the same) there was scarcely any sickness among them. It was not until the troops of the eastern, middle and southern states met at New York and Ticonderoga, in the year 1776, that the typhus became universal, and spread with such peculiar mortality in the armies of the United States.[26]

Rush later bitterly confirmed Tilton's observations:

Hospitals are the sinks of human life in an army. They robbed the United States of more citizens than the sword... should war continue to be the absurd and unchristian mode of deciding national disputes, it is to be hoped that the progress of science will so far mitigate one of its greatest calamities, as to produce an abolition of hospitals for acute diseases.[27]

Long before the Battle of Yorktown, Rush had made one of the war's most important contributions to medicine, his *Directions for Preserving the Health of Soldiers.* It was first published in a Philadelphia newspaper in April 1777, shortly after Rush had been made Surgeon General of the Middle Department of the Army. Rush's recommendations, reissued at the request of the Board of War less than a year later in pamphlet form, were prompted by his observation that "a greater proportion of men perish with sickness in all armies than fall by the sword." (Although we've seen that this estimate was true for the entire Revolutionary War period, the actual proportion was not so dramatic as Rush wanted his readers to believe.) To fight the disproportionate incidence of contagious disease, he emphasized the importance of personal cleanliness, diet (he favored vegetables over meat), appropriateness of dress, and suitability of encampment sites, so as to avoid the swamps and marshes, where intermitting fevers were most prevalent.[28]

When Benjamin Church issued his new regulations, designed to implement his reorganization of the medical services available to the regiments from New Hampshire and other colonies, General Sullivan was horrified at both their means and their ends:

> This [sending the troops to the general hospital in the rear lines, at Cambridge] filled [the men] with such fearful apprehensions that more than half of them refused to go, Declaring they would rather Die where they were, and under the care of those Physicians they were acquainted with, than be removed from their friends under the care of Physicians they never saw. I found it vain to attempt Reasoning them out of those Sentiments, but Dr. Church gave orders to the Commissary not to supply them with one article, & ordered all the persons unfit for duty to be removed to Cambridge, paying no regard to the Regimental Surgeons, and Refused to supply them with Medicine, & even with Bandages to Dress the Wounded, but ordered in case of any person being wounded he should be sent to be dressed at Cambridge at three or four miles Distance, which has Completely put our Regimental Surgeons out of employ [including Jackson] & raised such a Clamor among officers and soldiers That I know not what will be the Consequence...I must beg Leave to say that I never read or heard of such a regulation in an Army. I have ever understood That they have a grand Hospital for Capital wounds & Disorders, & Infirmaries & flying [mobile field] Hospitals for those that are Slightly wounded or Indisposed...You well know the prejudice of our people in favor of their own Physicians. The Terrible Ideas they form to themselves of an hospital Regulated by Strangers where there is scarce a face they know, & in order to bring them there they are even Denied a Little meal to work a Cathartic, Throw off a Disorder, or mutton to make them broth or any other thing, so that they must even in Case of a Common Cold go to the Hospital, or have nothing to take except Salt Beef and Pork. I must beg that some method may be taken to Quench the growing flame already at too great a heighth...I know Dr. Church complains of those Regimental Hospitals as having been very expensive,

which the Regimental Surgeons Deny, & say he cannot prove the assertion.[29]

Sullivan was hoping that Congress might establish brigade hospitals to accompany each fighting unit in the field. He was known to his contemporaries for his interest in the health of his men; a few months later he seems to have become familiar with Dr. John Jones's advocacy of the judicious use of regimental hospitals scattered throughout the armies in order to avoid crowding and consequent epidemics.

Six months after the Battle of Lexington, Jones (1729–1791), Professor of Surgery at King's College in New York, rushed into print with the first book on surgery published in America. His *Plain Concise Practical Remarks on the Treatment of Wounds and Fractures* was expressly "designed for the Use of young Military Surgeons in North America." The book was not only a very good first aid manual, but also a detailed exposition of surgical procedures commonly required in the field; it emphasized the necessity of fresh air for optimum care in military hospitals. Another authority on military medicine with whose ideas Sullivan might also have been familiar was Richard Brocklesby (1722–1797), who had called upon his observations in the French and Indian War when formulating recommendations for improving military hospitals. He was convinced that the practice of general medicine was more important to the health of armies than was the provision of emergency surgery.[30]

Sullivan's request to the Congress seems to have been inspired by a petition from the New Hampshire field grade officers who pointed out that:

> When we first Engaged in the service, and Enlisted our Men, in reciprocation of their promising Obedience We Solemnly Engag'd our utmost exertion for, and Constant attention to, their safety, their Comfort, and Satisfaction...But Alas—when our Men most need the Care of their officers, when Dispirited with Excruciating diseases, They must be Halled away by Cart loads; far distant from our Camps and Exposed to the inclemency of the Weather, in a manner Derogatory to human nature. The bare thoughts of being removed from the presence of friends, will naturally damp the spirit of A man, in the perfect Enjoyment of Health, but much more so the spirits of Men struggling with diseases scarcely supportable...If we are unhappily and Suddenly seized with the most dangerous Symptoms, we must be immediately mov'd to Cambridge Hospital, or expire unassisted by medicines, or Medicinal Art, for we are not allow'd Brigade Hospitals, nor can we be sufficiently supplied with proper necessaries for the Sick....Must the wounded tho' far Distant, Mangled Lacerated and Bleeding by the Hostile Ball be Carried to Cambridge To Suffer Amputation, when their Blood has deserted their Empty Veins; and nothing but the Painful Operation is necessary to put a Period to Life...We are furnish'd with surgeons of approved Skill, and Integrity, and with a Gentleman Who has

> Generously at the Request of many of the Gentlemen of the Province to which he belongs and satisfaction of the officers in this Brigade Voluntarily served as Surgeon, and Physician, Whose Character is too well known to need a Recommendation [i.e. Hall Jackson].

The officers concluded by asking Sullivan to persuade Washington to permit them to establish a brigade hospital and to have adequate medical supplies; they felt that Jackson was already meeting their medical needs.[31]

Ten days after writing to the New Hampshire delegates to Philadelphia, enclosing the officers' petition, Sullivan received the following enigmatic message from Benjamin Church, a week after Washington had ordered a full-scale investigation of charges brought by the regimental surgeons against Church's administration:

> Doctor Church presents his most respectful Complements to General Sullivan and most heartily felicitates himself on receiving so honorary a Testimonial of General Sullivan's Approbation as He met with the last Evening at Head Quarters. The Doctor esteems himself peculiarly happy that the undeserv'd Prejudice against him is so totally remov'd, which from frequent Intimations, He was apprehensive had possessed the General's Mind. He flatters himself that his whole Conduct during the present unhappy Contest will bear the strictest Scrutiny. Regard to Place, Popularity or the more detestable Motive of Avarice never influenc'd his Conduct in Publick Life— The sole Object of his Persuit, the first Wish of his Heart was ever the Salvation of his Country.
>
> The Doctor nevertheless in justice to himself, and with Respect to the Man who behind the Curtain has influenced and took the Lead in opposition to him must declare, that altho' He cou'd never stoop to act the Parrasite, play the Buffoon, or become the Herald of his own Eminence in his Profession, would feel the Indignation of conscious Merit shou'd He put in Competition with the Person who vainly endeavours to supplant him.

Because both Sullivan and Church were expert politicians, because Sullivan had not only received information which he must have felt was trustworthy from his officers but also had transmitted it and his own opinions to the New Hampshire members of Congress, because Sullivan's regiment had led the call for the investigation, and because Church is now known to have been both avaricious and uncommitted to the salvation of his country, it would seem that the two men had perhaps only exchanged ironic pleasantries with each other at the Headquarters dinner, presumably under Washington's scrutiny. Although he mentioned no name, Church was probably trying to undermine Hall Jackson's influence with Sullivan; nevertheless, Jackson and Sullivan remained good friends for many years afterward. Jackson was ambitious, but he was not the summer soldier and sunshine patriot that Church proved to be. In fact, Church may well have felt that Jackson was a real threat to his undercover work, that Jackson could potentially unmask the Director-General's efforts to facilitate an eventual British victory. Five days later the court of inquiry were "Unanimously of opinion, that the Complaints against the Director Gen¹ have arisen from a misunderstanding in the Regimental Surgeons, not distinguishing between supplies for Regimental Hospitals, and such as are for the sick in Camp, and that the Conduct of the Director Gen¹ Justly merits approbation and applause." Notwithstanding, the next day Church submitted his resignation, claiming preoccupation with family affairs; but General Washington was unwilling to part with a good officer.[32]

Sullivan had already proposed the obvious candidate for surgeon to his own brigade of New Hampshiremen to that province's representatives in Congress:

> I would humbly Recommend an Hospital to each Brigade, and some person of Integrity to Superintend each. Doctor Hall Jackson, who is now with me, was Superintendent of mine & gave great satisfaction. I need not say any thing to you of his great abilities as a Surgeon & Physician, & though he has out of Tenderness to his Countrymen attended the Army at his own Expense, Dressed the wounded & Treated the Sick, he has had no appointment but others have preferred whole Regiments of which would not serve the Army so much in Dressing the wounded or performing Chyrurgical operations. I wish for the good of the Army he might have some appointment, & if agreeable that he might be Chief or Superintending Surgeon to my Brigade.[33]

Jackson himself wrote to Langdon the next day, not only to urge Langdon to support his candidacy for the job of brigade surgeon, but also to explain why he needed the appointment:

> I had established a Hospital for General Sullivan's Brigade [in Charlestown] had near a hundred Patients for more than a month, under as good regulations as could be desired, provided with every necessity that prudence and economy would dictate. When all of a sudden they were hurried *Volens Nolens* to a general Hospital at Cambridge without a single compliment paid either to them, or their former attendants.
>
> As every Idea of an establishment in the Army was at an end, you may well conclude that I would have no inclination or desire to tarry at the expense of 20 or 30 Lawfull Mon'y p'r week, besides the loss of my Business at Portsmouth, which is infinitely more valuable than any thing I can expect in the Army. Yet I am still forced contrary to my inclination to tarry. General Lee, General Sullivan... will not suffer me to hint an intention to leave them; as not a Surgeon in the whole Brigade has ever had the small Pox, or ever performed a Capital Operation. Some Officers in the Army have offered me a substitution equal to anything I would expect, but this

I should dispise, their pay being little enough to support their own Commissions with Honour and decency. Gratitude to them, obliges me to continue with them, until the pleasure of the Continental Congress is known, after which I am at liberty to do as I shall think proper, I can assure you, that I have no great inclination to be employed, I am heartily sick of the din and confusion of War.[34]

A few days later Jackson wrote again to Langdon, expressing an opinion of the general hospital like Sullivan's. He bitterly detailed his expenses: "I have paid 12-L.M. p week for my board and 7-L.M. for my house, besides other contingent charges, add to this my extensive family at home, Doctors Cutter and Brackett & Little running away with all my business at Portsmouth." [35]

Knowing his former partner's political opinions, Jackson must have been particularly galled at the loss of his patients to a Tory brother-in-law. Dr. Stephen Little (1745–1800) had been apprenticed to Jackson's father, and married his preceptor's daughter Sarah. A convinced loyalist, he finally escaped to British protection in May 1777 and fled to London a year later after he had been banished by the state of New Hampshire. Little worked as a surgeon in a London hospital and in the Royal Navy, to supplement the small pension awarded him for his losses in support of his king and country, but he died the proprietor of an apothecary shop. Although he was proscribed from returning to Portsmouth, his family never joined him in England.[36]

By mid-September, Jackson's view of the war itself had been further colored by Benjamin Church:

The arts, contrivance, and hypocricy, of some of M------usetts Patriots is dam-able to the last degree. "A Struggle for Liberty"! —good God! my Soul abhors the Idea! If methodically to kill the wounded; to starve the sick, and languishing because they cannot Diet on Salt Pork, or will not submit to be severed from their dearest friends and relations, if these (my Dear Friend) are the Characteristicks of an Army raised for the defence of Liberty, I frankly confess I have no claim to an employment in the glorious Cause.[37]

Jackson's quarrel with Church was over within another month, when it was discovered that perhaps since before the beginning of the war Church had been providing information about the patriot leaders and, later, their army, to the British. He had probably lobbied to obtain his appointment as Director General harder than he might otherwise have done, on the assumption that the British would reward the enemy army's most senior physician more generously than they would a mere regimental surgeon. Perhaps the emotional side effects of the war, or the unfulfilled promise of the medical service in Cambridge, contributed as much to the political atmosphere of Church's court-martial as the treasonable letter that led to his unmasking, although no testimony to Church's professional activities was brought to his military or civil trials.[38]

General Sullivan illustrated the damage Church had done to the army and to Hall Jackson in a letter to Langdon and Bartlett on October 4, 1775:

You will by this Post Receive Intelligence from head-Quarters of Dr. Church'es having been detected in holding a Treasonable Correspondence with the Enemy—his Behavior Towards our Sick & wounded long since Convinced me that he either was void of humanity and Judgement, or that he was Determined by untimely Removal and Neglect of Duty to Let all those under his care breathe their Last within the walls of his detestable General Hospital—his Conduct with respect to my Brigade has been very regular, for he has Regularly Killed most of all those he has taken from us [to the General Hospital]. I will mention Two Instances of the wounded: one was the well known instance of Mr. Simpson, who was shot in the foot—an amputation was necessary—Doctor Jackson, who every one must allow to be Infinitely his Superior, was there, & had every thing prepared to take off the Limb—Doctor Church happened to come in—forbid him to proceed & ordered the man to be sent to the Hospital—he went home himself—Eat his Dinner—Drank his Glass—then went to meet the wounded voluntier who, by the loss of Blood, The Tearing and Lacerating his flesh by the Fractured Bone had become happy by growing Insensible of his pain—Jackson had fortold this, but Church Determining to Kill the man Secundem Artem, called his *Subs* around him—assigns each one his post, and then requests Jackson to take off the Limb—he Refused, Informing them that the only reason was the Man's life could not be saved by amputating the Limb or by any other methods, & agreeable to his predictions the Man Died on the Second day. The other was an instance of a man in my Brigade who, while we were throwing up our last Redoubts, was wounded in the Leg—Dr. Jackson was by—said his Leg must be taken off, but he did not dare to do it till Church was sent for—he sent down two of his Subs, who Complimented Jackson with the Liberty of using the Saw—one of them was to cut the flesh—the other to take up the Arteries. The first failed, leaving some of the muscles untouched, & the other would not if left to himself have taken up the Arteries till the man had Bled to Death—Jackson was obliged to take the knife from one & the needle from the other—performed the operation—Drest the man & tended him three Days—every symptom was favourable & Doubtless the man would have soon Recovered, but on the Fourth day Doctor Church sent for him & ordered him to the Hospital. Jackson told them that the fourth being the Day on which the Inflammation was at the highest he would assuredly die if removed—he was not regarded—the man was removed & died accordingly.[39]

It is not clear to what extent the rank and file of regiments from other colonies shared the feelings of the New Hampshire troops about the inhumanity of being separated from their friends and neighbors when they were sent to the General Hospital in Cambridge, but Sullivan's opinion was not an isolated one. It has been argued, with considerable force, that Church's efforts to consolidate the seriously ill patients into the General Hospital were justified and productive, as were his attempts to limit the autonomy of the many regimental surgeons. After all, the British army, for a long time, had chosen between regimental and general hospital services as local military circumstances dictated. And it cannot be argued successfully that considerations of friendship and a common provincial background should outweigh the necessity of ensuring the health of an entire military command. Church was unwise, however, and he probably prepared the way for a downfall more certain than otherwise might have befallen him, in three respects: it was inefficient, at best, to force even mild cases of illness to go to the rear lines; withholding food and treatment from men who would not go to the rear lines was easily interpretable as blackmail; and regardless of the merits of his system, Church's failure to take morale into account was guaranteed to impede the successful implementation of his medical goals. Later in the war, admission to the General Hospital was only by referral from regimental surgeons. In the face of Hall Jackson's previously demonstrated competence as a surgeon, Church's failure to cooperate with him must be regarded as a political or personal vendetta, perhaps coupled with a fear that Jackson might eventually expose him, and not as a bona fide attempt to provide optimal medical care to the troops on Winter Hill or elsewhere around besieged Boston.[40]

The astonishing circumstances of the loss of the new army's chief medical officer shocked the civilian population as well as the military. The story filled newspapers and diaries throughout New England. But the greatest damage had been done, of course, on the outskirts of Boston. When Dr. John Morgan (1735–1789) arrived in Cambridge in December 1775 to reorganize the shambles left by Church and his temporary successors, he found the General Hospital in a hopeless mess. One of his first acts was to take an inventory. Of the 120 items in it he wrote:

> many were useless, or in little demand, and of no value, and many, especially of the articles in most demand, were but in very small quantities... The quantities of [drugs essential to a military hospital] were in general so small, that... there was little more than a sufficiency of these for one good regimental medicine chest, and of some of them, not a sufficiency for even one... And these to supply an army of twenty thousand men! The blankets were brought in by the sick men, and carried out by them when they recovered. Of sheets, none, or but very few, and of straw beds, scarcely a sufficiency for about 500 patients that were at that time in the different Hospitals. In the whole of the General Hospital I did not find above two hundred bandages, and but few dressings, or materials for dressings of any kind... In those twenty-five battalions, were found six sets of amputating instruments, only two pocket cases of common incision knives, and but three sets of lancets in the whole, all

private property. In two battalions only were found a good assort-
ment of medicines. In the remaining twenty-two, none, or only in
a very small quantity.[41]

It was fortunate that these shortages were most acute at the time of the
siege of Boston, during which there were few additional battle injuries.
The infectious diseases that occurred during the winter were probably the
same as those that were found commonly in many army camps, such as
at Ticonderoga in August 1776, including the "bilious, remitting, and
intermitting fevers, with some of the putride kind; dysenteries, diar-
rhoeas, and rheumatick complaints."[42]

At that time the surgeons at Ticonderoga compiled "A Catalogue of
Medicines Most Necessary for the Army." For one battalion, perhaps
200 men, they recommended as minimum supplies 20 pounds of Peruvian bark, 4 pounds of gum camphor, 2 pounds of gum opium, 3
pounds of powdered ipecac, 4 pounds of powdered jalap, 2 pounds of
powdered rhubarb, 15 pounds of Epsom salts, and 3 pounds of tartar
emetic, among others. Using these and other average minimum requirements as a baseline, it can be calculated that the Cambridge General
Hospital, designed to serve many battalions, was left with the following
proportions of the amounts recommended, for one battalion, of the nine
drugs most commonly prescribed for Revolutionary War soldiers: bark,
11 percent; jalap, 5 percent; ipecac, one percent; rhubarb, 179 percent,
purging salts (Epsom or Glauber's), 21 percent; tartar emetic, one percent; Spanish flies, or cantharides, for blistering plasters, 66 percent;
camphor, one percent; and opium, 0 percent. It is unlikely, however,
that any Director General could have ensured adequate drug supplies
for the American army, because the British were blockading all shipping
routes.[43]

Hall Jackson realized that he had been Church's dupe since they first
met in Cambridge and Charlestown:

> I waited impatiently for some appointment, that would keep the pot
> boiling at home, whilst I exerted myself abroad, for good of my
> Country. Church pretended to be my friend, was mighty sorry that
> I was left out of the general hospital, beg'd General Sullivan and
> all the officers, to use their interest to retain me in that army whilst
> he would have a mistake in the matter satisfyed, all the time the
> dirty dog was plotting against me, and was as great an enemy to me,
> as he was to his own Country and made up the hospital upon some
> mercenary plan of his own.[44]

As Church lost his big gamble, so Jackson lost his. On October 18,
1775, John Adams wrote from Philadelphia: "Yesterday they [the Continental Congress] chose a successor [to Dr. Church], Dr. Morgan an eminent Surgeon of this city. We as usual had our men to propose, Dr. Hall
Jackson and Dr. [Isaac] Forster [of Charlestown, who had been chief
surgeon of the General Hospital in Cambridge] ... But Dr. Forster's sufferings and services and Dr. Jackson's great fame, experience and merits

were pleaded in vain." That Jackson was even considered for the senior military medical post attests to his surgical and other professional skills, but his candidacy was doomed to failure, largely for political reasons. He returned home to Portsmouth.[45]

The Provincial Congress of New Hampshire tried to save face both for Dr. Jackson and for itself. On November 11, 1775, it voted to send to the Continental Congress and General Washington "a Recommendation of Doctor Hall Jackson to be Chief Surgeon of the Northern Division of the Continental Army or to appoint him in any other way according to his merit." But the Continental Congress had already appointed John Morgan a month before, and the best that could be done for Jackson was to make him chief surgeon to the New Hampshire troops.[46]

Eighteen months later Jackson still held his vitriolic opinions of both Congress and Church. In May 1777 he wrote to some member of Congress, perhaps Langdon, from Marblehead, where he was running that town's second attempt at an inoculation hospital:

> That the Congress would be prejudiced against me it was natural to expect since there is One whose election I opposed for no other reason, but because I was convinced that pride, arrogance, self interest, added to desperate circumstances, were not the wished for qualifications—of your aguish Assembly... Doctor [Matthew] Thornton [the third signer of the Declaration of Independence for New Hampshire]... will know how much I have exercised my self in the common cause, even to the loss of my Business, which all most wholly fell into the hands of those, I now see promoted while I find myself neglected, but I rather think this circumstance was designed (by some) as an agravation to me.[47]

By that time, Congress had been convinced that Jackson should be appointed Senior Surgeon of the Middle Department of the Continental Army. But Jackson refused the belated offer, saying that he would accept it

> was I not engaged in a general Inoculation in this unhappy place [Marblehead]... I have 1600 Patients of all Ages, Constitutions, and Circumstances, under my care, and it is impossible to say how long I shall be detained nor am I convinced that after this perplexing affair I shall not be a more proper subject for a Bedlam or Lunatic Hospital than the one you so kindly recommend me to.[48]

As it turned out, the Continental Congress and General Washington had nothing but trouble with their principal physicians in the field. Drs. Church, Morgan, Shippen, and Rush were all to leave the service under clouds of treason, fiscal irresponsibility, or personality difficulties.[49]

Although Jackson had finally been recognized by Congress, however modestly, he was never rewarded with promotion, or even with pay for services actually rendered. Collecting his and others' back pay became almost an obsession with him until shortly before his death. Despite his continued protests throughout the war and afterward, however, he was never in serious financial straits. He was annoyed most that others were cutting into his practice at home while he was providing the army professional services for which he never received any compensation from the United States, in whose behalf he had fought with both drugs and cannon.

Late in October 1775, while in charge of a 42-man field artillery company in Portsmouth, Jackson displayed the bitterness that was to outlast the war, in a letter to the New Hampshire Provincial Congress. He seems to have been refuting a recent attack on his character and integrity:

> Gentlemen: It having been insinuated that I have been absent from the army a considerable part of my time since my first entering, I beg leave humbly to inform the Congress, that arrived at the army 19th of June I tarried until the 29th...On the 13th of July I return'd to the Army, and have never been absent but eight days, on command to recruit the Medicine Chest, which I did at Salem and Portsmouth. I have now been home fifteen days, my whole time has been taken up in laying out fortifications at Kittery and New-Castle, in making Cartridges, Cannasters, and port-fires, for the Field Pieces, in raising and exercising the Artillery Company, in hearing and administering to the innumerable complaints of the Soldiers in regard to their healths.
>
> The honourable Congress will please to observe, that I first perform my Business, then Ask for such a reward as they shall judge reasonable, while others, conscious of their own inabilities, would not venture their performances upon the same issue, but insist on large and remarkable Stipends before they enter the Service.
>
> If there is the least objection in Congress to grant me the commission [in the New Hampshire troops] asked for, I am so little anxious to continue in the service, that I beg leave to retract the request.[50]

On November 14, too late to really gratify him, the Provincial Congress finally voted:

> that Doctor Hall Jackson be paid out of the Public Treasurey of this colony in full for his good services to this Colony from the 19 June to the 4th of August last the sum of £15 per month and that he receive a Commission from this Congress as Chief Surgeon of the New Hampshire troops in the Continental Army.

Not only did they pay him a total of only about 22 pounds, but the Congress considered that he had worked for them only until August 4, although Jackson had provided a detailed timetable for his activities. He continued to point out that he had parted with his usual annual income of 350 pounds, or 1600 contemporary dollars, to honor a specific request from the Provincial Congress. His friends in that Congress also tried to augment his income. In March 1776 it voted Jackson a monthly salary of seven and a half pounds, and appointment as "Surgeon of our Troops at Piscataqua [Portsmouth Harbor]," although it is not clear from the records whether either term of the vote was to be retroactive, or if the new vote was to supersede that of five months earlier, when he was made Chief Surgeon of all New Hampshire troops at fifteen pounds a month. In December 1776 he was paid twenty-eight pounds for his professional services at Portsmouth for the period from June 10 to December 16, plus another twenty-three pounds for medicines. He continued to provide medical care for the New Hampshire troops stationed near Portsmouth over the next four years, often supplying them with medicines from his own stocks. The new state's government curtly refused to pay him more than 48 pounds, after considering his bill for yet another four years.[51]

Jackson even petitioned appropriate Congresses for monies owed to other people who had served the war effort. On September 15, 1777, while at Portsmouth, he certified that:

> the Wife of Morris Fitzgerald has faithfully nursed, washed, and taken care of all the Sick of Col. Long's Regiment, as also those of Forts Washington, & Sullivan, that have been carried to the Hospital on Adam's Island; as also a number of Sick belonging to the Company lately raised and marched for Providence, and also three men belonging to an Armed Schooner brought in by Capt. Pincum one of which tarried three months in the Hospital. The whole of which amounting at least to 90 Patients. That she has not received any pay or compensation for her services since October 1776.

A year later Jackson certified that Brigadier General James Reed of New Hampshire had become blind while on active duty in 1777 and was therefore incapable of employment. Three years later, Jackson certified that Simeon Fernald had died as a result of a hemorrhagic illness contracted on an expedition into Maine; presumably some form of compensation depended on the certification.[52]

As late as 1792, eleven years after Cornwallis' surrender at Yorktown, Jackson, General William Heath, and four others signed a printed circular addressed to the United States Congress at Philadelphia:

> We have had the honour to be appointed a Committee, by the Officers of the Massachusetts line of the late Army, to attend to and prosecute their memorial to the Congress of the United States, on the subject of compensation for the losses sustained by them and the soldiers who served during the war, in consequence of the singular manner in which their services have been acknowledged and requited by the United States...

The signatories went on to say that although they realized that for the first few years after the peace the country would have been unable to afford the funds owed her defenders, the present state of affairs should now allow the government to pay its legitimate debts.[53]

During the war and afterward, Congress was notorious for not compensating the Continental Army. General John Glover of Marblehead went unpaid for at least twenty months but at the same time was not allowed to resign his commission.[54] Although Jackson's own bad luck with Congress probably was the result of congressional inattention to his applications, perhaps tainted by long political memories, it is not likely that such inattention could have prevented the entire Massachusetts manpower contribution to the war effort from being compensated. Jackson thought that he had personal enemies in Congress, but he may have flattered himself in this respect.

He continued to contribute to the war effort for a year after he was refused a Continental Army medical position. Late in 1775 he wrote to Langdon that he had returned to Portsmouth because the town was in danger of a British attack. He goes on to tell Langdon that he has been drilling the local militia because he cannot practice much medicine, having used up all his own medical supplies while in the army:

> I have given up all prospects, and turn'd drill corporal again...I carried all the little Stock of Medicines into the army and have expended them, so that I have nothing to work with, but my knife and glyster pipe [a syringe for administering enemas and similar medications], no medicines to be had in New England.

Jackson described his drill methods, and sketched the fortifications of Portsmouth harbor. His military specialty was artillery; his map of the harbor defenses accurately reflects current thinking on effective defenses.[55]

The surgeon's expertise in designing fortifications was respected even by his commanding general, Sullivan. On November 1, 1775, while stationed in Portsmouth to protect the port facilities from possible British attack, Sullivan ordered:

> Col° Wingate is desired to call upon Doct' Hall Jackson to lay out a Redoubt upon the Summit of the Hill upon the North part of Great Island, who will mark out the same agreeable to the directions given him...The Redoubt which is to be thrown up is to have a re-entering angle in the middle of each Curtain [wall] in order to flank the Enemy of which Doct' Jackson is to take notice.[56]

When Jackson drew up general orders for his first Portsmouth Artillery Company, he specified that the men exercise from 8:00 to 9:30 each morning and from 4:00 until sunset each afternoon. During the interim one half the company was to form a working party, on alternate days, to improve the town's defenses against British attack. Jackson described his own activities with the ordnance captured on December 14–15, 1774, from the garrison at Fort William and Mary in Portsmouth Harbor:

> When the Brass Field Pieces fell into our hands, no person understood the method of constructing the Carriages amongst us. I under-

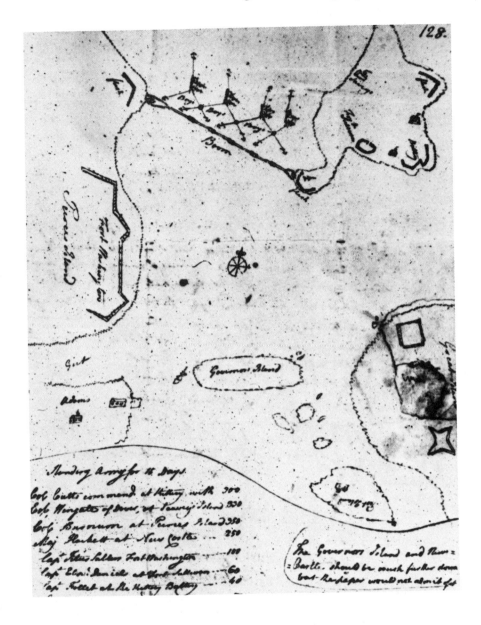

III. *Proposed defenses for Portsmouth Harbor, sketched by Dr. Hall Jackson in 1776. (By permission of the Houghton Library)*

took the business, and spent thirteen Days in mounting them, and I will venter to say they are as well executed as any on the Continent ...I spent near as much more time (gratis) in making Cartridges, Cannasters, Tubes, Vents, and Port Fires for them. I wrote to Col. Burbeck of the Laboratory, and Col. Gridley of the Train, who made me (a personal) present of a gross of Vents and a large quantity of Port Fires ready charged. These with what I made up myself are full sufficient for the Pieces in any emergency, and are not much short of a hundred pounds L.M. value tho' they did not cost the Colony one quarter of that sum.[57]

Jackson was pleased with the results of his training program and the newly refurbished artillery:

I rais'd the first Artillery Company and commanded it, and got my men in such perfection that we could discharge with great ease 11 times in a minute. A Cannister contains 48 musket Balls, so that we could every minute discharge out of the three pieces 1434 musket Balls (more than a whole Regiment could do) and these will do execution 500 yards.

However, the outbreak of war caused Jackson to relinquish his command to a Captain Turner, "as good a man for the Business as any on the Continent." During Jackson's absence the local militia, now grown to three companies, had been disbanded as the result of disagreements between Turner and one or more local officials. In March of 1776 Jackson pleaded with the House of Representatives to reestablish a Portsmouth militia company, even on a part-time basis. It would not merely provide employment to the poor men of the town; it would also provide protection to the community at large.[58]

The medical experiences of the 800 men sent from all over New Hampshire to help defend Portsmouth were distressingly like those at Winter Hill. An epidemic of diarrhea broke out among the troops stationed around the Piscataqua. Because they were dispersed throughout the many towns on the river, Jackson had to hire other physicians, including his father, to assist in their care. He blamed the outbreak on crowding, inadequate food supplies, and inadequate clothing and bedding:

That the Troops stationed at Piscataqua in proportion to their numbers have been equally, if not more sickly, than those at Cambridge, owing to the following causes. It is well known that animal substance of all kinds, if exposed for the shortest time in a degree of heat equal to the Blood will tend so far to putrifaction as to be unfit for food, and to be perfectly unwholsom, whilst Vegetables (especially those of the root kind) will remain unalterable for many months if not years. For some reasons our Soldiers have not been supplied with a due proportion of Vegetables, but have in lieu thereof been served with a double allowance of Beef. The clothing of many of the Soldiers are thin, being destitute of Beding they lodge hard, and cold, perspiration (the greatest out-let of the Body) is obstructed, the Habit soon becomes loaded with the juices of the animal Food, and a Fever of the inflammatory kind is the consequence. Some small evacuation, with a proper diluting diet, with the Benefit of...to promote perspiration would soon remove the complaints, but the unhappy Soldier is destitute of all these. The stagnated juices soon become putrid, and a fever of a more fatal kind takes place, viz, what is commonly called the Camp, Jail, or Malignat Fever, which are all of one kind. According to the degree of putridity they become more or less contagious, and is communicated from one to another, untill a general Sickness takes place, which often spreads into the Country and sweeps off great numbers of the Inhabitants. Certainly this is a matter of the highest concern to the community. For those that have been Sick, I have borrowed, begged, and even hired Beding, at an extravagant price, for as many as I could, whilst others have been obliged to linger out a month or six weeks Sickness on a little straw, upon a hard Board, with only a small wornout Blanket to cover them—and this in the heart of a populous Country.

The congress seems to have thought it could save money by doling out a few pence each day to each sick man, rather than establish a comissary from which supplies could be drawn for all at once. This only increased the men's suffering, because each then had to go shopping for his daily rations each day. To Jackson, the penny-pinching insufficiency of supplies for his patients was inconsistent with the goals of the revolution. Even worse, the troops at Winter Hill had fared better than those closer to home were able to do.[59]

By January 1776 Jackson, too, had fallen seriously ill of the current epidemic. Even by March he was barely able to use his hands to write legibly. He had tried to operate an efficient hospital system at Portsmouth (perhaps, however reluctantly, modeled on the General Hospital at Cambridge), and he had tried to promote the establishment of a dependable military defense for the town. But by that time the Provincial Congress was preoccupied with its own declaration of independence and establishing a government for the first state on the Continent, and the sense of urgency that Jackson tried to convey fell on deaf ears. In fact, the immediate threat to New Hampshire had passed in the fall of 1775, although Jackson's own illness and that of the men under his care left only him to campaign for greater attention to the purely medical and humanitarian needs of the Piscataqua area. He had every reason to feel frustrated, for the second time in his military career.

The medically trained artillery man was at least able to smile at himself and his varied interests. To Langdon he joked: "I think I begin to see you smile at my vanity and say *jack of all trades and good at none*..." Most of his letters written in the heat of war are filled with misspellings and poor constructions, as he knew. He excused himself to Langdon: "I don't care one grat [groat] about the bad English, bad spelling, and bad writing. When War-noise and confusion is over, I will then study correctness, and learn to write better." [60]

In April 1777 Jackson wrote to one of his former employers at Marblehead, Elbridge Gerry (1744–1814), who was later to be James Madison's Vice-President, about the apprehension of a gang of four counterfeiters of Tory persuasion. Apparently they had devised one of the earliest weapons in the history of biological warfare:

> I am also informed that these diabolical wretches had concerted a scheme for spreading the Small Pox thro' the Country by infecting these counterfeit Bills with this distructive disorder, and it is more than probably, they have succeeded in their indeavor, as the Small Pox is breaking out in every place in the most mysterious manner...

The plan might well have worked, as was probably recognized by Josiah Bartlett, the physician who was one of the three justices of the peace who signed the writ committing the offenders to jail. [61]

It has been reported that Jackson participated in Ethan Allen's daring capture of Ticonderoga on May 10, 1775, and that he accompanied Colonel Pierse Long's ill-fated expedition to relieve the garrison there in February 1777. [62] We have already seen, however, that Jackson was at home in May 1775, and he refused to go with Long as regimental surgeon, even if he had been enlisted in that capacity, because neither the state legislature nor Col. Long could guarantee that Jackson would be reimbursed for his expenses or his loss of professional income. Had he gone to Ticonderoga, he would not have been able to inoculate at Marblehead that spring. [63]

Jackson probably participated in running a military hospital for the last time in the fall of 1778. He arrived just in time for the siege of Newport, beginning on August 8, until General Sullivan was forced to retire from Newport Island to Providence twenty days later. From the hospital he established there in University Hall at Brown University, for the care of 137 men wounded on August 29, as well as the 4500 men who had not deserted Sullivan that day, Jackson wrote to Elbridge Gerry on September 20:

> I left home the 4th August with Col. Langdons Company of Independent Greens of which I have the honor of being second in command, on our arrival at Rhode Island Being all well mounted we were formed into a Company of Light Horse, in this I did duty some days—the Army being large and few Surgeons of consequence arrived, I was ordered to join Dr. Tillotson and form a General Hospital...I am distressed to get home as my business suffers greatly, and my expences here are beyond measure, such a place God never suffered before to stand, and I fear to say no worse, that it will soon be destroyed, for its want of humanity—and it's unparalleled extortions—I refer you to Dr. Hutchinson for a sight of such Bills, for the necessities of the wounded that will astonish you especially

when you consider the pay of those worthy Men who so gloriously fought, and suffered for the defence of these infamous Harpy's.

Jackson did not exaggerate the high prices charged by the people of Providence for food and supplies; civilian profiteering led to widespread stealing by the soldiers from military stores.[64]

The realities and necessities of war often have led to improvements in both military and civilian medical care, and the War for American Independence was no exception. At least twelve to fourteen hundred physicians, surgeons, and apothecaries—about one quarter to one third of all American health care professionals—played political or military roles, or both, in the Revolution.[65]

As early as 1810 Dr. Josiah Bartlett (1759–1820) of Massachusetts (not Hall Jackson's colleague from Kingston, New Hampshire) could evaluate some of his profession's gains from the conflict, gains of direct or potential benefit to patients and their care. Bartlett realized that the Revolution had:

> opened a new field of medical investigation, and the formation of an army, collecting the faculty from every part of the country, promoted a social intercourse... The establishment of military hospitals, afforded extensive opportunities for observations and experiments; important operations in surgery were rendered familiar; while the diseases and casualties of camps were constantly occurring. Anatomy was greatly improved by a frequent inspection without fear of detection of the organs of the body; physiology was more accurately comprehended, and a laudable spirit of inquiry, was assiduously cultivated.[66]

In addition to the increased communication between members of the profession, as well as the new learning gained, other side effects of the war resulted in improved medical care. The army's requirements for the best possible medical treatment had necessitated the first systematic procedures for examining military physicians (a process in which Jackson participated), the first American surgical text (Jones's), the first medical handbook designed to promote the effectiveness of fighting men (Rush's), and the 1778 pharmacopoeia written by Rush's successor as Physician General of the Middle Military Department, Dr. William Brown, which introduced a hitherto unknown degree of uniformity into the hospital system.[67]

It is, of course, difficult if not impossible to assess with much precision the impact of the regimental or regular army surgeons and physicians on the health of the Continental Army encamped around Boston. In the eight months following the Battle of Bunker's Hill, only 28 men were killed and another 26 wounded in confrontations with the enemy or its long-range artillery. Consequently, the monthly tallies of from 1185 to 2417 enlisted men who were sick and present in their camps must represent chiefly the effects of contagious diseases (officers' sick lists are not available). These numbers strained the available hospital buildings to their utmost, and forced Dr. Church to return sick men to their camps before he felt it really advisable to do so.[68]

The numbers of American troops bivouacked around Boston Harbor varied with public enthusiasm for the revolutionary cause. The initial wave of patriotism after Bunker Hill had brought over 20,400 officers and men to the siege by the end of July and over 23,100 by a month later. These numbers must have more than doubled the population of "suburban" Boston as well as doubled the demands for food, supplies, and services. As winter approached and any promise of military success faded, so did patriotic fervor at the same time that the first six-months enlistments began to expire, without replacements.[69]

It is not likely that sickness discouraged reenlistments. Morbidity rates were falling, after reaching their peak of 16.7 percent in August, long before the first enlistments were up, reaching a low of about 10 percent by December (including those on sick leave). In fact, as will be shown in Chapter 3, Americans could usually expect peak incidences of illness and death from September through November, the months during which the morbidity rates among the Continental troops were falling.

The increased crowding associated with the concomitantly increasing troop concentrations was probably responsible for the increase in the sick lists in the usually relatively healthy summer months. That is, a greater fraction of men was likely to be ill when the army was larger than when it was smaller—the expected effect of crowding. Certainly these relationships were apparent to John Morgan and his successors, for most of their efforts were directed toward obtaining adequate supplies of all kinds, and toward general measures designed to help control the spread of disease. Chapter 3 will show that late eighteenth-century physicians were aware of the relationship between population density and death rates.

The extent to which the crowded general hospital buildings around Boston contributed to the morbidity rates cannot be assessed. Benjamin Church should not be held responsible for the increasing rate of sickness during the first month of his directorate of the Hospital Department, nor is implementation of his reorganization of the Department likely to have been responsible for the decreasing morbidity in the second month of his administration. John Morgan did not arrive in Cambridge until December, two months after his formal appointment by the Congress, so even his massive efforts to reorganize the Medical Department could not have contributed substantially to the health of Washington's men; by then morbidity had already fallen to a low point.

Cash lists 43 individual physicians with the troops at Boston (although he does not include Hall Jackson, who never received a Continental Army commission). The 43 are probably representative of all American physicians who were there. Their ages averaged 26 years, ranging from 16 to 53. Two thirds were in their twenties; 14 percent were under 21, 19 percent were in their thirties, and one was 53. Half had attended college, all but two at Harvard. All had received their medical training as apprentices, but two also earned medical degrees (at Philadelphia and Edinburgh).[70]

Taking into account probable fluctuations and replacements, as well as other physicians known to have been at the siege of Boston, Cash's data permit us to estimate that on the average the Americans employed approximately forty physicians to attend an average 17,900 troops, which included an average monthly sick list of 2400 during the ten months' encampment. The ratios of one physician to 450 troops (approximately one to each of the 36 regiments investing Boston by July 1775), and to 60 sick and wounded are about one third better than those for contemporary New England civilian populations in peacetime.

One of the major difficulties in assessing the health and health care of the Continental Army, at Boston or during the rest of the Revolutionary War, is the lack of systematically collected data pertaining to morbidity and mortality among the troops when not on the battlefield. Previous studies have had to rely chiefly on anecdotal overviews of disease among the troops, or on only rough numerical estimates of the prevalence of selected diseases. Such data are useful for reconstructing the health hazards to which soldiers in Revolutionary America were exposed, but they are less than optimum.

However, Thomas Dickson Reide, surgeon to the First Battalion of the First (or Royal) Regiment of Foot, compiled a detailed account of the health statistics of his command during the eleven years (1776–87) that it was stationed in the St. Lawrence River area. His *View of the Diseases of the Army* provides detailed information about the military medicine of the British Army which, since disease knows few political barriers, can probably be taken as representative of military medicine in the Continental Army at the same time.[71]

The First Regiment embarked from Chatham Barracks in February 1776 and after a "healthy" voyage arrived in Quebec in the spring. It spent most of its tour of duty at Montreal, Quebec, Fort St. John, and, for its last two years, at Fort Niagara. The regiment fought Americans only in a small skirmish at Trois Rivières in June 1776 and in General Burgoyne's abortive campaign along Lake Champlain in September and October of the following year. Because Reide did not join the regiment until after Burgoyne's surrender at Saratoga, he reports no detailed data on battle casualties or garrison sick lists prior to November 1777.

During the eight wartime years, his regiment had an average strength of 511 rank and file, of whom about 5 percent were sergeants and 3 percent were drummers. There were probably about 100 officers. After the peace of 1783 the average regimental strength fell to 297 men; it was still falling as they left for home.

Table 3 lists the diagnoses made in the First Regiment of Foot during the 103 months following Reide's arrival. The 3248 cases represent an average of about one a day for the entire period. Sixty-one, or 1.88 percent, of the sick died. The most prevalent disorders were infectious dis-

Table 3.
Diagnoses made by Dr. Thomas Dickson Reide Among Men of the
British First Regiment of Foot during Eight Years in North America

| Diagnosis | Fraction of All 3248 Diagnoses | Fraction of All 61 Deaths | Fraction of All Men with Diagnosis Who Died |
|---|---|---|---|
| Remitting Fever | 19.92% | 18.03% | 1.70% |
| Dysentery | 18.93 | 27.87 | 2.76 |
| Inflammatory Fever | 10.13 | 0 | 0 |
| Lues Venerea | 3.57 | 0 | 0 |
| Rheumatism | 3.48 | 0 | 0 |
| Scurvy | 3.20 | 0 | 0 |
| Sore Eyes | 2.89 | 0 | 0 |
| Consumption | 2.87 | 27.87 | 18.28 |
| Cutaneous Eruption | 2.09 | 0 | 0 |
| Stomach Complaints | 1.82 | 0 | 0 |
| Vertigo | 1.17 | 0 | 0 |
| Sore Throat | 1.14 | 0 | 0 |
| Diarrhea | 0.89 | 0 | 0 |
| Erysipelas | 0.80 | 0 | 0 |
| Cough | 0.65 | 0 | 0 |
| Cholera Morbus | 0.58 | 1.64 | 5.26 |
| Ear Ache | 0.58 | 0 | 0 |
| Epilepsy | 0.55 | 0 | 0 |
| Hemmorrhoids | 0.49 | 0 | 0 |
| Worms | 0.49 | 0 | 0 |
| Small Pox, Inoculated | 0.37 | 0 | 0 |
| Colic | 0.34 | 0 | 0 |
| Pain in Side, Breast, or Back | 0.31 | 0 | 0 |
| Lumbago | 0.25 | 0 | 0 |
| Peripneumony | 0.25 | 13.11 | 100 |
| Gravel and Stone | 0.22 | 0 | 0 |
| Bowel Inflammation | 0.15 | 0 | 0 |
| Jaundice | 0.15 | 0 | 0 |
| Bladder Inflammation | 0.12 | 4.92 | 75.00 |
| Contusions of Side, Breast, or Back | 0.12 | 0 | 0 |
| Head Ache | 0.09 | 0 | 0 |
| Insane | 0.09 | 0 | 0 |
| Asthma | 0.06 | 0 | 0 |
| Gun Shot Wound | 0.06 | 3.28 | 100.00 |
| Hernia Humoralis | 0.06 | 0 | 0 |
| Palsy | 0.06 | 0 | 0 |
| Scrophula | 0.06 | 0 | 0 |

Table 3. (*continued*)

| Diagnosis | Fraction of All 3248 Diagnoses | Fraction of All 61 Deaths | Fraction of All Men with Diagnosis Who Died |
|---|---|---|---|
| Chronic Complaints of Old Age | 0.06 | 0 | 0 |
| Dropsy | 0.03 | 0 | 0 |
| Pleurisy | 0.03 | 1.64 | 100.00 |
| Inflammation of Brain due to large Quantity of Rum | 0.03 | 1.64 | 100.00 |
| Sores, Wounds, Accidents, etc. Requiring Surgical Treatment (Includes the two men listed above as having suffered gunshot wounds) | 20.84 | (3.28) | 0.30 |

SOURCE: Thomas Dickson Reide, *View of the Diseases of the Army . . .* (London, J. Johnson, 1793), passim.

eases, but relatively few men died of them. Only two deaths occurred among the 677 who had surgical procedures performed (both were for gunshot wounds); no amputations or other major operations were recorded. Reide also inoculated at least 234 loyalist civilian refugees because of smallpox epidemics raging in nearby Montreal and Niagara in the fall of 1783 and winter of 1785. No deaths occurred among those inoculated.

Dr. Reide was responsible for a regimental hospital, and when necessary he sent a few patients (all of whom died) to the general hospitals at Montreal and later at Fort Niagara. During the First Regiment's stay in North America, at least 145 men died (Reide did not know how many died in the campaign that ended at Saratoga). Of the 98 deaths that occurred during his tour of duty, about 80 percent died in the regimental hospital, 14 percent in the general hospitals, 3 percent in accidents, and 3 percent "suddenly" in the garrison. One important factor that probably contributed to the death rates in the British garrison regiment was the uncertain, even dwindling, food supply, a factor that had also contributed to the British decision to abandon Boston several months before Washington's men placed their threatening cannons on Dorchester Heights.[72]

The diagnoses for the 449 men in the General Hospital in Albany, New York, on August 20, 1777, shown in Table 4, suggest that the First

Table 4.
Diagnoses of 449 Men Hospitalized in the General Hospital at Albany,
New York, on August 20, 1777, Compared with the Incidences of the
same Diagnoses Among Thomas Dickson Reide's British Patients

| Diagnosis | Fraction of All 449 Patients | Fraction Among Reide's Diagnoses |
|---|---|---|
| Dysentery | 18.04% | 18.93% |
| Intermittent Fever | 17.59 | 19.92 |
| Diarrhea | 13.59 | 0.89 |
| Cough | 5.57 | 0.65 |
| Rheumatism | 4.90 | 3.48 |
| Convalescent | 3.79 | |
| Debility | 3.79 | |
| Lues Venerea | 3.12 | 3.57 |
| Fever | 2.90 | |
| Whooping Cough | 2.23 | |
| Head Itch | 2.00 | |
| Measles | 1.78 | |
| Putrid Fever | 1.34 | |
| Bilious Fever | 0.89 | |
| Dropsy | 0.89 | 0.03 |
| Scorbutic | 0.89 | 3.20 |
| Pleurisy | 0.67 | 0.03 |
| Nephritis | 0.67 | (? 0.22) |
| Scrofula | 0.67 | 0.06 |
| Jaundice | 0.45 | 0.15 |
| Rupture (Hernia) | 0.45 | 0.45 |
| Hemoptus (Hemoptysis) | 0.45 | |
| Paralysis (Palsy) | 0.45 | 0.06 |
| Hemorrhoids | 0.22 | 0.49 |
| Asthma | 0.22 | 0.06 |
| Cholera | 0.22 | 0.58 |
| Hypochondria | 0.22 | |
| Ophthalmia | 0.22 | 2.89 |
| Surgical patients | 11.80 | 20.84 |

SOURCES: "Hospital Patients—New York, 1777," *Morbidity and Mortality Weekly Report*, 25 (July 2, 1976, no. 25), 4. See also Table 3.

Regiment's experience was, indeed, typical of the medical experience on
both sides during the American Revolution. If modest allowance is made
for seasonal fluctuations in morbidity attributable to specific infections,
the causes of illness in the two camps were very much alike.

The data in Tables 3 and 4 present the experiences of one military
physician over a long period of time, and of one hospital on one day,
respectively. Tables 5 and 6 summarize the monthly reports of about

twenty military hospitals in 1781–82, as collated by Dr. John Cochran (1730–1807), the fourth Director General of the Continental Army's Medical Department. As Table 5 shows, it is hazardous to interpret corresponding data from more than one hospital—which also implies the contributions of more than one physician—over many months. Although the overall frequencies of these rather limited diagnoses are not unlike those made in more detail by Reide and at Albany, the fluctuations in monthly returns reflect the influence of the seasons on certain infectious diseases, the influence of engagements with the enemy on the incidence of wounded men who required hospitalization, and the sporadic nature of epidemics, like those of smallpox, whose incidence is not especially related to climatic conditions. A probable major source of inconsistency among these data is that they originate from about twenty hospitals scattered along the seaboard from New Hampshire to Virginia, none of which submitted reports for the entire period. Not only the severely limited number of disease categories but also the wide fluctuations in unspecified diagnoses impair our interpretations of the data.

It is even difficult to reconcile with other data the number of wounded listed in Cochran's returns, as shown in Table 6. For instance, in ten months he listed more wounded men than are represented in the returns from orderly rooms throughout the entire command, but in only one month did the deaths reported by Cochran outnumber those reported through field commanders. Some of these discrepancies seem to arise from the hospital commanders' habit of reporting not new admissions but all patients with any given condition at the end of each reporting period, regardless of how long the men had been hospitalized. Thus, the influence of the five major actions listed in Table 6 presumably carries over for some months beyond the times of the original admissions for wounds after each battle.

Deaths are more easily related to other factors, because each death is a discrete event, with no possibility of becoming a prolonged process, which might result in recovery from wounds or an infectious disease. The numbers of deaths reported from both field commanders and hospitals are highly correlated ($r = 0.923$, $P < 0.01$), as are the fractions of men on both sick-list aggregates (which must have overlapped to a now undistinguishable extent) who died ($r = 0.677$, $P < 0.01$). Overall, 2.3 percent of those hospitalized died each month (range, 0.3 to 8.3 percent), while an average of 4.7 percent on the camp sick lists died in the same period (range, 1.7 to 11.8 percent).

Similarly, the number of hospitalized men reported by Cochran is correlated with the number of men reported to army headquarters as sick and present ($r = 0.565$, $P < 0.05$; for the data in Table 6, the value of $r$ increases to 0.628, $P < 0.01$, if the men who underwent smallpox inoculation in February 1782 are included). The incidence of deaths among hospitalized troops reported to Cochran was not proportional to the number of hospitalized troops ($r = 0.353$, $P > 0.05$); but the number of deaths in the entire command was proportional to the number on sick lists in the command ($r = 0.800$, $P < 0.01$), although the number on sick

Table 5.
Diagnoses Listed on Monthly Continental Army Returns from about
Twenty Military Hospitals, Compiled by Dr. John Cochran, Director
General of the Hospital of the United States, over Twenty-One Months
during 1781–1782 (percentages)

| | *1781* | | | | | | | | |
|---|---|---|---|---|---|---|---|---|---|
| | Apr | May | Jun | Jul | Aug | Sep | Oct | Nov | De |
| Wounded | 7 | 7 | 3 | 28 | 6 | 6 | 7 | 12 | 8 |
| Ulcers | 6 | 5 | 2 | 8 | 8 | 4 | 1 | 4 | 9 |
| Convalescent | 29 | 18 | 13 | 11 | 13 | 5 | 20 | 12 | 14 |
| Lame & casual hurts | 9 | 14 | 17 | 5 | 4 | 3 | 3 | 2 | 1 |
| Various chronic diseases | 9 | 12 | 17 | 12 | 13 | 9 | 3 | 11 | 11 |
| Rheumatism | 8 | 9 | 11 | 8 | 8 | 11 | 3 | 7 | 9 |
| *Fevers* | | | | | | | | | |
| Inflammatory | 4 | 7 | 6 | 1 | 1 | 1 | 5 | 9 | 12 |
| Intermitting & remittent | 8 | 6 | 8 | 4 | 11 | 11 | 26 | 6 | 10 |
| Bilious & putrid | 8 | 2 | 5 | 6 | 16 | 19 | 5 | 3 | 1 |
| Nervous | 0 | 1 | 2 | <1 | 1 | 0 | 2 | 4 | 2 |
| Dysentery | 1 | 3 | 3 | 2 | 4 | 22 | 10 | 8 | 4 |
| Diarrhea | 3 | 3 | 4 | 3 | 8 | 3 | 11 | 7 | 7 |
| Lues venerea | 9 | 11 | 7 | 8 | 7 | 7 | 4 | 4 | 6 |
| Smallpox | 0 | 3 | 2 | 5 | 0 | 0 | <1 | 13 | 10 |
| N | 572 | 361 | 462 | 360 | 677 | 657 | 1260 | 854 | 614 |
| % All hospital patients with unrecorded diagnoses | 0 | 0 | 0 | 0 | 3 | 34 | 30 | 16 | 13 |

* Of these, 1177 men were inoculated for smallpox "East of the Hudson River"; of them,
3.0 percent died, while among the men who developed smallpox in the natural way, about
61 percent died. If the men who were inoculated were subtracted from the totals for this
month, smallpox would account for only about 63 percent of the diagnoses made, but the
incidences of other diagnoses would not be substantially affected.
SOURCE: Morris H. Saffron, *Surgeon to Washington: Dr. John Cochran, 1730–1807*
(New York, Columbia University Press, 1977), pp. 181–200.

| '82 *n* | Feb | Mar | Apr | May | Jun | Jul | Aug | Sep | Nov | Dec | Total Period |
|---|---|---|---|---|---|---|---|---|---|---|---|
| 0 | 1 | 2 | 4 | 1 | 1 | 1 | 1 | 1 | 1 | 1 | 3.7% |
| 9 | 1 | 1 | 7 | 3 | 3 | 2 | 1 | 10 | 6 | 5 | 3.7% |
| 5 | 8 | 25 | 13 | 15 | 19 | 14 | 19 | 18 | 17 | 18 | 15.0% |
| 1 | 1 | 6 | 4 | 19 | 17 | 13 | 13 | 2 | 20 | 20 | 8.0% |
| 9 | 2 | 6 | 11 | 10 | 12 | 11 | 9 | 9 | 13 | 12 | 8.5% |
| 6 | 2 | 7 | 6 | 5 | 6 | 5 | 4 | 3 | 8 | 9 | 5.5% |
| 12 | 2 | 6 | 8 | 1 | 4 | 3 | 3 | 2 | 6 | 9 | 4.3% |
| 17 | 2 | 5 | 18 | 17 | 18 | 28 | 19 | 23 | 5 | 3 | 11.8% |
| 2 | 2 | 9 | 3 | 1 | 2 | 3 | 13 | 10 | 7 | 4 | 5.9% |
| 0 | 0 | 1 | <1 | 0 | 0 | 1 | 0 | 0 | 0 | 0 | 0.6% |
| 4 | 1 | 1 | 2 | 1 | 5 | 6 | 6 | 8 | 5 | 3 | 4.7% |
| 6 | 1 | 3 | 6 | 4 | 4 | 9 | 7 | 9 | 5 | 5 | 5.0% |
| 6 | 1 | 4 | 14 | 8 | 8 | 6 | 5 | 5 | 5 | 8 | 5.4% |
| 4 | 77 | 24 | 3 | 16 | 3 | 0 | 0 | 1 | 1 | 5 | 17.9% |
| 63 | 3173* | 917 | 312 | 764 | 865 | 1025 | 1215 | 1025 | 971 | 874 | 17,321 |
| 9 | 0 | 3 | 23 | 0 | 8 | 6 | 5 | 4 | 4 | 4 | 8.6% |

Table 6.
Incidence of "Wounded, Sick and Deaths" in Hospitals Reporting to
Dr. John Cochran during 1781–1782 and in Reports of Field
Commanders for the Same Period

| | | Cochran's Returns | | |
| | | Wounded | | |
| Month | Total Number | Number | Fraction of Total | Number of Deaths |
|---|---|---|---|---|
| *1781* | | | | |
| Apr | 572 | 41 | 7.2% | 2 |
| May | 361 | 25 | 6.9% | 1 |
| Jun | 462 | 15 | 3.2% | 5 |
| Jul | 360 | 102 | 28.3% | 13 |
| Aug | 700 | 42 | 6.2% | 5 |
| Sep | 990 | 37 | 5.6% | 12 |
| Oct | 1806 | 88 | 7.0% | 28 |
| Nov | 1012 | 101 | 11.8% | 51 |
| Dec | 702 | 46 | 7.5% | 131 |
| *1782* | | | | |
| Jan | 399 | 35 | 9.6% | 50 |
| Feb | 1996 | 16 | 0.8% | 78 |
| Mar | 948 | 16 | 1.7% | 79 |
| Apr | 405 | 13 | 4.2% | 9 |
| May | 764 | 11 | 1.4% | 10 |
| Jun | 935 | 6 | 0.7% | 11 |
| Jul | 1088 | 8 | 0.8% | 8 |
| Aug | 1285 | 10 | 0.8% | 11 |
| Sep | 1062 | 0 | 0.9% | 25 |
| Nov | 1010 | 14 | 1.4% | 14 |
| Dec | 913 | 8 | 0.9% | 21 |

Men who were inoculated are omitted from the above data. See legend for Table 5 for details.
SOURCES: Morris H. Saffron, *Surgeon to Washington: Dr. John Cochran, 1730–1807*
(New York, Columbia University Press, 1977), pp. 181–200. Howard H. Peckham, *The
Toll of Independence: Engagements and Battle Casualties of the American Revolution*
(Chicago, University of Chicago Press, 1974), pp. 83–98. Charles H. Lesser, ed., *The
Sinews of Independence: Monthly Strength Reports of the Continental Army* (Chicago,
University of Chicago Press, 1976), pp. 200–241.

| Commanders' Reports of Number Wounded (Major Engagements) | Returns for Washingtons' Command (Numbers) | | |
|---|---|---|---|
| | Total Army | Sick List | Deaths |
| 135 (Hobkirk's Hill, SC) | 7,223 | 369 | 12 |
| 31 | 8,514 | 406 | 23 |
| 93 (Ninety-Six, SC) | 10,445 | 199 | 11 |
| 199 (Kingsbridge, VA) | 10,265 | 286 | 17 |
| 19 | — | — | — |
| 465 (Eutaw Springs, SC) | 6,087 | 411 | — |
| 128 (Yorktown, VA) | 16,769 | 1233 | 21 |
| 19 | — | — | — |
| 1 | — | — | — |
| 5 | 10,687 | 1676 | 119 |
| 0 | 10,510 | 1752 | 139 |
| 7 | 14,339 | 1070 | 126 |
| 0 | 10,547 | 736 | 35 |
| 20 | 10,566 | 677 | 32 |
| 9 | 11,681 | 756 | 18 |
| 0 | 12,392 | 903 | 25 |
| 33 | 12,519 | 792 | 16 |
| 0 | 11,640 | 725 | 30 |
| 5 | 12,240 | 656 | 14 |
| 5 | 12,224 | 715 | 23 |

report in the entire army was not related to the size of the army ($r = 0.443$, $P > 0.05$), which was then dispersed and moving, unlike the situation at the siege of Boston.

In aggregate, then, the available data suggest that death rates provide one of the most reliable indices to health among Revolutionary troops even though they are subject to various influences, not the least of which is the accuracy and completeness of contemporary official reports. The incidences of infectious diseases are subject to so many influences that, in fact, they provide useful information only when they can be relatively isolated in both time and place. Nevertheless, the few data from returns such as those used to compile Tables 3 through 6 do confirm our a priori assumption, one often reinforced by anecdotal accounts, that infections were responsible for about half of the total sick lists in both armies, even if relatively few—unexpectedly few, from today's standpoint—died of those diseases. The remaining morbidity among both armies was associated with many different kinds of illness and accident, none of them with special predilections for army camps but to be expected among men of military age in the late eighteenth century.

Hall Jackson had the care of the survivors among the 86 New Hampshire men killed or wounded at Bunker Hill, who represented 9.5 percent of the colony's troops who participated in the battle. We lack data pertaining to survival rates among the wounded, even when treated; none of the American prisoners of war held by the British in Boston survived amputation of wounded limbs.[73]

At Winter Hill, north of Charlestown Neck, where Sullivan's three regiments comprising a monthly average of 1780 men were encamped, from 13 to 25 percent of the New Hampshire troops were on the sick list during the four months Jackson was there. At the same time, the overall Army sick list ranged only from 12 to 17 percent. The sickness rate among the New Hampshire troops was consistently about 5 percent greater than that among other Continental troops until January 1776. It may have been the greater burden of sickness among Sullivan's regiments that increased the sense of frustration that he, his officers, and his chief surgeon, Hall Jackson, experienced when Church began to reorganize the Hospital Department. It seems unlikely, from this distance, that we can determine just what might have accounted for the seemingly disproportionate morbidity rates among the New Hampshire men; differences in the quality of medical care rendered then are unlikely to be documentable.[74]

Altogether, the regimental or regular army doctors appear not to have altered the patterns of health and disease among the Continental Army besieging Boston in 1775–76. As Applegate has pointed out, "there is little evidence to show that remedial medicine effectively reduced the death rate."[75] Jackson may even have returned to Portsmouth in October 1775 as evidence of the expected annual autumnal decline in morbidity failed to materialize. Although he may have had good reason to leave in high dudgeon as the result of his quarrel with Church and his failure to achieve a suitable rank, the rest of his professional career suggests that it might not have been characteristic of him to have left if his services were, in fact, actually needed by the army.

We might know more of Hall Jackson today had he not become so embroiled in medical politics in 1775, a fight he could not have won. He was to put his best professional foot forward only after the war, when he introduced digitalis to America. The new wonder drug would have come across the Atlantic anyway, probably through Philadelphia, but not until later. Even so, Jackson's introduction of the foxglove was hardly heralded by fireworks and a brass band. The thwarting of his military ambitions permitted him to return to his civilian practice long before the war was over.

In the next chapter we will examine the characteristics of the population from which his patients came, and the reasons why they sought his help. By the time Withering's book on a new treatment for dropsy, which had seemed so refractory to treatment, appeared in Portsmouth, Jackson was able to assess the new drug's therapeutic potential. All in all, his work as patriot, physician, surgeon, and pathologist (see Chapter 4), when taken in conjunction with his attempts to spread the gospel of a new drug whose usefulness could be proved by scientific methods, reveals him as a true disciple of the Age of Enlightenment.

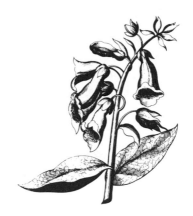

# CHAPTER THREE

# Portsmouth: 'As Healthy a Place as Any in America'

## A CASE STUDY OF AN EARLY

## AMERICAN PATIENT POPULATION

WHAT WAS the medical milieu in which Hall Jackson practiced in New England or William Withering in old England? What kinds of diagnoses did they make, and how often? What difference did the discovery of the effect of the foxglove on dropsy make to their individual patients or to the health of the public?

Although the Age of Enlightenment was, above all else, characterized by the emergence and development of increasingly scientific methods of study of both natural and social phenomena, it produced few immediate dividends related to health care delivery during its own life span. The concept of medical progress that is now popular even among politicians was in its infancy then. In spite of Hall Jackson and his colleagues, the people of America and the rest of the world continued to be born, to live, to become ill, and to die. The differences among the rates at which people in different places accomplished these tasks were the results not of specific medical efforts, but of changing social and economic milieus.

Jackson's opinion that Portsmouth was as healthy as any place in the world was not merely parochial or patriotic. Similar assessments of Portsmouth and its region were made by contemporary observers, mostly travelers, and the available data confirm their opinions in all respects—geographical, meteorological, cultural, and social, as well as medical.

For instance, the Reverend Timothy Dwight (1752–1817), then President of Yale College in Connecticut, journeyed up the coast to New Hampshire and Maine in 1795–96. In his journal describing the trip, he observed that "New England is the healthiest country in the United States, and probably inferior in this respect to few in the world." He supported this generalization with data showing that a newborn infant had one chance in two of living to the age of 5 in Europe, while he had the same chance of living to the age of 17 in New England. Dwight also calculated that the people of Connecticut had a greater life expectancy than did those of Virginia, Georgia, and the Carolinas.[1]

He was not impressed, however, by the physical appearance of Hall Jackson's Portsmouth. In his usual encyclopedic fashion Dwight described the face of the city:

> There are in Portsmouth thirty-one streets, thirty-eight lanes, ten alleys, and three public squares. The squares are not remarkable either for their size or their beauty. A few of the streets are wide and pleasant; most of them are narrow and disagreeable. The town was laid out without any regard for regularity...The statehouse is barely a decent structure.

Only grudgingly did Dwight admit that "a delightful assemblage of objects" could be seen from a church steeple, mostly the harbor and the opposite shore.[2]

One of Dwight's purposes in setting down his observations and data was the detailed documentation of the growth of the new republic and the spread of its frontiers. The works of man are Dwight's measuring

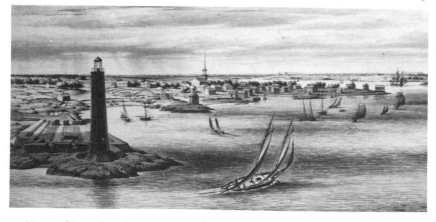

IV. *View of Portsmouth in 1778. Watercolor by Pierre Ozanne. (National Museum of Blérancourt, 02, France)*

Table 7.
Prevalences of the Major Categories of Occupations in Portsmouth,
Compared with Those in All New Hampshire, in 1820

|  | Portsmouth % | All New Hampshire % | Portsmouth Compared with New Hampshire |
|---|---|---|---|
| Agriculture | 1.79 | 21.45 | 0.08 |
| Commerce | 5.90 | 0.43 | 13.72 |
| Manufacturing | 8.64 | 3.56 | 2.43 |
| Population | 7,481 | 244,161 | 0.031 |

SOURCE: *Census of the United States for 1820, Book I* (Washington, D.C., Gales and Seaton, 1821).

sticks. Thus he tells us that in 1798, the year after Hall Jackson's death, there were 626 houses in Portsmouth. Of these, 86 had one story, 524 had two stories, and 16 had three stories. Their aggregate assessed value for tax purposes was $916,731, which Dwight thought underestimated their true worth. Their average value was, then, $1464.[3]

Dwight also provides economic data to help him describe life in Hall Jackson's Portsmouth. In 1791 the city's marine commerce involved about 250 seamen on 27 schooners and 20 boats engaged in cod and whale fishing, bringing in over two and a half million pounds of fish that year. Ten years later the number of ships working out of Portsmouth had more than doubled, and annual customs revenues at the port of entry had doubled to about $90,000. In 1789–91, approximately $300,000 worth of exports, chiefly lumber, dried fish, and beef, cleared the port on 277 vessels, heading mostly for France and her colonies. At the same time, 223 ships brought raw sugar, molasses, rum, salt, nails, and other manufactured items valued at over $1,000,000 to Portsmouth from the French West Indies and England.[4]

If we assume that the way of life in Portsmouth had not changed much in relation to that in New Hampshire as a whole, Table 7 demonstrates the port city's, and Hall Jackson's patients', preoccupation with trade and manufacturing. Portsmouth provided an economic lifeline to the otherwise primarily agricultural state. Because of the city's growing commercial role, its population grew more rapidly than that of the state as a whole after the Revolution, whereas before the war Portsmouth's population had increased only as rapidly as that of the entire state.[5]

In 1790 Jeremy Belknap, the first historian of New Hampshire, asked the state's leading practicing physician for data about its population, health, and native medical plants. Jackson sent him the results of the

Portsmouth census of 1767, taken just after he had begun his own practice:

Total Number of Inhabitants in the State or
Province of New Hampshire 1767                          52,700

Inhabitants in the Town of Portsmouth 1767
    Unmarried Men, from 16 to 60                    440
    Boys from 16 years of age, & under              700
    Unmarried Females                              1340
    Married Men, from 16 to 60 years of age          641
    Married Females                                 677
    Men 60 and upwards                               61
    Male Slaves                                     124
    Female Ditto                                     63
                                      4466 [sic]

These statistics describe the population from which most of the doctor's patients came, although he also treated inhabitants of other New Hampshire communities. As will be seen later, the population of Portsmouth had increased by 17 percent by the time of the 1790 census, distributed among 873 separate households.[6]

The President of Yale was almost surprised to find that he enjoyed the company of his New Hampshire hosts, even if he found their capital city unattractive: "The people of Portsmouth have ever been friendly to literature...The manners of the inhabitants are of the same polished, pleasing character so extensively seen along this coast." Hall Jackson and Timothy Dwight may have met during Dwight's brief visit to Portsmouth but if they did, Dwight does not mention it. He names very few of the men he met in his travels, mostly those who happened to tell him a good story.[7]

Jeremy Belknap agreed with Dwight's estimate of the quality of life in Jackson's Portsmouth, where "there is as much elegance and politeness of manners, as in any of the capital towns of New-England. It is often visited by strangers, who always meet with a friendly and hospitable reception." It has been estimated that about one third of Portsmouth's population consisted of artisans, and about one eighth of merchants or shopkeepers; their combined proportion was less than that found in other New Hampshire towns, which were almost entirely rural and agricultural. About a quarter of Portsmouth's men were employed at sea, and Hall Jackson belonged to the tenth that included the professions. Although most of the wealth of the state was controlled from Portsmouth, there was more poverty in the seacoast town than in the interior, and, consequently, more disease.[8]

In 1781, the last year of Revolutionary War hostilities, the Marquis de Chastellux (1734–1788), a major general in the French Army under Rochambeau, visited Portsmouth. Among the many American physicians he met during his three-year stay in this country was Hall Jackson's colleague Joshua Brackett, in Portsmouth, but he does not mention Jackson in his memoir of those years. A professional soldier, the Marquis regarded Portsmouth from both military and economic points of view:

> [Portsmouth] was in a pretty flourishing state before the war, and carried on the trade of ship timber, and salt fish. It is easy to conceive that this commerce must have greatly suffered since the commencement of the troubles, but notwithstanding, Portsmouth is, perhaps, of all the American towns, that which will gain the most by the present war. There is every appearance of its becoming to *New-*England, what the other Portsmouth is to the *Old*: that is to say, That this place will be made choice of as the depot of the continental marine, The access to the harbor is easy, the road immense, and there are seven fathoms water as far up as two miles above the town;...This circumstance, joined to its proximity to the timber for ship-building, especially the masts,...will doubtless determine the choice of Congress. But if a naval establishment be thought necessary at Portsmouth, the quays, the rope-walks, the arsenals, &c. must be placed in the islands, and not on the continent; for it would be easy for an enemy's army to land there, and take possession of the town, the local situation of which would require too considerable a development of fortification to shelter it from insult...
>
> It has happened in New-Hampshire, as in the state of Massachusetts, that the losses of commerce have turned to the advantage of agriculture; the capitals of the rich, and the industry of the people having flowed back from the coasts toward the interior of the country, which has profited rapidly from the reflux...
>
> When I was at Portsmouth the necessaries of life were very dear, owing to the great drought of the preceding summer. Corn [wheat, according to the translator] costs two dollars a bushel (of sixty pounds weight), oats almost as much, and Indian corn was extremely scarce. I shall hardly be believed when I say, that I paid eight livres ten sols (about seven shillings and three pence) a day for each horse. Butcher's meat only was cheap, selling at two-pence halfpenny a pound. That part of New-Hampshire bordering on the coast is not fertile; there are good lands at forty or fifty miles distance from the sea, but the expense of carriage greatly augments the price of articles, when sold in the more inhabited parts. As for the value of the landed property it is dear enough for so new a country. Mr. Ruspert, my landlord, paid seventy pounds currency per annum (at eighteen livres, or fifteen shillings the pound) for his inn. Lands sell at from ten to sixteen dollars per acre. The country produces little fruit, and the cider is indifferent.

The American editor of Chastellux' book noted, in 1828, that "The anticipations of Portsmouth becoming a great naval depot, have not been realized. It is too far distant from the seat of government and centre of commerce and naval resources. Although we have a number of navy-

yards, the Portsmouth of England has as yet been found at New-York."
New Hampshire's only port has, of course, been a prominent naval base
in more recent years, laid out, as the Marquis had recommended, on the
islands in the harbor.[9]

A few years later the noted French republican apologist Jacques Pierre
Brissot de Warville (1754–1793) visited Portsmouth in 1788 while tour-
ing the United States. Brissot came to America to gather financial information for French investors, to look for a place in which he might some-
day settle himself, and, mostly, to observe the quality of life in a country
that had just won its liberty from an oppressive form of government. He
took his lessons home with him, but for his efforts died on the guillotine
soon after.

Brissot was no more enchanted with Portsmouth than was Timothy
Dwight, but he left more than his impressions of the town's outward
appearance with which to support his judgement:

> Situated on the swift and deep Piscataqua River, Portsmouth has
> a fine port which is always ice-free as far as four or five miles above
> the town...Everybody here is involved either in trading or in
> building...The inhabitants are also beginning to engage in fishing,
> but they have not as yet been very successful...Portsmouth is less
> active than the other towns I have described and everything shows
> signs of being in a state of decline. The population is small, many
> of the houses are dilapidated, and I saw a good number of women
> and children in rags, a sight I had never before encountered in Amer-
> ica. Yet there are some handsome houses [as Chastellux had noted,
> but Dwight denied]; I was told that labor is so cheap that a charm-
> ing three-story house cost to build no more than 12,000 to 15,000
> livres [approximately $1000 to $1400, consistent with Dwight's
> figures]. People are complaining about the scarcity of money. They
> are beginning to export horses and wood to the West Indies. I heard
> that there are a lot of land jobbers and that they have caused many
> people to lose money.
> ...I stayed at a very good inn run by a Mr. Greenleaf. I found
> a neatness and cleanliness rarely met with in France—good beds,
> pretty wallpaper, substantial and inexpensive food...
> In New Hampshire the cold sets in early and the winters are long
> and rigorous, beginning in November and ending in May. When I
> visited the state in October I was forced to have a blazing fire...It
> is to the cold air that may be attributed the good health enjoyed by
> inhabitants of this state...Nevertheless, unbelievable as it may
> seem, there is a great deal of consumption...At Portsmouth there
> were twenty-five persons suffering from the terrible illness all at one
> time.

The bills of mortality for Portsmouth will suggest that Brissot's estimate
was about right. Belknap, relying largely on information supplied to him
by Hall Jackson, among others, thought that the prevalence of consump-

tion was increasing, and that it had both heritable and contagious causes.[10]

Some years later, while investigating the prevalence of malaria in New England, Dr. Oliver Wendell Holmes wrote to Dr. Thomas Chadbourne of Concord, New Hampshire, to ask, "Are there any particular spots in your vicinity, or in New Hampshire, noted for unhealthiness?" Dr. Chadbourne, who had assembled bills of mortality for Concord, replied: "There are none. There probably is no State in the Union that enjoys a greater exemption from disease than New Hampshire." Although it may be correct, Chadbourne's opinion cannot be confirmed with much confidence from contemporary data, because we have no numerical information pertaining to the prevalence and morbidity of disease, regardless of whether it led to death, in New Hampshire, or, for that matter, elsewhere in the country. In the absence of prevalence data, however, mortality data provide at least one valid measure of the public health, and it may well have been mortality data on which Chadbourne based his estimate.[11]

We will see shortly that, in terms of life expectancy and of overall death rates, all these casual observers of Hall Jackson's New Hampshire were right in their opinions of the relative healthiness of the state. And we will see as well that the eighteenth-century population of New Hampshire died of the same diseases, and in the same relative proportions, barring epidemics, as did populations elsewhere in the United States and Europe.

About a century before Jackson began to practice medicine, the scientific as well as the sociopolitical relevance of bills of mortality had first been appreciated. In the year following Jackson's death, Thomas Robert Malthus published the first edition of his pioneering *Essay on the Principles of Population, as it Affects the Future Improvement of Society*, in which he explored thoroughly the social implications of differences among the health of people and their habitats. Thus today's dictum relating health and the social characteristics of society is not a new discovery.[12]

Much can be learned about the health of Portsmouth at the turn of the eighteenth century from the unusually detailed bills of mortality published yearly from 1801 to 1811 by Dr. Lyman Spalding (1775–1821), who practiced there from 1799 to 1812, and who later was one of the authors of the first *United States Pharmacopoeia*. From 1818 to 1820, Dr. Richard Thurston (1787–1835) carried on the bills for Portsmouth.

Although the Spalding-Thurston bills of mortality cover fourteen of the twenty-three years after Hall Jackson's death, they can be taken as representative of much of Jackson's own professional experience. He would have had to cope with much of the same spectrum of disease as did the next generation of Portsmouth's physicians, because no major improvements in disease prevention or cure occurred between his death and the last of the bills of mortality—or at least none gained common acceptance and use among the profession during those years. Citing only some of Benjamin Rush's most radical treatments as evidence, Shryock even asserts that "From the present viewpoint, American therapy... went from bad to worse between 1750 and 1800." Fortunately, Rush's therapeutic methods did not become as popular in New England as they did in the Middle Atlantic states, and other evidence to support Shryock's contention is lacking.[13]

Jackson himself was responsible for introducing one major new treatment, for dropsy, but its prevalence, as we will see, was insufficient for the cure to have altered significantly the overall life expectancy of the community. Also, Jenner's new vaccination for smallpox was introduced to Portsmouth by Lyman Spalding, shortly after Jackson's death, but the data will suggest that Jackson's own earlier efforts to eradicate the disease by the technique of inoculation had already reduced the incidence of smallpox to a practical minimum in the Portsmouth area.

In 1801 Dr. David Ramsay (1745–1815) of Charleston, South Carolina, presented a contemporary view of the medical advances of the preceding century. The most important factors, Ramsay believed, involved increased understanding of how the body works in health and disease— a view now shared by historians looking back over an even greater distance. Ramsay included only a few drugs in his list of the most valuable new therapeutic methods developed over the century just ended (e.g., Peruvian bark, antimony, opium, mercury, uva ursi, colombo root, and

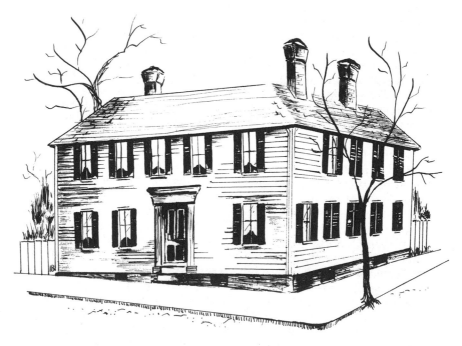

v. *Hall Jackson's house in Portsmouth. Original drawing by Irene Buonopane from photographs made in 1900 and 1937.*

digitalis, among others), and he mentioned improvements in hospital care. But none of these first appeared between Jackson's death and the end of the Portsmouth death statistics, and none could have reduced mortality significantly.[14]

A number of problems are associated with eighteenth-century data and sampling techniques. We will beg the question of the validity of at least some of the diagnoses presented here, partly because it is most likely that the answers to our questions would not be altered substantially with "better" data, which are not readily available in any case, and partly because we are interested chiefly in viewing the health of eighteenth-century Portsmouth through eighteenth-century eyes. The data to be examined are those, or are like those, which were available to Jackson and his colleagues, and only upon such data could they have based any of their own conclusions; where possible, of course, we will use those data in ways that were not then available, and with all the advantages of informed hindsight, but without the necessity of "translating" from eighteenth to twentieth century terminologies. We can then proceed to examine Jackson's own data, insofar as they are comparable, in the light of these community, national, and international "standards."

In order to construct the most accurate life tables, it is necessary to use data pertaining to the number of deaths in each age category as well as to the number of persons at risk in the same age categories in the population being studied. In addition, it is not realistic to accept a stationary model for each population studied in colonial America or even in the contemporary European communities to be used as standards of comparison. The questions we will explore in this chapter, however, are not so much concerned with changes in death rates or life expectancy over a period of time, much less with their mathematical precision, as with assessing these and other aspects of public health in several communities during approximately the same period. The raw data used appear to meet Vinovskis' criteria for completeness, although it is not possible to verify this assumption satisfactorily, and the method used for computing life expectancy does imply a stationary population. No other method is possible, given the nature of the data available, and we will therefore have to recognize this limitation; the method will permit us to make comparisons of the kind needed here even though it may not be suitable for precise actuarial purposes, and it will help us to answer the questions posed about the health of Hall Jackson's Portsmouth, and about his perceptions of it, by using the same kind of raw data and computation in every case. Similar methods were used in Jackson's own day; although he could not have appreciated their limitations, the conclusions to be drawn from these data were known to him and his colleagues.[15]

The population of Portsmouth at the three United States censuses taken during the period covered by the Spalding-Thurston bills of mortality is characterized in Table 8 by age, sex, and race. Although the smaller proportions of men among the older age groups might suggest that women lived longer than men, we will see later that the life expectancies of the two sexes were about the same.

Table 8.
The Population of Portsmouth in 1800–1820, Characterized by Age Group, Sex, and Race

| | Free Whites | | | | | |
| | 1800 | | 1810 | | 1820 | |
| Age Group | % of Total | % Males | % of Total | % Males | % of Total | % Males |
| --- | --- | --- | --- | --- | --- | --- |
| Under 10 | 32.1 | 49.7 | 30.2 | 51.1 | 26.3 | 51.5 |
| 10–15 years | 20.1 | 51.2 | 14.3 | 47.7 | 14.9 | 47.1 |
| 16–25 years | 22.1 | 54.7 | 21.7 | 48.5 | 20.3 | 48.4 |
| 26–44 years | 13.8 | 43.5 | 22.7 | 47.6 | 22.2 | 51.5 |
| Over 44 years | 11.9 | 40.1 | 11.0 | 38.3 | 16.3 | 45.8 |
| TOTAL | | 49.1 | | 47.9 | | 49.3 |
| Population | 5200 | | 6803 | | 7321 | |

* There were no slaves in Portsmouth at the times of these censuses.
SOURCES: *Population Schedules of the Second Census of the United States, 1800,* microcopy No. 2, Roll 20, "New Hampshire" (Washington, D.C., National Archives, 1960); *Census of the United States for 1810* (Washington, D.C., 1813); *Census of the United States for 1820, Book I* (Washington, D.C., Gales and Seaton, 1821).

The increase in the proportion of people aged 26 to 44 between 1800 and 1810 suggests that families were moving to Portsmouth during that time, a change consistent with Dwight's data demonstrating the growth of maritime industries in the city. The relative deficits of men in that age group in 1800 and 1810 also suggest that a number of men had been lost to the population during the Revolution, confirming Brissot's observation of women and children in rags five years after the war had ended. The data for the free Negroes—there were no slaves in Portsmouth at the time—strongly suggest that a few Negro families had emigrated from Portsmouth: there had been more in 1767.

Table 9 shows that over the years 1801–20 there was no consistent change in any of the three kinds of death rate which can be computed from the Portsmouth bills of mortality when they are taken in conjunction with the United States census figures for the same years. Because the rate neither increased nor decreased significantly over the first twenty years of the nineteenth century, it may be reasonable to infer that there had been little if any measurable change in the overall state of the health of Portsmouth during at least a number of the preceding years, when Hall Jackson was in practice. Later, in Table 13, we will see that about a half of all deaths were attributed to infectious diseases, a group of diseases that could be treated with specific therapy no better in the twenty

| *Free Negroes** | | |
| --- | --- | --- |
| *1810* | *1820* | |
| | *% of Total* | *% Males* |
| — ⎫ | } 26.3 | 45.2 |
| — ⎭ | | |
| — | 15.0 | 50.0 |
| — | 36.3 | 63.4 |
| — | 22.5 | 38.9 |
| 130 | 160 | |

years after Jackson's death than during the twenty years before. As has long been known, the prevalence of infectious disease is "the great index to the health of a people." [16]

Only the birth rate changed constantly during the period over which Drs. Spalding and Thurston reported the medical facts of life in Portsmouth. The gradual decrease over that time span was about the same as the decrease that can be calculated for the entire United States, although the Portsmouth birth rate and fertility rate (the birth rate per 1000 women aged 15 to 44) have been less than those of the country as a whole for the past 170 years. [17]

The average marriage rate in Portsmouth 150 years ago, 9.8 per 1000, was about three fourths of that for the 1960's but greater than those for other contemporary communities, such as Paris (6.2/1000), rural France (8.2/1000), and Salem, Massachusetts (7.8/1000). Conversely, the birth rate 150 years ago was about twice the current birth rate, a biologically useful adjustment for maintaining a growing population but not for one that has reached its spatial limits. [18]

The fetal death rate per 1000 live births was the same then as it is now, which might be expected if adverse effects on the fetus were no more prevalent in either period. The newborn death rate, on the other hand, will be seen in subsequent tables to have been extraordinarily high a cen-

Table 9.
Selected Vital Statistics for Portsmouth, 1801–1820 and 1956–70

| Year | Total Population | Marriage Rate per 1000 Population | Birth Rate per 1000 Population | Fetal Death Rate per 1000 Live Births |
|------|------|------|------|------|
| 1801 | 5511 | | | |
| 1802 | 5600 | | | |
| 1803 | 6000 | | 35.5 | 14.0 |
| 1804 | 6050 | 10.5 | 48.4 | 20.4 |
| 1805 | 6200 | 10.8 | 47.5 | 6.7 |
| 1806 | 6400 | 9.8 | 40.0 | — |
| 1807 | 6500 | 9.5 | 43.6 | — |
| 1808 | 6660 | 8.4 | 41.2 | 18.1 |
| 1809 | 6835 | 10.1 | 42.2 | 3.4 |
| 1810 | 6933 | 9.2 | 36.3 | 11.9 |
| 1811 | 7000 | 9.9 | 36.2 | 7.8 |
| 1818 | 7380 | | 32.1 | 16.8 |
| 1819 | 7435 | | 31.3 | 12.8 |
| 1820 | 7481 | | 25.3 | 31.5 |
| Mean for 1801–20 | 6570 | 9.8 | 38.3 | 14.4 |
| 1956–70 | 19804 | 13.8 | 17.7 | 14.6 |

Only the Birth Rate per 1000 population is significantly correlated (negatively) with time.
SOURCES: *Population Schedules of the Second Census of the United States 1800*, microcopy no. 2, roll 20, "New Hampshire" (Washington, D.C., National Archives, 1960). *Census of the United States for 1810* (Washington, D.C., 1813). *Census of the United States for 1820, Book I* (Washington, D.C., Gales and Seaton, 1821). Lyman Spalding and Richard Thurston, *Bills of Mortality for Portsmouth, New Hampshire*, 1801–1811 and 1818–1820. U.S. Bureau of the Census, *Statistical Abstract of the United States 1970* (Washington, D.C., 1970).

tury and a half ago, when compared to modern figures. Of the 3131 births recorded by Spalding and Thurston, one half were males and one half were females, as would be expected.

The overall death rate for Portsmouth has been almost halved since 1820. The increased mean ratio of deaths to births since then is consis-

| Death Rate per 1000 Population | Deaths per 100 Births | Total Increase in Population Minus Births |
|---|---|---|
| 17.9 | | |
| 26.0 | | |
| 24.1 | 69.0 | 332 |
| 17.6 | 37.5 | −136 |
| 21.6 | 45.4 | − 11 |
| 18.5 | 46.5 | − 63 |
| 18.3 | 41.9 | − 65 |
| 16.2 | 39.3 | − 67 |
| 12.2 | 29.4 | 29 |
| 16.0 | 44.0 | − 43 |
| 15.7 | 43.3 | − 77 |
| 15.9 | 49.8 | |
| 14.6 | 46.8 | − 69 |
| 19.2 | 77.9 | 10 |
| 18.1 | 47.6 | − 14 |
| 10.2 | 62.1 | |

tent with the present lower birth rate and with the larger proportion of the population of child-bearing age in the first decades of the nineteenth century. In Table 11 it will be seen that in the twentieth century the proportion of young people in the population has grown smaller, as the older, nonreproducing population has grown larger. Again, the lower

Table 10.
Deaths in Portsmouth, N.H., by age group

| Age Group | Percent of All Deaths in Ports- mouth, 1801–20 | Cumulative Probability of Dying by end of age interval | |
| | | Portsmouth, 1801–20 | U.S.A., 1956–61 |
| --- | --- | --- | --- |
| Stillbirths | 3.52 | 3.52 | |
| Premature Births | 0.88 | 4.40 | |
| 1 day–7 days | 1.46 | 5.86 | |
| 8 days–28 days | 2.75 | 8.61 | |
| 1 months–6 months | 7.21 | 15.82 | |
| 7 months–12 months | 7.74 | 23.56 | 2.59 |
| 1 year–10 years | 12.91 | 36.47 | 3.00 |
| 11 years–20 years | 7.62 | 44.09 | 3.45 |
| 21 years–30 years | 9.33 | 53.42 | 4.48 |
| 31 years–40 years | 9.80 | 63.22 | 5.86 |
| 41 years–50 years | 8.50 | 71.72 | 8.62 |
| 51 years–60 years | 7.80 | 79.52 | 15.29 |
| 61 years–70 years | 7.86 | 87.38 | 28.85 |
| 71 years–80 years | 7.57 | 94.95 | 51.83 |
| 81 years–90 years | 4.34 | 99.29 | 66.42 |
| 91 years–99 years | 0.71 | 100.00 | 99.99 |

SOURCES: Lyman Spalding and Richard Thurston, *Bills of Mortality for Portsmouth, New Hampshire, 1801–11 and 1818–20*. National Center for Health Statistics, *United States Life Tables by Causes of Death 1959-61* , U.S. Public Health Service publication 1252, Vol. 1, No. 6 (Washington, D.C., 1968), 15.

ratio of deaths to births 150 years ago would be expected in a rapidly growing new country in which the average family size ranged from 5.7 to 9.5 (in Portsmouth it was 6.1), of whom about three were children; in 1970 the average family comprised only 3.2 persons.[19]

For each of the eleven years for which data are available, the annual number of births less the annual number of deaths exceeded the total increase in the population of Portsmouth during the year by the negative numbers in the right-hand column of Table 5. These data suggest that, for instance, in 1803 a substantial number of immigrants settled in Portsmouth, but subsequent years witnessed a trickle of emigration away from the city. Brissot had observed that emigration away from port cities like Portsmouth was probably minimal.[20]

Table 10 lists the probabilities—individually and cumulatively—of dying within certain age limits in Portsmouth. The remarkably high likelihood of dying in the first year of life reflects the prevalence of infectious diseases in infants, as will also be seen in Table 13. The mean age at death was 34 years, and one half of all deaths occurred by the age of 29. It is no surprise, then, that the median age of the entire population of the United States during those twenty years was about 16; today, the median age is just over 30 years, and the mean age of death is about 79.[21]

From Tables 10 and 11 it is apparent that the first ten years of life carried a disproportionate risk of death, compared to that among older persons. This situation has not changed substantially in the past fifteen decades, in terms of the number of children at risk in the youngest age group, although today a smaller fraction of all deaths occurs before the age of ten. Once a person survived those first dangerous years, however, the next fifteen years carried very little risk of death. The very low death rates among people aged 26 to 44 in 1810 reflects the unusual scarcity of infectious disease among that group, as noted anecdotally by Lyman Spalding in a footnote to that year's bill of mortality.

The data in Table 12 confirm the opinion shared by Jackson, Dwight, Chadbourne, Belknap, and Brissot that New England, and New Hampshire in particular, was at least "as healthy a place as any in America." Some of the data in the Table probably were known to them; for instance, Brissot included portions of the same data in his account of America.[22]

Table 11.
Selected Vital Statistics for Portsmouth in the Early Nineteenth and Mid-Twentieth Centuries

| | *Percentage of Total Population of Portsmouth* | | *Age-Specific Death Rates per 1000 Population of Portsmouth* | | | |
| --- | --- | --- | --- | --- | --- | --- |
| *Age Group* | *1801–20\** | *1969\*\** | *1801* | *1810* | *1820* | *1967\*\** |
| Under 10 years | 29.3 | 20.3 | 17.3 | 22.8 | 21.0 | 18.0 |
| 10–15 years | 16.1 | 10.5 | 2.9 | 3.0 | 8.9 ⎫ | 1.5 |
| 16–25 years | 21.3 | 16.5 | 6.1 | 7.4 | 5.7 ⎭ | |
| 26–44 years | 20.1 | 21.9 | 27.8 | 9.7 | 21.9 | 2.6 |
| Over 44 years | 13.2 | 30.8 | 64.6 | 46.9 | 33.3 | 25.0 |
| TOTAL | | | 19.0 | 16.3 | 16.7 | 10.6 |

* Means for time period.
** Based on data for all New Hampshire.
SOURCES: *Population Schedules of the Second Census of the United States 1800*, microcopy no. 2, roll 20, "New Hampshire" (Washington, D.C., National Archives, 1960). *Census of the United States for 1810* (Washington, D.C., 1813). *Census of the United States for 1820, Book I* (Washington, D.C., Gales and Seaton, 1821). Lyman Spalding and Richard Thurston, *Bills of Mortality for Portsmouth, New Hampshire* (1801–11, 1818–20). U.S. Bureau of the Census, *Statistical Abstract of the United States, 1970* (Washington, D.C., 1970).

Table 12.
Selected Vital Statistics for Portsmouth and Other Cities and Towns in the United States and Europe in the Eighteenth and Mid-Twentieth Centuries

| Place | 1700–1800 | | 1976 |
| --- | --- | --- | --- |
| | Number of Deaths per 1000 Population | Number of Deaths per 100 Births | Number of Deaths per 1000 Population |
| Rochester, N.H. | 8.3 | | |
| New Jersey frontier counties | 10.0 | 33.0 | |
| Concord, N.H. | 10.3 | | |
| Andover, N.H. | 11.6 | | |
| Mason, N.H. | 12.8 | 43.5 | |
| Kingston, N.H. | 13.8 | | |
| 25 New England towns with populations of 380 to 5946, mean ± S.D.* | 14.4 ± 6.7 | 46.0 ± 28.2 | |
| Amherst, N.H. | 14.8 | | |
| Shrewsbury, Mass. | 18.0 | 49.1 | |
| Hampton, N.H. | | 50.9 | |
| New Market, N.H. | | 58.4 | |
| PORTSMOUTH, N.H. | 18.1 | 46.2 | ca. 10.2 |
| Salem, Mass. | 21.2 | 49.1–75.2** | |
| Philadelphia, Pa. | 22.2 | 50.0 | |
| New York, N.Y. | 27.8 | | |
| Trois Rivières, Quebec, Canada | 34.4 | 56.3 | |
| Boston, Mass. | 36.6 | 98.6–117.2** | |
| Charleston, S.C. | | 122.0 | |
| All UNITED STATES | | | 8.9 |
| Worcestershire, England | 26.7 | 76.9 | |
| Holy Cross Parish, near Shrewsbury, England | 30.3 | | |
| All ENGLAND | 28.4 | 80.0 | 12.2 |
| Nottingham, England | 34.6 | 86.7 | |
| Norwich, England | | 100.0 | |
| Northampton, England | 37.7 | 123.2 | |
| Edinburgh, Scotland | 40.0 | | 12.5 |
| London, England | 48.1 | 124.9 | |
| Pays de Vaud, Switzerland | 22.2 | | 8.8 |
| A country parish in Brandenburg | 22.2 | | 14.0 |

Table 12. (*continued*)

| Place | 1700–1800 | | 1976 |
| | *Number of Deaths per 1000 Population* | *Number of Deaths per 100 Births* | *Number of Deaths per 1000 Population* |
|---|---|---|---|
| All FINLAND | 25.4 | 61.9 | 9.4 |
| All SWEDEN | | 72.9 | 11.0 |
| Narke, Sweden | 26.8 | 79.5 | |
| Paris, France | 30.7 | 76.9–112.1** | 10.5 |
| Breslau, Silesia [now Wroclaw, Poland] | 35.7 | 119.5 | 8.8 |
| Berlin, Prussia | 37.7 | 131.0 | 14.0 |
| Vienna, Austria | | 121.4 | 12.6 |
| Amsterdam, Netherlands | | 169.6 | 8.3 |

* Standard Deviation.
** These data represent two or more mortality compilations for the period studied.
SOURCES: Jeremy Belknap, *History of New Hampshire*, 2nd ed., 3 vols. (Boston, Bradford and Read, 1813), Vol. 3, pp. 179–184. J. Farmer and J. B. Moore, *Collections, Topographical . . . New Hampshire*, 3 vols. (Concord, Hill and Moore, 1822), Vol. 1, pp. 24, 80–83. Lyman Spalding and Richard Thurston, *Bills of Mortality for Portsmouth, New Hampshire* (1801–11, 1818–20). U.S. Bureau of the Census, *Statistical Abstract of the United States 1970* (Washington, D.C., 1970). Lemuel Shattuck, *The Vital Statistics of Boston* (Philadelphia, Lea and Blanchard, 1841). William Barton, "Observations of the Probabilities of the Duration of Human Life . . .," *Transactions of the American Philosophical Society*, 3 (1793), 25–62. United Nations, *Statistical Yearbook 1964* (New York. United Nations, 1965). "Bill of Mortality for Rochester, N.H.," *Collections of the New Hampshire Historical Society*, 1 (1824), 283–284. O. Pearson, "Mortality in Kingston, N.H. from 1725 to 1832," ibid. 5 (1837), 250–252. Daniel Adams, ed., *Medical and Agricultural Register*, 1 (1806–07), 284–285. D. V. Glass and D. E. C. Eversley, eds., *Population in History* (Chicago, Aldine, 1965), pp. 241, 351–352, 404, 441, 506, 538, 555, 658–659. Robert V. Wells, *The Population of the British Colonies in America Before 1776* (Princeton, Princeton University Press, 1975), p. 68. John Duffy, *History of Public Health in New York City 1625–1866* (New York. Russell Sage Foundation, 1968), pp. 575–578. Francisco Guerra, *American Medical Bibliography 1639–1783* (New York, Lathrop C. Harper, 1962), pp. 460–476, 509, 532–536, 543–545. Metropolitan Life Insurance Company, New York, *Statistical Bulletin*, 59 (April/June 1978), 14.

In the late eighteenth and early nineteenth centuries, Portsmouth, the largest city in New Hampshire, had a death rate up to twice as large as that of other, smaller towns in that state and in the less densely populated parts of New Jersey, as might have been expected. Salem, across the border from Portsmouth in Massachusetts, was comparable in size, population, and death rate to Portsmouth; Shrewsbury was a smaller town (Table 12). Boston and Philadelphia were, of course, the metropolises of America, and the population of peninsular Boston was confined to a smaller land mass than was that of mainland Philadelphia.

Contemporary English and Scottish death rates were up to twice as large as that of Portsmouth. Northampton and Norwich have always been busy manufacturing centers. The lowest documented death rates were those for rural English populations. The death rates for a country parish in Brandenburg, now Prussia, in East Germany, and for the Pays de Vaud in western Switzerland, north of Lake Geneva, were like those for Portsmouth and Salem. It is surprising, perhaps, that the death rate for Paris at the same time was as low as the available data suggest; Paris was not known as the "City of Light" under the *ancien régime*, nor for the health of her population, and it is likely that the vital statistics for the great city were not as complete as contemporary data for England and her colonies.

All these data support the hypothesis that overall death rates in the more densely populated urban areas are likely to be greater than in the less populated or rural areas, as has also been found, in terms of age-specific death rates, for American communities during 1826–35. This hypothesis was not new in the late eighteenth century, however, when Malthus began to apply it to the study of social problems and their solutions. During the eighteenth century the basis of the principle had become grounded in scientific observation for the first time, but it was also incorporated into the new attitude now called Romanticism. That is, the relative healthiness of rural areas could now be proved, thus providing an acceptable rationale for the Romantic's delight in the rural life.[23]

The ratio of deaths to births provides one estimate of the rate of growth of a population. When births outnumber deaths by two to one, as in Portsmouth, Salem, and Philadelphia, it can be inferred that not only is the population being replenished rapidly, but also that a substantial proportion of the population consists of persons in the usually more vigorous and productive years, which coincide with the reproductive years. As the ratio approaches one, as at Norwich, Paris, and Boston, it would appear that something like zero population growth has been achieved, at least when immigration is not taken into account. As the ratio of deaths to births further increases to more than one, as was true for eighteenth-century Berlin and Amsterdam, the resulting picture might be one of at least stagnation if not actual decline. But as Malthus pointed out in 1798, a high birth rate might be favorable to developing nations like America, but it might also be unfavorable to older, established, nations.[24]

The conditions to which the Portsmouth physicians ascribed their patients' deaths are listed in Table 13, in which the diagnoses are arranged according to both modern nosologic concepts and the frequencies with which the diagnoses were made. These include diagnoses that Hall Jackson made. No estimate of their precision is possible in terms of modern pathophysiological concepts. In fact, the imprecision of the Portsmouth diagnoses is self-evident. We are concerned, however, more with eighteenth-century physicians' concepts of disease than with modern concepts of the diseases found in eighteenth-century America. Where the earlier concepts and diagnoses were similar to ours today will be evident in many cases, and instructive, but they are of less practical consequence to our study of medical practice in colonial America.

The last two columns of data in Table 13 are from reports compiled by a leading London physician, Robert Willan (1757–1812) for his own public dispensary and private patients in 1769 and 1797–1800. As we study Willan's 1801 volume, we cannot help being impressed by his powers of observation and his ability to systematize his thinking, and after reading the work we are not surprised to learn that he was the first English physician to develop a clear classification of dermatological diseases. Comparing the Portsmouth data (and, later in this Chapter, the diagnoses that Hall Jackson made) with Willan's data provides good evidence that the diagnoses in Jackson's Portsmouth were consistent with those being made by a busy practitioner at one fountainhead of American medical knowledge. Willan's data are also especially helpful in that they provide information about the diseases a late eighteenth-century physician might expect to see among his patients who did not die; too often we have had to rely only on causes of death in assessing the health of historically remote populations.[25]

Infectious disease, especially consumption (tuberculosis), was the leading cause of death in Portsmouth. In his note to the 1801 Bill of Mortality, Lyman Spalding drew attention to the high prevalence of consumption, and cried out, echoing Jeremiah, "IS THERE NO BALM OF GILEAD? IS THERE NO PHYSICIAN THERE?" (Although the prophet was concerned with his people's dependence on graven images rather than on the Lord, and not with their medical problems, the imagery fit Dr. Spalding's lamentation very nicely: "For the hurt of the daughter of my people am I hurt;...*Is there* no balm in Gilead; *is there* no physician there? why then is not the health of the daughter of my people recovered?...Go up into Gilead, and take balm, O virgin, the daughter of Egypt: in vain shalt thou use many medicines; *for* thou shalt not be cured.")[26]

The data for smallpox confirm that inoculation and, later, vaccination, had caught on in New England more readily than in London and Philadelphia. Both Portsmouth and Boston had had vigorous inoculation programs for many years, and Hall Jackson had participated in such programs in both places.

Eighteenth-century medicine did not understand central nervous system disease in the same ways we do now—if at all. Most of the conditions listed in the second section of Table 13 were then associated with lesions in the brain, although most are now recognized to be symptoms of other diseases. Most deaths ascribed to convulsions, for instance, probably were of infectious origin, and most cases of palsy and apoplexy resulted from cerebrovascular accidents (strokes). In the absence of more reliable information about the patients listed in the bills of mortality,

Table 13.
Causes of Death as Given in the Portsmouth Bills of Mortality for 1801
to 1811 and 1818 to 1820

| Causes of Death* | Age at Death, in Years, Mean (Range) | Cause-Specific** Death Rates per 100,000 |
|---|---|---|
| Number in Tabulations | | |
| (Infectious Diseases) | | 958.8 (45.8) |
| CONSUMPTION (Tuberculosis) | 41 (5–84) | 390.3 (3.5) |
| DISEASED VERTEBRAE (Pott's Disease?) | — 24 | 1.1 |
| SCROPHULA (Lymphatic tuberculosis) | 18 (4–48) | 8.7 |
| CHOLERA INFANTUM | 1 (1w–65y) | 88.1 |
| PULMONIC FEVER (Pneumonias) | 43 (1w–80y) | 73.9 ⎫ |
| PERIPNEUMONIA | — 81 | 1.1 ⎬ (27.0) |
| INFLUENZA | 26 (2–76) | 7.6 ⎭ |
| TYPHUS or TYPHOID FEVERS | 30 (1–87) | 60.9 |
| PNEUMONIA TYPHODES | 46 (3–70) | 4.3 |
| SCARLET FEVER or CANKER RASH | 10 (1m–37y) | 43.5 |
| [W]HOOPING COUGH | 3 (10d–9y) | 41.3 |
| BILIOUS REMITTING FEVER (Yellow Fever) | 29 (6m–76y) | 38.1 |
| QUINSY (Streptococcal?) | 4 (4m–22y) | 29.3 |
| APHTHA (Thrush) | 3 (10d–2y) | 22.8 |
| DYSENTERY | 15 (4m–75y) | 20.7 |
| CROUP (Laryngitis) | 10 (1–74) | 17.4 |
| ERYTHEMA (?) | 9w (1w–6m) | 14.1 |
| MEASLES | 4 (7m–20y) | 12.0 |
| PHRENITIS (Encephalitis?) | 26 (8–63) | 9.8 |

| Per Cent of All Deaths in: | | | | Willan's London Practice in 1769 and 1797–1800, Per Cent of All: | |
|---|---|---|---|---|---|
| Portsmouth 1801–20 | Boston 1811–20 | Philadelphia 1746–75 | London 1770 | Deaths | Diagnoses |
| [1654] | [8491] | [1798] | [21463] | [394] | [12571] |
| 21.70 | 22.27 | 15.18 | 22.40 | 25.38 | 3.61 |
| 0.06 | | | | | |
| 0.48 | 0.12 | | 0.06 | 1.02 | 0.90 |
| 4.89 | 0.76 | | | 0.76 | 0.47 |
| 4.11 | 4.82 | | | 3.55 | 11.89 |
| 0.06 | 0.30 | 4.28 | 0.06 | 1.27 | 0.55 |
| 0.42 | 0.05 | | | | |
| 3.38 | 6.39 | | | | |
| 0.24 | | | | | |
| 2.41 | 0.16 | | 0.005 | 2.28 | 1.95 |
| 2.29 | 0.91 | 1.27 | 1.16 | 1.52 | 1.23 |
| 2.11 | 0.82 | | | 0.51 | 1.05 |
| 1.57 | 1.09 | | 0.02 | | |
| 1.26 | | | 0.32 | 0 | 0.95 |
| 1.14 | 1.13 | 5.39 | | 0.25 | 0.74 |
| 0.96 | 0.45 | | | | |
| 0.78 | | | | 0 | 0.15 |
| 0.66 | 0.36 | 2.55 | 0.53 | 2.03 | 2.08 |
| 0.54 | 0.23 | | | | |

| Causes of Death | Age at Death | Death Rate |
| --- | --- | --- |
| (Hepatitis?) | | 9.7 (0.4) |
| BILIOUS COLIC | 31 (17–42) | 4.3 |
| JAUNDICE | 41 (27–56) | 4.3 |
| INFLAMMATION OF LIVER | — 17 | 1.1 |
| MALIGNANT FEVER (?) | 30 (3–47) | 8.7 |
| PUERPERAL FEVER | 34 (18–44) | 7.6 |
| INFLAMMATION OF STOMACH or BOWEL | 32 (7m–68y) | 7.6 (3.8) |
| ABSCESS (Staphylococcal?) | 36 (8–86) | 5.4 |
| HERPES | 18 (9w–66y) | 4.3 |
| LOCKJAW, or TETANUS | 23 (4–38) | 4.3 |
| SMALLPOX, NATURALLY ACQUIRED | 26 (20–33) | 4.3 |
| SMALLPOX, INOCULATED | — 1 | 1.1 |
| INFLAMMATORY FEVER (?) | 14 (4–24) | 4.3 |
| FEVER DUE TO WORMS (Hookworm) | 4 (2–6) | 4.3 |
| SYPHILIS | 34 (26–39) | 3.3 (1.2) |
| INTERMITTENT FEVER WITH AGUE (Malaria) | 27 (18–33) | 3.3 |
| ERYSIPELAS (? Streptococcal) | 16 (5m–31y) | 2.2 |
| MALIGNANT SORE THROAT (Diphtheria) | 3 (2–3) | 2.2 |
| SCALD HEAD (Ringworm) | — 1 | 1.1 |
| PETECHIAL FEVER (?) | — 9 | 1.1 |
| CARIOUS ULCER (?) | — 70 | 1.1 |
| [All FEVERS] | | |

| Portsmouth | Boston | Philadelphia | London | Deaths | Diagnoses |
|---|---|---|---|---|---|
| 0.54 | 0.67 | | | | |
| 0.24 | 0.03 | | | 0 | 1.04 |
| 0.24 | 0.35 | | | 0.25 | 0.53 |
| 0.06 | | | | 0 | 0.06 |
| 0.48 | 0.55 | | | 5.08 | 4.50 |
| 0.42 | 0.74 | 2.53 | 0.80 | 0.76 | 1.22 |
| 0.42 | 0.02 | | 0.36 | 0.51 | 11.79 |
| 0.30 | 0.15 | | | 0.25 | 0.14 |
| 0.24 | | | | 0 | 0.21 |
| 0.24 | 0.09 | | | 0.51 | 0.02 |
| 0.24 | 0.08 | 16.68 | 7.73 | 6.09 | 1.81 |
| 0.06 | | | | 0 | 0 |
| 0.24 | 0.61 | | | 0 | 0.74 |
| 0.24 | 0.25 | | 0.03 | 0 | 0.79 |
| 0.18 | 0.22 | | 0.30 | | |
| 0.18 | 0.02 | | 0.005 | 0 | 0.53 |
| 0.12 | 0.01 | | | 0 | 0.24 |
| 0.12 | 0.21 | | 0.10 | 0.76 | 0.17 |
| 0.06 | 0.22 | | | 0 | 0.19 |
| 0.06 | | | | 1.02 | 0.21 |
| 0.06 | 0.01 | | 0.11 | | |
| 13.63 | | 11.73 | 10.59 | | |

| Causes of Death | Age at Death | Death Rate |
|---|---|---|
| (*Central Nervous System Disorders*) | | 269.7 (< 0.1) |
| CONVULSIONS (many probably secondary to infectious diseases) | 9 (1d–68y) | 100.0 |
| DROPSY OF BRAIN (Hydrocephalus?) | 4 (1m–18y) | 70.7 |
| PALSY | 61 (19–87) | 53.3 |
| APOPLEXY | 59 (28–45) | 35.9 (102.2) |
| EPILEPSY | 18 (4w–64y) | 9.8 |
| (*Cardiovascular Diseases*) | | 108.7 (588.0) |
| DROPSY (Congestive Heart Failure) | 49 (3–89) | 59.8 |
| MORTIFICATION (Gangrene) | 37 (7m–90y) | 39.1 |
| ANGINA PECTORIS | 53 (18–73) | 5.4 |
| *** ANEURYSM | 42 (26–57) | 2.2 |
| *** MORTIFICATION DUE TO OSSIFIED ARTERY | — 77 | 1.1 |
| *** OSSIFICATION OF AORTIC VALVES | — 39 | 1.1 |
| CONGENITAL MALFORMATIONS | | 8.8 (8.8) |
| *** PATENT FORAMEN OVALE | 10 d (2d–17d) | 3.3 |
| *** OF HEART, Unspecified | 7 (6d–13y) | 2.2 |
| SPINA BIFIDA | 7m (3m–10m) | 2.2 |
| Unspecified | — 8d | 1.1 |
| (*Genitourinary Diseases*) | | 9.8 (4.8) |
| NEPHRITIS | 52 (34–74) | 5.4 (5.0) |
| GRAVEL (Calculi) | 51 (41–60) | 2.2 |
| STRANGURY (Dysuria) | 41 (20–61) | 2.2 |

| Ports-mouth | Boston | Phila-delphia | London | Deaths | Diagnoses |
|---|---|---|---|---|---|
| 5.56 | 0.71 | 14.23 | 26.68 | 0 | 0.04 |
| 3.92 | 1.01 | | 0.10 | 2.54 | 0.19 |
| 2.96 | 0.64 | | 0.32 | 0 | 0.25 |
| 1.99 | 1.29 | 1.66 | 1.03 | 2.03 | 0.33 |
| 0.54 | 1.61 | | | 0 | 0.41 |
| 3.32 | 2.29 | 3.11 | 4.77 | 5.58 | 2.17 |
| 2.17 | 0.81 | | 0.92 | 0.25 | 0.02 |
| 0.30 | 0.10 | | | | |
| 0.12 | 0.02 | | | | |
| 0.06 | | | | | |
| 0.06 | | | | | |
| 0.18 | | | | | |
| 0.12 | | | | 0.25 | 0.01 |
| 0.12 | | | | | |
| 0.06 | | | | | |
| 0.30 | 0.02 | | | 0 | 0.06 |
| 0.12 | 0.05 | | 0.10 } | 0.25 | 1.01 |
| 0.12 | 0.01 | | | | |

| Causes of Death | Age at Death | Death Rate |
|---|---|---|
| CANCER | 61 (42–76) | 10.9 (193.3) |
| *** SCIRRUS BLADDER (Carcinoma?) | — 74 | 1.1 |

| Other Diseases | | |
|---|---|---|
| SCIRRUS LIVER (Cirrhosis?) | 49 (25–65) | 9.8 (14.1) |
| ASTHMA (Asthma?) | 53 (40–77) | 3.3 |
| GOUT | 59 (50–74) | 3.3 |
| RHEUMATISM | — 55 | 1.1 |
| STRANGULATED HERNIA | — 55 | 1.1 (5.0) |
| ILIAC PASSION (Ileus) | — 95 | 1.1 |
| CHLOROSIS (Iron deficiency anemia) | — 13 | 1.1 |

| Casualties | | 71.9 (53.1) |
|---|---|---|
| Less probable poisonings & shipboard drownings) | | 53.6 |
| DROWNING | 35 (2–78) | 34.8 |
| BURNS AND SCALDS | 19 (8m–75y) | 15.2 |
| FALL | 32 (17–76) | 8.7 |
| FALLING EARTH (Landslide?) | — 35 | 1.1 |
| FROZEN | 69 (38–86) | 3.3 |
| SMOTHERED | 21 (1m–62y) | 3.3 |
| RUN OVER BY A WAGGON | 25 (5–45) | 2.2 |
| CHOAKED | — 5 | 1.1 |
| FRACTURE | — 72 | 1.1 |
| CONCUSSION OF BRAIN | — 35 | 1.1 |
| OPIUM POISONING (Chiefly paregoric) | 6 (4m–22y) | 4.3 |

| Ports-mouth | Boston | Phila-delphia | London | Deaths | Diagnoses |
|---|---|---|---|---|---|
| 0.60 | 0.37 | | | 0.19 | |
| 0.06 | | | | 0.76 | 0.06 |
| | | | | | |
| 0.54 | 0.01 | | 0.01 | 2.79 | 0.39 |
| 0.18 | 0.03 | | 2.74 | 0 | 0.11 |
| 0.18 | 0.13 | | 0.42 | 0 | 0.13 |
| 0.06 | | | 0.01 | 0 | 5.37 |
| 0.06 | 0.09 | | 0.05 | 1.27 | 0.18 |
| 0.06 | | | | | |
| 0.06 | | | | 0 | 2.23 |
| 5.59 | 2.79 | | | | |
| 4.03 | | | | | |
| 1.93 | 1.40 | | | | |
| 0.90 | 0.30 | | | | |
| 0.48 | | | | | |
| 0.06 | | | | | |
| 0.18 | 0.01 | | 0.03 | | |
| 0.18 | 0.05 | | | | |
| 0.12 | | | | | |
| 0.06 | | | | | |
| 0.06 | 0.01 | | | | |
| 0.06 | | | | | |
| 0.24 | 0.07 | | | | |

| Causes of Death | Age at Death | Death Rate |
|---|---|---|
| DRUNKENNESS, DEBAUCHERY, MANIA TEMULENTA (Alcoholism) | 38 (25–58) | 15.2 |
| SUICIDE | 33 (18–51) | 9.8 (10.8) |
| *(Unassignable)* | | |
| HEMORRHAGE, FROM LUNGS | 43 (14–61) | 4.3 |
| HEMORRHAGE, ELSEWHERE | 37 (1–69) | 12.0 |
| HYSTERITIS (Disease of uterus) | — 45 | 1.1 |
| INFANTILE COMPLAINTS | 17d (6d–4w) | 2.2 |
| PHRENZY AND INSANITY | 41 (24–48) | 4.3 |
| SUDDEN DEATH | 42 (2d–80y) | 18.5 |
| ATROPHY | 19 (2d–91y) | 120.7 |
| BEDRIDDEN | 86 (84–87) | 2.2 |
| MARASMUS (Wasting) | 39 (5m–71y) | 3.3 |
| OLD AGE | 82 (60–99) | 127.2 (12.2) |
| UNKNOWN | 18 (3w–63y) | 12.0 |
| STILLBIRTHS | | |

Shown are the mean ages and their ranges at death of patients dying from each reported cause; the respective cause-specific death rates during 1801–20 and in the midtwentieth century; and the frequencies with which each diagnosis appears as a cause of death in the bills of mortality for Portsmouth as well as for near-contemporary Boston, Philadelphia, and London, and among the morbidity and mortality records of Robert Willan, a London physician. All ages are given in years, except when noted otherwise (d = days, w = weeks, m = months, and y = years).

* When possible, approximate modern equivalents are given in parentheses.
** The numbers given in parentheses are comparable values for the United States or New Hampshire in 1960–1970.
*** Causes of death that most likely could be diagnosed only at autopsy.
**** It is probable that many or most of these deaths resulted from infectious diseases.
SOURCES: Lyman Spalding and Richard Thurston, *Bills of Mortality for Portsmouth, New Hampshire* (1801–11, 1818–20); Lemuel Shattuck, *The Vital Statistics of Boston* (Philadelphia: Lea & Blanchard, 1841), pp. xxxviii–xl; E. B. Krumbhaar, "The State of Pathology in the British Colonies of North America," *Yale Journal of Biology and Medicine* 19 (1947): 801–815; Robert Willan, *Reports on the Diseases in London. . .* (London: R. Phillips, 1801); Roger Hart, *English Life in the Eighteenth Century* (New York: G. P. Putnam, (1970), p. 76.

| Ports-mouth | Boston | Phila-delphia | London | Deaths | Diagnoses |
|---|---|---|---|---|---|
| 0.78 | 0.76 | | | | |
| 0.54 | 0.34 | | | | |
| | | | | | |
| 0.24 | 0.02 | | | 2.28 | 1.26 |
| 0.66 | 0.27 | | | | |
| 0.06 | | | | | |
| 0.12 | 18.69**** | | | | |
| 0.30 | 0.21 | | 0.42 | 0 | 0.79 |
| 1.02 | 1.80 | | | | |
| 6.71 | | 8.78 | | 0 | 5.89 |
| 0.12 | | | 0.005 | | |
| 0.18 | 1.18 | | | 0 | 0.02 |
| 7.07 | 4.58 | | 7.04 | 1.78 | 0.06 |
| 0.66 | 11.41 | | | | |
| 3.50 | 5.28 | | 3.24 | | |

these diagnoses cannot be reassigned to other categories in the table with any greater certainty. Hydrocephalus, on the other hand, generally is an unequivocal diagnosis which can be made with ease. One wonders why its prevalence was so remarkably high in Portsmouth, Boston, and among Willan's patients, unless its diagnostic criteria have varied with time and place.

If all the deaths attributed to palsy and apoplexy, as well as those ascribed to sudden death—and, say, 75 percent of those attributed to atrophy, bedridden, marasmus, old age, and unknown causes—are added to the deaths that are known to be referable to the cardiovascular system, the cause-specific death rate for all cardiovascular disease in Portsmouth would come to about 420 per 1000, a rate more consistent with, but still less than, current rates. The astonishingly low prevalence of cancer is undoubtedly an underestimate, some cancer deaths being obscured by diagnoses such as atrophy, marasmus, old age, even jaundice, and, perhaps, others.

That tuberculosis was a world-wide scourge is readily seen from comparable figures from America and London. Its lower incidence among causes of death at Philadelphia probably reflects only the relatively greater prevalence of other infectious diseases there. Brissot noted that consumption, which he knew to be the greatest killer in the United States, must have been brought from Europe by the early American settlers. Timothy Dwight provides a glimpse of what he and his contemporaries thought about the sources of the dread disease:

> The causes of its prevalence are both natural and artificial. The natural causes are the severity and especially the frequent and sudden changes of the weather. The artificial ones are intemperance, prevailing to a considerable extent among people of the lowest class, and unhappily not altogether confined to them; a sedentary life continued to such an extent and so much unaccompanied by exercise as to leave the constitution too feeble to resist the attacks of a cold … A young lady dressed *à la Grecque* in a New England winter violates alike good sense, correct taste, sound morals, and the duty of self-preservation.[27]

Cholera infantum, Portsmouth's second most frequent killer, caused six times as many deaths there as in Boston, though typhus and typhoid fevers, which were not then distinguishable, were twice as often responsible for death in the larger city. All of the differences among frequencies of diagnoses in the four cities may be attributed to varying endemic and epidemic conditions—rates that are not measurable as long as morbidity data are not available. However, for one disease that was probably endemic—but hardly epidemic—at a relatively constant rate, namely puerperal fever, the data show that childbirth was less risky in Portsmouth than in other large English-speaking cities. Even so, Willan noted in 1801 that childbed fever was less often fatal than commonly thought. In support of his contention he cited the decline in its incidence since

1749, and the fact that one of his colleagues who had had 2982 pregnant patients over fifteen years had lost only 0.02 percent of them to puerperal fever (and only 1.01 percent of them to any perinatal cause of death).[28]

Many of the cardiovascular diagnoses listed in the Portsmouth bills of mortality could have been made only at autopsy. It is certain that diagnoses such as patent foramen ovale could have been made only after detailed dissections. Post-mortem examinations cannot have been rare even in Hall Jackson's practice. A clinicopathologic correlation in which he presented his findings at the dissection of the heart of one of his patients (see Chapter 4) will demonstrate that he could bring considerable intellectual insight to such problems. Seven of the nine cases of scirrus liver occurred in the years preceding Laennec's 1819 description of cirrhosis; presumably the adjective "scirrus" implies that the liver had been examined and found to be hard, either before or after death.

One death associated with angina pectoris was reported in Portsmouth in 1805, some seven years before John Warren's paper on the subject appeared in the first issue of the *New England Journal of Medicine and Surgery*. It can be inferred, then, that earlier descriptions of angina, by Heberden, Parry, and others were known to the physicians of Portsmouth. The 63-year-old man who died of angina in Portsmouth in 1808 was the Reverend James Neal of Greenland, New Hampshire, who was autopsied by Spalding and Joshua Brackett. Warren printed Brackett's report of the autopsy as an example of angina in which ossification of the coronary arteries was *not* responsible for the symptom complex. (The principal post-mortem findings were extensive pleural and pericardial adhesions, cardiac hypertrophy, severe atherosclerosis of the aorta, and tricuspid valve disease, probably stenosis.)[29]

Although there was some public opposition to the practice of post-mortem dissection in colonial and federalist America, as in all ages, the 27 autopsies published in American newspapers in the middle half of the eighteenth century suggest widespread interest in their results. The reported post-mortem findings included renal stones, bronchial obstruction, liver disease, worms in the brain, arsenic in the stomach, dropsy, and heart disease. Some of these were formal "anatomies," performed for instructional as well as diagnostic purposes. Although post-mortem dissections were not rare events, very rarely do we have their results. In 1807 an anonymous oration published in a Massachusetts journal designed for both doctors and farmers put the case for autopsy as well as it could be now:

> With a view to enlarge our knowledge of the nature of diseases, we ought to open dead bodies as often as it may be convenient...We know that the most rational method of treating diseases is founded on a knowledge of their seats and proximate causes; and it has been long confessed that the...history of the phenomena discovered on opening bodies...is of the last consequence in acquiring that knowledge.

In order to rebut what must have been the principal objection to autopsies then, as it is sometimes now, the orator concluded:

> It is to be hoped, my friends, that a superstitious veneration for the relics of the dead will ere long be done away, and that physicians will be permitted unreservedly to explore an avenue so highly important towards the investigation of the nature of diseases.[30]

Comparison of the 1801–20 data with twentieth-century data shows some similarities that corroborate both the skills of the Portsmouth physicians and the relatively unchanging prevalence of some causes of death. The decline in mortality from infectious diseases in the past 150 years is, of course, the greatest single triumph of recent medical preventive and therapeutic efforts. The apparent increases in the death rates from cardiovascular disease and cancer are only factitious, to a degree, reflecting largely our increasing understanding of those disease processes, as well as the declining prominence of infectious disease among the causes of death. Other Portsmouth diagnoses are, it is obvious, only guesses, or result from the lack of any other information; "old age" and "marasmus" tell us only that the Portsmouth physicians had an imperfect understanding of pathology.

The prevalence of primary renal disease as a cause of death seems not to have changed much in 150 years, nor has the incidence of congenital malformations. The latter, of course, would be expected to remain fairly constant in the absence of some major catastrophe, or of some massive change in the size and quality of the population's gene pool. Accidental deaths, too, seem not to have decreased if the kind of fatal accident that is likely to be peculiar to a port city—drowning—is subtracted from the overall total. In all probability drug poisonings are now about as frequent as they were in Hall Jackson's Portsmouth, after removing the current predisposition to use drugs for nonmedical purposes from the comparable data. Even suicide continues at about the same rate, perhaps an irreducible minimum. Unlike London and other large cities, no murders were reported in Portsmouth during the period of the bills of mortality.[31]

As cancer and cardiovascular disease are the medical conditions of greatest concern to both the profession and the public in the twentieth century, so the infectious diseases played that role in the eighteenth century—in fact until well into the present century. The most complete epidemiologic data for Hall Jackson's day are for the diseases now known to be transmitted by microorganisms, probably because their symptoms are easily categorized and because of the disproportionate number of children who were their victims.

The death of children was particularly disturbing in a growing country whose future depended on the survival of succeeding generations. The available information about epidemics in British North America has been summarized many times in recent years. Ernest Caulfield's painstaking detective work on the concurrent epidemics of diphtheria and scarlet fever in New England in 1735–40 provides a first-hand view of the fear inspired by diseases that we now see only infrequently. He quotes a 1736 poem, *Lamentation*, that expresses not only the colonists' horror at the deaths of so many children, but also the New Englanders' conviction that epidemic diseases were God-sent punishments for their sins, in the tradition of the Old Testament, and especially as preached by Cotton Mather (see above, Chapter 1):

> Both Young and Old, come mourn with me
>   with bitter Lamentation,
> Here is a Call from CHRIST above,
>   to th' rising Generation.
> For GOD above, in Righteousness,
>   an Angel sent with Power,
> Who with a Sword already drawn
>   our Children to devour.
> GOD smitten hath with sore Plagues,
>   our Children young and small,
> Which makes me weep exceedingly,
>   and on CHRIST's Name to call.
> What tears apace, run from our Face,
>   to hear our Children crying
> For help from pain, but all in vain,
>   we cannot help their dying.
> New England's Sins have greater been
>   than Sins of Heathen round,
> Such breach of Laws, is the grand Cause,
>   GOD's Judgments do abound.[32]

Another literary effort which illustrates the popular impact of health conditions was intended as preventive medicine for the souls of children themselves:

> Your Souls affair, Children take care,
>   you don't procrastinate;
> O now begin, to turn from sin,
>   before it be too late.
> O may this Call, awaken all
>   you Children to amend
> Your sinful Lives: O now be wise
>   and mind your latter end.[33]

Twelve year old Peter Thacher's thanksgiving for his deliverance from smallpox inoculation in 1765 (Chapter 1) is an echo of this pediatric theology.

Sin was not the only cause of pestilential disease in New England, in spite of the persuasiveness of pastors like Mather. The concept of contagion, the transmissibility of disease, was known in the eighteenth century, but the concept of infection, by microorganisms, would not be established until the mid-nineteenth century, again in spite of Mather's unprovable precognition. Noah Webster (1758–1843), who is now remembered more as a doctor of words than of people, nevertheless held that epidemics were the natural accompaniments of natural disasters such as comets, volcanic eruptions, and extremes of weather. His dogmatism, however, was not itself contagious, although others, such as Dwight, and perhaps Hall Jackson, as we will see, agreed that bad weather might predispose to disease. Webster accumulated vast amounts of meteorological data to support his hypothesis. About dysentery, for instance, he concluded:

> The acquiescence of all descriptions of men, learned and unlearned, in the opinion that epidemic diseases are to be ascribed solely to infection of specific contagions, has proven extremely injurious to philosophy and medicin. [Dysentery] is infectious, but it originates in any place, in particular seasons, whether in peace or war; and ends at the command of the elements and seasons.

Webster was not alone in his theories. Dr. Edward Augustus Holyoke, from whom we will hear more later, included meteorological data in his description of the health of Salem in 1786. Dr. Benjamin Rush of Philadelphia thought that death could be caused by drinking cold water, a diagnosis completely absent from the Portsmouth bills of mortality but not from those of other cities and towns in the same time period.[34]

Table 14 shows the seasonal fluctuations in death rates for Portsmouth in the early nineteenth century. In general, deaths were more likely to occur in the fall and least likely in the spring, a differentiation found in Boston at the same time and in Salem in 1781–82. Although Spalding provided no data from which morbidity rates for each disease can be computed, he did provide notes about the duration of certain epidemics. The table shows that each of these diseases produced more deaths in the years in which epidemics occurred than in the whole span of the bills of mortality, as expected. Such outbreaks would have been recognized as epidemics, of course, only when they erupted from the endemic to the epidemic state, and especially when the numbers of deaths attributable to them increased over usual numbers.[35]

Everyone in early America knew what each season would bring in the way of diseases:

> I in prophetic numbers could unfold
> The omens of the year; what seasons teem
> With what diseases; what the humid south [wind]
> Prepares, and what the demon of the east:
> But you perhaps refuse the tedious song.[36]

Data pertaining to the health of eighteenth-century Americans, other than birth and death statistics, are very few. For a more accurate picture of the complaints that patients brought to their doctors, such as that provided by Robert Willan in London, physicians' day books will have to be examined in detail. But we do have a few clues.

For instance, dietary components are potential indicators of the health of a population. Travelers like Brissot occasionally tell us what they had to eat in a certain place, but such menus may be unusual ones, offered

Table 14.
Profile of Deaths and Epidemics in Portsmouth by Month and Year, from 1801 to 1820 (percentage of deaths for the year in each month)

| YEAR | JAN | FEB | MAR | APR | MAY | JUN | JUL | AUG | SEP | OCT | NOV | DEC |
|------|-----|-----|-----|-----|-----|-----|-----|-----|-----|-----|-----|-----|
| 1801 | 10 | 3 | 6 | 6 | 4 | 10 | 4 | 8 | 9 | 15 | 12 | 12 |

←——————————————— Bilious Remitting Fever (10%) ———————————————→

Cholera Infantum (7%) ←————————→

Hooping Cough (11%) ←————→

| YEAR | JAN | FEB | MAR | APR | MAY | JUN | JUL | AUG | SEP | OCT | NOV | DEC |
|------|-----|-----|-----|-----|-----|-----|-----|-----|-----|-----|-----|-----|
| 1802 | 7 | 7 | 10 | 3 | 11 | 5 | 5 | 16 | 8 | 8 | 8 | 11 |

Hooping Cough (5%) ←——————————————————→

Measles (8%) ←————————→  Bilious Remitting Fever (9%) ←————→

Scarlet Fever (5%) & Cholera Infantum (9%) ←————→

| YEAR | JAN | FEB | MAR | APR | MAY | JUN | JUL | AUG | SEP | OCT | NOV | DEC |
|------|-----|-----|-----|-----|-----|-----|-----|-----|-----|-----|-----|-----|
| 1803 | 13 | 8 | 13 | 6 | 8 | 10 | 11 | 8 | 5 | 9 | 4 | 7 |
| 1804 | 6 | 9 | 7 | 10 | 7 | 6 | 6 | 4 | 10 | 13 | 11 | 11 |

Cholera (5%) ←——————————————————→

Hooping Cough (4%) ←——————————→

Quinsy (4%) ←————————→

| YEAR | JAN | FEB | MAR | APR | MAY | JUN | JUL | AUG | SEP | OCT | NOV | DEC |
|------|-----|-----|-----|-----|-----|-----|-----|-----|-----|-----|-----|-----|
| 1805 | 16 | 4 | 9 | 9 | 7 | 8 | 8 | 4 | 8 | 8 | 9 | 10 |
| 1806 | 15 | 7 | 10 | 7 | 8 | 7 | 7 | 11 | 5 | 10 | 8 | 3 |
| 1807 | 6 | 11 | 5 | 6 | 6 | 8 | 8 | 8 | 16 | 8 | 8 | 10 |

Influenza (6%) ←——————————————————————————————————→

Typhus (1%) ←————————→

| YEAR | JAN | FEB | MAR | APR | MAY | JUN | JUL | AUG | SEP | OCT | NOV | DEC |
|------|-----|-----|-----|-----|-----|-----|-----|-----|-----|-----|-----|-----|
| 1808 | 6 | 7 | 1 | 10 | 11 | 9 | 7 | 11 | 8 | 7 | 17 | 4 |
| 1809 | 9 | 11 | 8 | 15 | 5 | 4 | 6 | 7 | 6 | 9 | 9 | 11 |
| 1810 | 6 | 9 | 12 | 8 | 5 | 5 | 10 | 10 | 8 | 12 | 8 | 6 |
| 1811 | 4 | 9 | 7 | 5 | 7 | 7 | 13 | 11 | 5 | 11 | 12 | 9 |
| 1818 | 9 | 8 | 7 | 9 | 9 | 3 | 12 | 6 | 10 | 9 | 10 | 8 |
| 1819 | 11 | 11 | 6 | 6 | 8 | 11 | 7 | 6 | 14 | 9 | 5 | 5 |
| 1820 | 9 | 5 | 4 | 7 | 3 | 5 | 3 | 13 | 18 | 15 | 7 | 11 |
| Rank Order | 4 | 7 | 10 | 9 | 11 | 12 | 8 | 5 | 2 | 1 | 3 | 6 |

Horizontal lines indicate duration of epidemics of specific diseases described in notes to the Bills of Mortality; the numbers in parentheses indicate the proportions of total deaths in the respective year caused by these diseases. Of all deaths in Portsmouth during these fourteen years, the following proportions were reported to have been caused by: Bilious Remitting Fever, 2.1%; Cholera, 4.9%; Hooping Cough, 2.3%; Measles, 0.7%; Scarlet Fever, 2.4%; Quinsy, 1.6%; Influenza, 0.4%; and Typhus, 3.4%.
SOURCE: Lyman Spalding and Richard Thurston, *Bills of Mortality for Portsmouth, New Hampshire* (1801–1811, 1818–1820).

Table 15.
Basic Weekly Diets of Americans, and of British in America, in the
Eighteenth Century

| Population | Calories per Day | Grain |
|---|---|---|
| Privateers, 18th-century Mass. and Early 18th-century Mass. | 4,748 | 1 pt. Rice<br>7 lb. Bread<br>1 qt. Peas |
| Militia: In garrison | 2,480 | 7 lb. Bread<br>3.5 lb. Peas |
| On the March | 2,688 | 7 lb. Bread |
| Acadians in Maryland, 1755 | 1,934 | 1 lb. Bread<br>5 lb. Flour |
| British Army in Canada | 2,736 | 7 lb. Flour<br>3 pt. Peas<br>0.5 lb. Flour |
| Convicts transported to America, about 1770 | 2,061 | 4.7 lb. Bread<br>1.7 lb. Oatmeal<br>1 lb. Peas |
| Continental Army rations: 1775 | 3,545 | 1 pt. Cornmeal<br>3 pt. Peas<br>7 lb. Bread |
| 1780 | 3,110 | 7 lb. Bread<br>7 lb. Flour<br>1.75 pt. Cornmeal |
| Slaves at Mt. Vernon, about 1790 | 3,752 | 14.4 lb. Cornmeal |

SOURCE: U.S. Bureau of the Census, *Historical Statistics of the United States* (Washington, D.C., 1965).

to guests but not part of the host's daily fare. Some are cited only for their unexpected qualities. The few available data reflecting the nutrition of eighteenth-century Americans are given in Table 15.

It is likely that the chief reason for the survival of these diets, on paper, is that they were designed for special groups, such as soldiers or prisoners, living under the restricted conditions for which logistic records were required. The diets were contrived for ease of transporting the food and of preparing it for large numbers of people, not for their culinary delight. Although not appetizing to us, they would have provided adequate ca-

| | Weekly Allowances | |
| Meat | Dairy | Liquor |
| --- | --- | --- |
| 3 lb. Beef<br>4 lb. Pork | | |
| 4.7 lb. Pork | | 1/6 gal. Molasses |
| 7 lb. Pork | | 7 gills Rum |
| 1 lb. Beef | | |
| 7 lb. Beef,<br>or<br>4 lb. Pork | 3/8 lb. Butter | |
| 0.7 lb. Beef<br>0.5 lb. Pork | 0.7 lb. Cheese | 1.25 lb. Molasses<br>0.33 gills Gin |
| 7 lb. Fish, or<br>7 lb. Beef, or<br>5.25 lb. Pork<br>7 lb. Beef, or<br>6.5 lb. Pork | 7/8 gal. Milk | 1.75 gal. Beer, or<br>0.36 gal. Molasses |
| 3.6 lb. Fish<br>0.6 lb. Meat | | |

loric nutrition; the daily dietary allowance recommended by the National Research Council in 1968 is 2900 calories. The actual mean caloric intake of young American adults in 1971–74 was, however, only 2300 calories, even among people officially above the poverty level (3000 calories for men and 1700 for women). The greatest deficiencies that might have been associated with the colonists' diets would have been of the vitamins.[37]

Benjamin Rush pointed out the contributions to the public health made by certain changes in the average American diet during the Revolutionary War. He noted that the consumption of meat tended to decrease, while that of vegetables not only increased, but remained more or less constant all year long, because of improved transportation facilities as well as changing tastes. Such dietary changes would, of course, have helped maintain vitamin intake at something more like optimum levels.[38]

Babies probably did not eat as well as their parents. Virtually all infants were breast-fed, and weaning did not occur until, on the average, the age of 17 months or the time of next pregnancy, whichever occurred first. "Dry nursing," or artificial feeding from a pewter or silver bottle, seldom was practiced in the colonies, but when it was, it provided no better nourishment than did breast feeding. After weaning, children ate almost anything their parents did.[39]

Although books of medical advice were often among the small collection of books in most colonial homes, and although the ratio of physicians to patients in the colonies was no smaller than it is now, many Americans appear not to have heeded the earliest signs and symptoms of disease until it was too late. This situation, which has not been entirely reversed even today, was summarized by a poetically inclined physician in 1807:

> ...But should the public bane
> Infect you, or some trespass of your own,
> Or flaw of nature hint mortality,
> *Soon as a not unpleasing horror glides*
> *Along the spine through all your torpid limbs,*
> *When first the head throbs, or the stomach feels*
> *A sickly load, a weary pain the loins,*
> Be [*a physician*] *called:* the fates come rushing on;
> The rapid fates admit of no delay.
> While wilful you, and fatally secure
> Expect to-morrow's more auspicious sun,
> The growing pest, *whose infancy was weak*
> And easily vanquish'd, *with triumphant sway*
> O'ERPOW'RS YOUR LIFE. For want of timely care
> *Millions have died of medicable wounds.*

The poet concludes by summing up some of the causes of disease known to him—overwork, sin, meteorological, and geological disasters:

> Ah! in what perils is vain life engag'd!
> ... Of indolence, of toil,
> We die; of want, of superfluity.
> *The all-surrounding heaven, the vital air,*
> IS BIG WITH *DEATH:* and though the putrid south [wind]
> Be shut, though no convulsive agony
> Shake from the deep foundations of the world
> Th' imprisoned plagues, *a secret venom oft*
> Corrupts the air, the water, and the land.[40]

Like many of his contemporaries, Jackson kept a journal. It was not a detailed record of either his professional or nonprofessional experiences, but a collection of data designed for a special use. It consists of two volumes bound in cardboard, containing one page for every month from December 1774 through June 1795. They were designed as a "Meteorological Register," as Jackson called it. For every day of all 246 months during which he made entries, he recorded the outdoor thermometer readings at sunrise, noon, and sunset, as well as wind direction, inches of snowfall, whether the Mill Pond froze, the occurrence of meteorological spectaculars like the aurora borealis or a solar eclipse, and many other phenomena that were unusual, as well as remarks on the weather in general. The right-hand column of each page was reserved for special events. Sometime after the Revolutionary War, Jackson went through the journal and inserted, in their proper places, the most important battles of the war, and a few significant political events. In this column he referred to himself in only a single entry: on March 25, 1786, he "began to make my Garden."

One wonders why Jackson omitted any other mention of himself in his data. In none of the few other traces of him that survive does he appear to be entirely selfless. Moreover, we do have good evidence, from his own hand, that he was at Cambridge several times in 1775, and at Providence in 1778; yet he included in his Register no mention of those journeys, or of his sojourn in Marblehead in early 1777.[41]

The clue probably lies in the fact that there is not a single omission from the table of temperatures for the entire twenty years of the journals. Because we have conclusive evidence that he was absent for several periods during the War, someone else must have collected the data for him, so that he could transcribe them at his convenience. In Chapter 6 we will see that the recording of such data had the expected practical implications for scientists, especially those whose interests included botany. Jackson did, in fact, own a farm, although he did not work it himself.[42]

We have noted that fluctuations in climate and weather sometimes were thought to be related to fluctuations in the health of populations, and Jackson probably kept his logs in order to collect data to corroborate —or reject—this hypothesis. That conclusion is supported by what, for our purposes, are the most interesting data in the journals, those relating to births and deaths. After the first few months, he began to label his right-hand columns "Bills of Births and Mortality," hinting that he might be trying to relate them to his meteorological data.

From 1737 to 1753 Dr. John Lining (1708–1760) of Charleston, South Carolina, collected data pertaining to the weather in an attempt to establish a definite correlation between weather and disease, although he finally admitted that he could find none for the sporadic yellow fever epidemics. Noah Webster was more concerned with the possible relationships between natural catastrophes on a grand scale and major epidemics than with those between everyday weather and diseases. Jeremy Belknap and Ezra Stiles were among Jackson's own correspondents

Table 16.
Summary of Outcomes of 511 Pregnancies Attended by Hall Jackson in the Full Years 1775–1794

| | Live Births | | | | | | |
| | Single Births | | | | | | |
| | Whites | | Negroes | | No. of Twins* | Still-births | |
| Year | Males | Females | Males | Females | and Sex | and Sex | TOTALS |
|---|---|---|---|---|---|---|---|
| 1775 | 10 | 7 | 1 | | | | 18 |
| 1776 | 7 | 4 | | | | | 11 |
| 1777 | 9 | 15 | 1 | 1 | 2 MM | 1 F | 29 |
| 1778 | 8 | 8 | | | | 2 FM | 18 |
| 1779 | 15 | 12 | | | | | 27 |
| 1780 | 14 | 11 | 1 | | | | 26 |
| 1781 | 18 | 5 | | | | 2 FF | 25 |
| 1782 | 12 | 4 | | | 2 FF | | 18 |
| 1783 | 13 | 9 | | | 2 ?? | 2 FF | 26 |
| 1784 | 14 | 9 | | 1 | | 2 FM | 26 |
| 1785 | 14 | 15 | | | | | 29 |
| 1786 | 16 | 19** | 1 | 1 | 2 ?? | | 39 |
| 1787 | 16 | 12 | | 1 | | | 29 |
| 1788 | 16 | 10 | 1 | | 2 ?? | 2 MM | 31 |
| 1789 | 16 | 16 | | | 2 ?? | | 34 |
| 1790 | 8 | 13 | | | | 1 F | 22 |
| 1791 | 16 | 12 | | 1 | | | 29 |
| 1792 | 13 | 9 | | | | | 22 |
| 1793 | 10 | 15 | | 1 | | | 26 |
| 1794 | 15 | 15 | | | 4 ???? | | 34 |
| TOTAL | 260 | 220 | 5 | 6 | 16 | 12 | 519 |

* All white    ** One of these girls was born with an imperforate anus.

who also exemplified what has been called "the scientific chauvinism of the Enlightenment." Jackson would probably have agreed with John Lining's rationale for collecting such data: "What first induced me to enter upon this Course, was, that I might experimentally discover the influence of our different seasons upon the Human Body; by which I might arrive at some more certain knowledge of the causes of our epidemic Diseases, which as regularly return at their stated Seasons, as a good Clock strikes Twelve when the Sun is in the Meridian." Perhaps Jackson was, in fact, taking John Arbuthnot up on his 1730 recommendation of "keeping a journal of the Weather and reigning Diseases, as a thing which might be of singular Use, especially to posterity." [43]

The average yearly numbers of births and deaths that Jackson recorded are about a fourth of those expected for the entire town of Portsmouth, as would be expected because Jackson was one of four doctors in the town. Thus even if the 519 births and 247 deaths do not provide a complete tally, any omissions are probably negligible. He included none of the patients he treated during the war or in Marblehead, but they could not be considered to be natives of Portsmouth. Of the 246 consecutive months for which Jackson recorded the vital statistics of his own practice, there are only ten, scattered randomly throughout, during which he recorded no births or deaths. Because there is no external evidence that he was elsewhere during those months, they presumably were only relatively uneventful months in the professional life of an otherwise busy practitioner, whose actual work load was based on about 1200 patients.

In the aggregate, Jackson's own data are entirely consistent with other evidence pertaining to the health of Portsmouth, and they seem to provide a valid sampling of the health statistics of that town, although we will see that he did select some data for inclusion, while purposely omitting others. The journals provide a rare first-hand glimpse of the vital statistics of the practice of an eighteenth-century physician, despite the lack of data about nonobstetrical and nonfatal cases—information that is lacking for most physicians of the time.

The 511 pregnancies attended by Dr. Jackson during the twenty years of his journals are tabulated by year, race, and sex in Table 16. He averaged about 25 deliveries a year—not an overwhelming patient load by twentieth-century standards, although the data may not be strictly comparable because of the previously noted increase in prenatal care of the present day.

Table 17.
Summary by Race and Sex, of Deaths among Hall Jackson's Patients for the Full Years 1775 to 1794 in Portsmouth, Including Still Births.

| | WHITES | | | NEGROES | | | |
| Year | Males | Females | Sex Unknown* | Males | Females | Sex Unknown* | TOTALS |
|---|---|---|---|---|---|---|---|
| 1775 | 5 | 7 | 1 | | | | 13 |
| 1776 | 16 | 9 | 3 | 1 | 1 | | 30 |
| 1777 | 8 | 6 | 1 | | | | 15 |
| 1778 | 12 | 11 | 1 | | | | 24 |
| 1779 | 3 | 1 | | | | | 4 |
| 1780 | 3 | 1 | | | | | 4 |
| 1781 | 2 | 3 | | | | | 5 |
| 1782 | 4 | 4 | 1 | | | | 9 |
| 1783 | 11 | 6 | 5 | | | | 22 |
| 1784 | 7 | 10 | | | | | 17 |
| 1785 | 6 | 2 | | | | | 8 |
| 1786 | 12 | 2 | 1 | 2 | | | 17 |
| 1787 | 11 | 2 | | | | | 13 |
| 1788 | 2 | 4 | | 1 | | 2 | 9 |
| 1789 | 3 | 6 | 1 | | | | 10 |
| 1790 | 7 | 5 | 2 | | | | 14 |
| 1791 | 5 | 4 | | | | | 9 |
| 1792 | 2 | 2 | | | | | 4 |
| 1793 | 8 | 5 | | | | | 13 |
| 1794 | 3 | 3 | 1 | | | | 7 |
| TOTAL | 130 | 93 | 17 | 4 | 1 | 2 | 247 |

* Identified only as "Child."

Table 18.
Summary, by Age, of Deaths Among Hall Jackson's Patients in
Portsmouth in the Full Years 1775–1794

| | Number of Deaths among Jackson's Patients | | | |
| Age | Males | Females | Sex Unknown | TOTAL |
| --- | --- | --- | --- | --- |
| Stillbirths | 4 | 8 | | 12 |
| 1 day–7 days | 3 | 1 | | 4 |
| 8 days–28 days | 4 | 2 | 4 | 10 |
| 1–6 months | 2 | | | 2 |
| 7–12 months | | | | 0 |
| 1–10 years | 9 | 6 | 2 | 17 |
| 11–20 years | 8 | 8 | | 16 |
| 21–30 years | 9 | | | 9 |
| 31–40 years | 7 | 4 | | 11 |
| 41–50 years | 8 | 2 | | 10 |
| 51–60 years | 6 | 1 | | 7 |
| 61–70 years | 3 | 2 | | 5 |
| 71–80 years | 8 | 6 | | 14 |
| 81–90 years | 8 | | | 8 |
| 91–99 years | | 1 | | 1 |

Of all the pregnancies, 2.31 percent resulted in stillbirths. Of the 507 live births, 51.28 percent were white males, 43.39 percent were white females, 0.98 percent were Negro males, and 1.18 percent were Negro females. The remainder were twin births, which occurred in 1.60 percent of the 499 pregnancies that resulted in live births. This incidence is about 25 percent greater than the 1.28 percent incidence of twin births in similar populations in the present century.[44] Although the discrepancy may not be statistically significant, if Dr. Jackson did indeed have a special reputation as an obstetrician, he would have been sought out for possibly difficult cases, as twins might have presented.

He noted that one of the babies he delivered had an easily recognizable congenital malformation, a girl with an imperforate anus. As many as six or seven anomalies would now be predicted among the 507 live births; that Jackson noted only one can be attributed to the less extensive knowledge of such conditions in his day.[45]

The low number of deliveries in 1776 may reflect the general social malaise that prevailed at the outbreak of the Revolution during the preceding year. He delivered the greatest number in 1786, after the peace with Britain had become well established, and during the height of speculation that Portsmouth might become the country's principal naval center.

Table 17 lists all the deaths in Hall Jackson's own bills of mortality;

| Cumulative Percentage of All Deaths | |
|---|---|
| *Jackson's Patients, 1775–1794* | *All Portsmouth, 1801–1820* |
| 9.52 | 3.52 |
| 12.69 | 5.86 |
| 20.62 | 8.61 |
| 22.20 | 15.82 |
| 22.20 | 23.56 |
| 35.69 | 36.47 |
| 48.38 | 44.09 |
| 55.52 | 53.42 |
| 64.25 | 63.22 |
| 72.18 | 71.72 |
| 77.73 | 79.52 |
| 81.69 | 87.38 |
| 92.80 | 94.95 |
| 99.14 | 99.29 |
| 100.0 | 100.0 |

as will be seen in Table 19, however, four of these may not have been his own patients. The average annual number of deaths among his patients is about twelve. The ratio of births to deaths among his patients is, then, about two, which is approximately the same as that for the whole town of Portsmouth (see Table 12) over the subsequent two decades— further evidence that Jackson's tabulation is a random sampling of some measures of the public health of late eighteenth-century Portsmouth.

It is not entirely clear why the greatest annual number of his patients, thirty, died in 1776. From the diagnoses given, the majority of deaths resulted from pneumonia and other infectious diseases, and may have been connected largely with the outbreak of the War and its associated hardships.

From the data in Table 18 it can be inferred that the distribution of the ages of the 126 patients whose age at death Jackson recorded was like that of all persons dying in Portsmouth in the next twenty years. However, Jackson does seem to have attended more deaths of children under six months of age than might be expected on the basis of the later overall population statistics. This, too, is probably associated with his reputation in obstetrical and, presumably, postnatal, care.

The causes of death among the 91 patients whose diagnoses Jackson listed show some of his special concerns as well as diseases that he may have taken for granted or had no special interest in. That only about a

Table 19.
Causes to Which Jackson Attributed the 91 Deaths Listed in His Journals for 1775−1794

| Diagnosis | Hall Jackson's Patients, 1775−94 | | Frequency in Portsmouth, 1801−1820 |
|---|---|---|---|
| | Number | Frequency | |
| Abcess | 1 | 0.40 | 0.30 |
| Angina | 1 | 0.40 | 0.30 |
| Apoplexy | 4 | 1.61 | 1.99 |
| Bayonet, killed by | 1 | 0.40 | 0 |
| Bleeding | 1 | 0.40 | 0.90 |
| Burnt | 1 | 0.40 | 0.90 |
| Cancer | 1 | 0.40 | 0.90 |
| Colic | 3 | 1.21 | 0.24 |
| Consumption | 5 | 2.02 | 21.70 |
| Convulsions | 6 | 2.42 | 5.56 |
| Diarrhea and Dysentery | 4 | 1.61 | 1.14 |
| Dropsy and Hydrops | 12 | 4.85 | 3.32 |
| Drowned (in well) | 1 | 0.40 | 1.93 |
| Fever, Malignant | 1 | 0.40 | 0.48 |
| Fever, Miliary | 6 | 2.42 | } 13.63 |
| Fever, Nervous | 1 | 0.40 | |
| Fever, Unspecified | 4 | 1.61 | |
| Hectic (a fever, sometimes accompanying tuberculosis) | 1 | 0.40 | 0 |
| Lightning, struck by | 1 | 0.40 | 0 |
| Mortification | 2 | 0.80 | 2.17 |
| Murdered | 1 | 0.40 | 0 |
| Peripneumonia and Pulmonic | 19 | 7.68 | 4.17 |
| Podagra (Gout) | 1 | 0.40 | 0 |
| Post-Amputation of thigh | 1 | 0.40 | 0 |
| Smallpox | 6 | 2.42 | 0.24 |
| Spasmodic | 1 | 0.40 | 0 |
| Tabes (Wasting) | 4 | 1.61 | 0 |
| Worms | 1 | 0.40 | 0.24 |

The frequencies are based on the total 247 deaths recorded in Jackson's journals, not on the 91 for which he gave causes. The four violent deaths (by burning, bayonetting, lightning, and murder) may not have occurred among his own regular patients; they appear to have been listed because they were unusual occurrences.

third of all the deaths tabulated in his journal were assigned diagnoses probably suggests some of his particular interests rather than his ignorance.

Table 19 shows that many of the causes of death listed in Jackson's notes occurred, among all 247 deaths, at frequencies like those found by Spalding and Thurston twenty years later. Although about half of the individual diagnoses involve infectious diseases, as is true for the Spalding-

Thurston data for the whole town, they amount to only about one fourth of all the deaths listed. Perhaps Jackson regarded such diseases as so common that they needed no particular emphasis. For instance, he recorded only about a tenth as many deaths fron consumption as might have been expected, although, as noted in Chapter 1, he was appalled at the rise in incidence of the disease in 1789. Neither does he include a single case of puerperal fever, in spite of his remark that it was rampant in the summer of 1784. We have already seen that he included no cases of malignant putrid sore throat, again in spite of the 1783–86 epidemic. It would also be possible to conclude from such negative data that Jackson was extraordinarily successful in reducing the mortality from infectious diseases among his patients, but that cannot be proved in the absence of data pertaining to the incidence of the diseases among his patients who did not die.

That Hall Jackson attributed deaths to the pneumonias more often than did his successors may reflect greater interest, as well as greater diagnostic accuracy or error, on his part or theirs. The 90 percent reduction in smallpox deaths after his own death is most likely the result of the introduction of vaccination in 1800, but in his journals he does not tell us whether the smallpox deaths he attended resulted from naturally acquired smallpox or from inoculations. (Jabez Dow's notes cited in Chapter 1 suggest the former possibility.) His use of the diagnosis of tabes does not imply tertiary syphilis, as it would today; "tabes" was then used to denote wasting or emaciation.

Jackson listed only what must have been a very small fraction of his other clinical experiences. As we noted earlier, he included only three of his amputations and none of his cataract operations. However, it is quite clear from his journal that he had already developed a special interest in dropsy some years before he learned of the new therapeutic advance that Dr. Withering published in Birmingham in 1785.

On February 2, 1778, Jackson "Tapped a girl of 5, 2 qts of green [illegible] water," which, while not indicating that she had dropsy, shows that Jackson used paracentesis to remove fluid from body cavities, a measure that Paré had reassured surgeons two centuries earlier was safe when done properly, even if many of his colleagues were reluctant to use such an extreme measure.[46] On April 2 and again on May 4, 1780, Jackson tapped Joseph Varney for dropsy, and five months later, on October 10, he tapped Thomas Lowd for the same reason. Neither of these men appears among the deaths listed by Jackson. Thus it is clear that, when Hall Jackson first learned of the usefulness of foxglove in the cure of dropsy, he was ready to try it out.

Life expectancy data provide yet another index of the health of populations. The technique was already in use in the eighteenth century, to permit comparisons among various cities in respect to their relative healthiness, as well as for life insurance purposes; J. Meyer of New York used Lyman Spalding's bills of mortality for Portsmouth in computing his table of annuities and premiums in 1811.[47]

Table 20 shows the average life expectancies in Hall Jackson's day of

Table 20.
Average Life Expectancies of White Populations, at Entry into Given
Age Groups, for Several Cities and Towns in Eighteenth- and Early
Nineteenth-Century America and Europe

| Place and Time | Life Expectancy, in Years, | | | |
|---|---|---|---|---|
| | 0–5 | 6–10 | 11–20 | 21–30 |
| Dover, N.H. (10 years in late 18th century)** | | | | |
| Rochester, N.H. (1776–1822) | 33 | 44 | 43 | 38 |
| Hingham, Mass. (50 years in Late 18th century)** | | | | |
| Hampton, N.H. (1735–92) | 20 | 24 | 43 | 39 |
| Harvard Graduates*** (1711–86)** | | | | |
| New England (18th century) | 30 | 42 | 41 | 35 |
| Concord, N.H. (1798–1821) | 29 | 42 | 40 | 34 |
| New England (1780's)** | 28 | 41 | 39 | 34 |
| PORTSMOUTH, N.H. (1801–11, by Meyer)** | 29 | 42 | 40 | 34 |
| PORTSMOUTH, N.H. (1801–11, 1818–20) | 32 | 41 | 37 | 32 |
| Salem, Mass. (1781–82) | 19 | 33 | 32 | 26 |
| Philadelphia, Pa. (18th century) | 24 | 36 | 34 | 27 |
| Philadelphia, Pa. (1821–30) | 16 | 20 | 33 | 25 |
| Boston, Mass. (1811–20) | 28 | 36 | 33 | 26 |
| Holy Cross Parish, England (18th century) | 34 | 45 | 45 | 38 |
| Norwich, England (18th century) | 24 | 41 | 41 | 35 |

| | | | | | | Total Experience, Compared with that of |
|---|---|---|---|---|---|---|
| *at Entry into Age Group* | | | | | | |
| 31–40 | 41–50 | 51–60 | 61–70 | 71–80 | 81–90 | Portsmouth* |
| 35 | 29 | 23 | 15 | 10 | 7 | 121% |
| 33 | 28 | 23 | 17 | 11 | 7 | 117% |
| 34 | 28 | 22 | 15 | 10 | 6 | 117% |
| 37 | 31 | 24 | 17 | 11 | 8 | 115% |
| 33 | 26 | 20 | 15 | 10 | 7 | 113% |
| 32 | 28 | 23 | 16 | 11 | 7 | 112% |
| 30 | 26 | 21 | 15 | 12 | 7 | 109% |
| 31 | 26 | 21 | 15 | 10 | 6 | 107% |
| 29 | 23 | 19 | 14 | 10 | 6 | 105% |
| 27 | 23 | 18 | 14 | 9 | 6 | 100% |
| 22 | 22 | 19 | 15 | 9 | 5 | 86% |
| 22 | 19 | 16 | 12 | 10 | 8 | 86% |
| 22 | 19 | 16 | 13 | 9 | 5 | 78% |
| 22 | 19 | 17 | 13 | 9 | 6 | 84% |
| 32 | 26 | 20 | 15 | 11 | 6 | 115% |
| 30 | 24 | 18 | 14 | 10 | 8 | 106% |

| Place and Time | Life Expectancy, | | | |
|---|---|---|---|---|
| | 0–5 | 6–10 | 11–20 | 21–30 |
| Northampton, England (18th century) | 26 | 41 | 41 | 33 |
| London, England (18th century) | 19 | 36 | 35 | 30 |
| Country Parishes in Brandenburg (18th century) | 33 | 45 | 45 | 39 |
| Annuitants in France (18th century)** | | | | |
| Annuitants in Holland (early 18th century)** | | | | |
| France (18th century)** | 29 | 43 | 41 | 34 |
| Breslau, Silesia (late 17th century)**** | 34 | 42 | 40 | 34 |
| Paris, France (18th century) | 28 | 42 | 41 | 34 |
| Vienna, Austria (18th century) | 17 | 36 | 37 | 31 |
| Pays de Vaud, Switzerland (18th century) | 37 | 47 | 38 | 31 |
| UNITED STATES, 1970** | 72 | 68 | 63 | 54 |

Except for the data marked with double asterisks (**), all life expectancies were calculated by the method outlined in Rose Sachs, "Life Table Technique in the Analysis of Response-Time Data from Laboratory Experiments on Animals," *Toxicology and Applied Pharmacology*, 1 (1959), 203–227.

* Calculated as years squared, the area under the life expectancy curves up to age 70, with the area under the Portsmouth curve taken as the standard, 100%.

** Life expectancies computed in the original sources; all others were newly computed as specified above. When availability of the original data permitted recalculation by the modern method, the old and new computations yielded life expectancies within one year of each other at each age interval (for Great Britain, Breslau, and Brandenburg).

*** These data are for all Harvard graduates, regardless of domicile.

**** Now called Wroclaw, in Poland.

SOURCES: Jeremy Belknap, *History of New Hampshire*, 2nd ed., 3 vols. (Boston, Bradford and Read, 1813), pp. 178–187. J. P. Brissot de Warville, *New Travels in the United States of America, 1788* (Cambridge, Harvard University Press, 1964), pp. 288–289. J. Farmer and J. B. Moore, *Collections, Topographical . . . New Hampshire* (Concord, Hill and

| *in Years, at Entry into Age Group* | | | | | | *Total Experience, Compared with that of Portsmouth** |
|---|---|---|---|---|---|---|
| 31–40 | 41–50 | 51–60 | 61–70 | 71–80 | 81–90 | |
| 29 | 23 | 18 | 13 | 9 | 6 | 102% |
| 25 | 19 | 16 | 12 | 9 | 6 | 88% |
| 32 | 25 | 18 | 13 | 8 | 6 | 112% |
| 32 | 27 | 20 | 14 | 8 | 5 | 111% |
| 31 | 25 | 19 | 14 | 9 | 5 | 105% |
| 29 | 23 | 18 | 12 | 8 | 5 | 103% |
| 27 | 22 | 17 | 12 | 8 | 5 | 100% |
| 27 | 22 | 16 | 12 | 8 | 6 | 98% |
| 25 | 20 | 16 | 12 | 9 | 6 | 90% |
| 24 | 17 | 12 | 8 | 6 | 5 | 89% |
| 44 | 35 | 26 | 19 | 12 | 7 | 157% |

Moore, 1822), pp. 24, 81–83. Lyman Spalding and Richard Thurston, *Bills of Mortality for Portsmouth, New Hampshire* (1801–11, 1818–20). Lemuel Shattuck, *The Vital Statistics of Boston* (Philadelphia, Lea and Blanchard, 1841). William Barton, "Observations of the Probabilities of the Duration of Human Life . . . ," *Transactions of the American Philosophical Society*, 3 (1793), 25–62. "Bill of Mortality for Rochester, N.H.," *Collections of the New Hampshire Historical Society*, 1 (1824), 283–284. Edward A. Wigglesworth, "A Table Shewing the Probability of the Duration . . . of Life . . . ," *Memoirs of the American Academy of Arts and Science* Vol. 2, pt. I (1793), 131–135. Joseph McKean, "Synopsis of Several Bills of Mortality," ibid., pt. II (1804), 62–70. J. Meyer, *Of Insurances on Lives and Life Annuities* (New York, D. & G. Bruce, 1811), pp. 78–79. G. Emerson, "Medical Statistics; Consisting of Estimates Relating to the Population of Philadelphia," *American Journal of the Medical Sciences*, 9 (1831), 17–46. D. V. Glass and D. E. C. Eversley, eds., *Population in History* (Chicago, Aldine, 1965), p. 494. National Center for Health Statistics, *Vital Statistics of the United States, 1970*, Vol. 2, U.S. Public Health Service publication (HRA) 74–1104 (Washington, D.C., 1974), pp. 5–8.

persons entering several age groups. In Figure 1 representative life-expectancy curves are presented graphically, so that data pertaining to Portsmouth in relation to those of other cities and towns may be more readily understood. In the right-hand column of Table 20 numbers that summarize the data in the curves in a convenient way are tabulated. In this column the total experience of life expectancy at entry into successive age groups was measured as the area under the life-expectancy age curves, in years squared. The area under the curve for Portsmouth was taken as 100 percent and all the other areas compared with it, in order to provide a rough assessment of the health of Portsmouth relative to that of other areas of the world.

Life expectancy in Portsmouth during the years of the Spalding-Thurston bills of mortality was about what would have been expected in a community of its size, consistent with the data presented in Table 12.

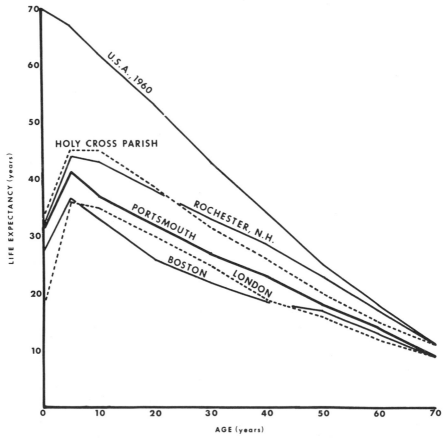

FIG. 1. *Representative life expectancy curves, taken from data in Table 20, for Portsmouth and for larger and smaller American and English cities and towns, compared with twentieth-century American data.*

That is, Portsmouth was about average, or on the median, in terms of healthiness measured by life expectancies, among all the cities and towns in America and Europe for which data are available. Residents of the large American cities, like Boston and Philadelphia, and of large European cities, like London and Vienna, had shorter life expectancies than did residents of Portsmouth. Conversely, inhabitants of smaller towns in both America and Europe had greater life expectancies than did those of Portsmouth. The two sets of data compiled for all New England, regardless of population density, are so similar as to suggest that differences in total life-expectancy experience of greater than, say 2 to 3 percent for any age interval are probably significant. The New England data also suggest that they were drawn from predominantly rural areas, in spite of the higher population concentrations along the coast. The greater life expectancy in France is somewhat difficult to accept at face value, a difficulty already mentioned; the discrepancy cannot be resolved easily except by assuming that the original data are not representative samples.

The chief distinction between eighteenth-century and twentieth-century life-expectancy curves is the lower life expectancy among children two hundred years ago. From the data we have already examined, this difference would be expected, because of the high prevalence of infectious diseases coupled with physicians' inability to provide definitive cures for them. At about the time these data were being collected, Malthus correctly attributed at least a portion of the difference between urban and rural dwellers to the increased mortality among children, especially the children of the poor, who were found in the greatest numbers in the larger cities. Thus the continuing extension of human life expectancy has resulted from the progressive decline in deaths occurring before the maximum achievable life span.[48]

In Table 21 the life expectancies of the populations of Portsmouth and contemporary European communities for which data are available are segregated by sex; some of these data are presented graphically in Figure 2. Although the greater life expectancy of twentieth-century women is well known, they did not have the same advantage in early nineteenth-century Portsmouth. Indeed, men had the advantage from the fourth decade of life on. The difference between Portsmouth and other contemporary societies cannot be attributed solely to the greater hazards of childbirth to which women were exposed in the earlier period. Not only have we already seen that the incidence of such complications was surprisingly slight at the time even to contemporary observers, but the data for Chester, Stockholm, and France suggest that Portsmouth may have been unusual in this respect. Only in Portsmouth did the difference between the sexes increase over the last decades of life; in the other populations, the life expectancies began to converge after about the age of 50. In the absence of other data, it may be inferred that the women of Portsmouth lived under some biological disadvantage that was not necessarily related to any sex-specificity of disease processes.

Brissot suggests one answer. He thought that American women were more likely to have consumption because they took less exercise than did

Table 21.
Average Life Expectancies at Entry into Given Age Groups for White
Male and Female Populations in Portsmouth and Contemporary
European Communities

| Place and Time | 0–5 | 6–10 | 11–20 | 21–30 | 31–4( |
|---|---|---|---|---|---|
| **Portsmouth, N.H. (1809–11)** | | | | | |
| MALES | 30 | 45 | 42 | 36 | 29 |
| FEMALES | 35 | 43 | 40 | 37 | 28 |
| **Chester, England (18th century)**\*\* | | | | | |
| MALES | | | | | 29 |
| FEMALES | | | | | 32 |
| **British Ducal Families (1730–79)**\*\* | | | | | |
| MALES | 45 | 51 | | 40 | |
| FEMALES | 48 | 51 | | 44 | |
| **Stockholm, Sweden (18th century)**\*\* | | | | | |
| MALES | | | | | 19 |
| FEMALES | | | | | 24 |
| **All Sweden (18th century)**\*\* | | | | | |
| MALES | | | | | 30 |
| FEMALES | | | | | 32 |
| **All France (1805–7)**\*\* | | | | | |
| MALES | 35 | 46 | 44 | 38 | 31 |
| FEMALES | 38 | 48 | 45 | 38 | 32 |
| **European Ruling Families (born 1700–99)**\*\* | | | | | |
| MALES | 36 | | | | |
| FEMALES | 38 | | | | |
| **UNITED STATES, 1970**\*\* | | | | | |
| MALES | 68 | 65 | 60 | 50 | 41 |
| FEMALES | 76 | 72 | 67 | 57 | 48 |

See Legend to Table 20 for footnotes.
SOURCES: J. P. Brissot de Warville, *New Travels in the United States of America, 1788*
(Cambridge, Harvard University Press, 1964), pp. 288–289. Lyman Spalding and Rich-
ard Thurston, *Bills of Mortality for Portsmouth, New Hampshire* (1801–11, 1818–20).
D. V. Glass and D. E. C. Eversley, eds., *Population in History* (Chicago, Aldine, 1965),
pp. 98, 359–361, 504–505. National Center for Health Statistics, *Vital Statistics of the
United States, 1970*, Vol. 2, U.S. Public Health Service publication (HRA) 74–1104
(Washington, D.C., 1974), pp. 5–8.

| 41–50 | 51–60 | 61–70 | 71–80 | 81–90 | Total Experience,* | |
|---|---|---|---|---|---|---|
| | | | | | Compared with Same Sex in Portsmouth | Compared with Males in Same Population |
| 25 | 20 | 14 | 11 | 5 | 100% | — |
| 24 | 17 | 10 | 8 | 5 | 100% | 93% |
| | | | | | | |
| 23 | 18 | 12 | 8 | 5 | 87% | — |
| 26 | 21 | 14 | 9 | 5 | 117% | 114% |
| | | | | | | |
| 26 | | 13 | | | 105% | — |
| 30 | | 16 | | | 123% | 110% |
| | | | | | | |
| 16 | 12 | 9 | 6 | | 61% | — |
| 19 | 15 | 10 | 6 | | 85% | 119% |
| | | | | | | |
| 24 | 18 | 12 | 8 | 4 | 88% | — |
| 25 | 19 | 13 | 8 | 4 | 113% | 109% |
| | | | | | | |
| 24 | 18 | 13 | 9 | 7 | 98% | — |
| 25 | 19 | 13 | 9 | 7 | 109% | 103% |
| | | | | | | |
| | 18 | | 7 | | — | — |
| | 18 | | 8 | | — | — |
| | | | | | | |
| 32 | 23 | 16 | 11 | 7 | 131% | — |
| 38 | 29 | 21 | 14 | 8 | 166% | 117% |

American men. Chi-square analysis of the raw data which were used to compute the percentages in Table 22 shows that the number of all females dying in Portsmouth was in proportion to the number of females in the town's population, and that insignificantly more females died of "old age" than males; but females suffered a disproportionately large number of deaths attributed to consumption (chi-square = 31.18, P < 0.01). Brissot used the observation that American women took what he thought was insufficient exercise to suggest that women were not the biological equals, and, by current standards of philosophical extrapolation, neither were they the intellectual or political equals, of their husbands. In spite of its contributions to the progress of man, the eighteenth century was very much dominated by traditional male attitudes, although the malignant epithet "chauvinist" cannot be hurled at men of that period.[49]

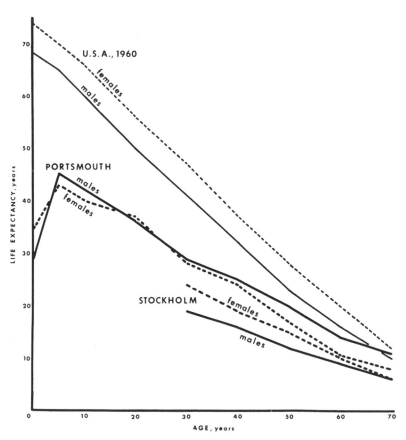

FIG. 2. *Representative life expectancy curves, taken from data in Table 21, for men and women in Portsmouth, contemporary Stockholm, and twentieth-century America.*

Table 22.
Population of Portsmouth, 1803–1811 and 1818–1820,
Characterized by Age Groups, Fractions Dying of
Consumption and Old Age, and Sex

|  | *Males* | *Females* |
|---|---|---|
| Total population | 48.5% | 51.5% |
| All deaths, 1803–11, 1818–20 | 47.5% | 52.5% |
| Population at greatest risk from consumption (age 26–44) | 47.5% | 52.5% |
| Death attributed to consumption | 36.2% | 63.8% |
| Population aged over 44 | 41.4% | 58.6% |
| Deaths attributed to old age | 41.7% | 58.3% |

Life expectancies were first calculated by some eighteenth-century medical statisticians. The idea had been proposed by William Petty in the late seventeenth century, but suitable data were not available for another hundred years. The uses of life tables were apparent to inquiring minds of the Enlightenment. When Edward Wigglesworth combined the mortality data from many towns in Massachusetts and New Hampshire in 1789, he was aware that the data could be used to predict the rate of growth of the population, something that had to be taken into account in long-range planning for the new republic. It was for this reason, among others, that the decennial United States census was required in the Constitution. Not only that, wrote Dr. Wigglesworth, but the data "would be of utility to the publick; and would afford entertainment to persons of a philosophical disposition, both in Europe and America."[50]

Longevity and how to achieve it were among the more fascinating intellectual pursuits of the Enlightenment. Brissot incorporated many European and American life expectancy data in his book about his travels. His data and conclusions conveniently and amply supported his political hypothesis that a republic is the best form of government. His logic ran as follows:

The general causes of longevity are:
1. A healthy climate
2. Abundant and nutritious food and drink
3. A regular, active, and happy life
   Moreover, one must take into account such external circumstances as a man's work, his morals, his religion, and the government under which he lives. Wherever property is concentrated in the

hands of a few and where employment is precarious, dependent, and uncertain, human life is briefer... Wherever government is arbitrary, where tyranny... stops only at the members of the lowest classes, to crush them all, there the life of the common people must be shorter. For such people are slaves, and a miserable slave, forever trodden under the feet of his masters, enjoys neither the material well-being, nor the regularity of existence, nor the inner contentment that are necessary to the sustenance of the principle of life. Nor is life long even for the power-hungry ruling class, for their days are shortened by excesses and worries.

If you apply these moral and political considerations to the United States you must conclude that there cannot be any country in which life expectancy is longer, for, in addition to all their natural advantages, the people enjoy the benefits of a liberty unequalled in the Old World, and it cannot be sufficiently stressed that it is liberty which is the source of health.[51]

Not all Europeans agreed with Brissot. Jeremy Belknap launched into a refutation of what must have been a series of European efforts to dissuade other Europeans from emigrating to the new Republic:

It has been confidently asserted by European writers... that the climates of America, under similar latitudes to those of Europe are unfriendly to health and longevity; that the general [maximum, not average] period of human life [in America] is from forty-five to fifty; and these pernicious effects are ascribed to putrid exhalations from stagnant waters; to a surface uncleared, uncultivated, and loaded with rank vegetation, which prevents it from feeling the purifying influence of the sun.

Although it is not clear whether Belknap was guilty of xenophobia or of having studied the available data, he did admit that the southern states were less friendly to health. He goes on to set the story straight:

If the authors profess to write as philosophers they should seek for information from the purest sources, and not content themselves with theorising on subjects, which can be determined only by fact and observation; or with forming general conclusions from partial reports. If they write as politicians, their aim may indeed be answered by stating facts in a delusive light; and by representing America as a grave to Europeans, they may throw discouragement on emigration to this country.

It may be too much to suppose that Belknap observed what would later be known as the principle of the survival of the fittest, but his observations are consistent with it, when applied to colonists and immigrants to a new world:

In that part of America which it falls to my lot to describe, an "uncleared and uncultivated soil," is so far from being an object of dread, that there are no people more vigorous and robust than those who labour on new plantations... This is true not only of the natives of the country, but of emigrants from Europe. It has been a general observation that the first planters in new townships live to a great age.

Belknap even postulated biological reasons for the advantages conferred on immigrants from Europe by the salubrious new land:

The tall and luxuriant growth which an European might call "rank vegetation", not only indicates strength and fertility of soil; but conduces to absorb noxious vapours... A profusion of effluvia from the resinous trees impart to the air a balsamic quality which is extremely favourable to health... To these observations it may be added, that the northwest wind is the grand corrector of every noxious quality which can exist in America; and whilst that wind prevails, it diffuses health and imparts vigour to the human frame.

He could recognize that all was not perfectly conducive to health, even in New Hampshire,

where vapour arising from land overflowed with fresh water, produces bilious and nervous diseases, and the inhabitants are subject to an early lassitude and debility; which is often increased by an injudicious use of spirituous liquors for medical purposes.

The final argument that Belknap hurled at the European doubters and detractors was derived from the hard data that eighteenth-century philosophes loved so well:

From the tables of mortality which I have collected and which are here exhibited, it appears that a very large proportion of people [in New Hampshire, at least] live to an old age, and that many of them die of no acute disease but by the gradual decay of nature. The death of adult persons between twenty and fifty years of age is very rare, when compared with the bills of mortality from European countries.

For instance, he points out that one in twenty Londoners die each year, but only one in seventy in New Hampshire, unless "some epidemic disorder prevails, which very seldom happens." [52]

The new republic differed in many respects from its mother country, but most of all in one outstanding respect, its very rapid growth rate, which was the net effect of its immigration, marriage, fertility, birth, and death rates; however, it has not yet been possible to assess the relative contribution of immigration to the American population at the time of Independence. The English had devised, however unconsciously, a number of measures to keep their population from getting out of hand. Their marriage rates varied with economic conditions, and marriage usually occurred later in life than ever before. Men were even reluctant to marry, partly because there were ample opportunities for sexual activity without having to assume the economic burden of a wife, and partly because of the restrictions imposed by marriage contracts. The English law of primogeniture sent younger sons into the less well compensated professions or trades, so that their economic readiness for marriage was long delayed. When women took jobs as servants, they felt no economic pressure toward marriage at all. And once babies were conceived, in or out of wedlock, their potential burden on the economy of individuals or the nation was reduced by the expedients of abortion, infanticide, or abandonment. On the Continent, celibacy was rampant, compared with England. Americans neither wanted nor needed, nor could they even afford, any of these expedients; in fact, America could not succeed as a country or as an idea, unless it reversed all of them. In doing so, it could advertise its own attractions to the potential immigrants who were needed to finish the job of settling the country.[53]

American and European newspapers, magazines, and journalists delighted in reporting examples of American longevity. The quest for more examples continues today, but now the questions to be answered are biological rather than political. In the eighteenth century the long life was equated with the good life, in terms of health, morals, and the ease of making a living in the American Eden. Books such as Luigi Cornaro's sixteenth-century best-seller, *The Probable Way of Attaining a Long and Healthful Life*, were popular in America, and among her propagandists. Hall Jackson probably knew Cornaro's book; it was reprinted, in part, in Portsmouth in 1788. Perhaps its greatest appeal to Romantic Americans lay in its implicit advocacy of the "simple life."[54]

Although James Cassedy has called detailed attention to both the intensity and the success of studies of the duration of life by late eighteenth-century American scientists, he also points out that the majority of Americans failed to understand that vital statistics might be of practical use to the commonweal. In fact, science in general then enjoyed much less public support or enthusiasm than it has over the past century, unless some direct appeal was involved—unless scientific endeavor could be related to patriotic, practical, moral, or religious ends. For instance, although a state official might enjoy collecting data that showed his state to be growing more rapidly than another and thus be entitled to a greater voice in the next Congress, he might still be equally reluctant to provide the federal government with the full census figures for the state because of the danger of having a greater tax burden imposed on his state. Apparently scientists (and not only physicians) and insurance companies realized the true value of the accurate enumeration of the population for assessing the relative health of the new country.[55]

When Brissot looked at the relatively greater life expectancy for Harvard graduates than for the general population, he exulted: "one can logically induce the causes of longevity: regularity of morals, an enlightened mind, independence of spirit, and freedom from want." That Harvard graduates were dispersed all over the thirteen United States, even in relatively unhealthy places, only bolstered Brissot's enthusiasm for his hypothesis—and his assumptions about certain characteristics of Harvard graduates.[56]

Timothy Dwight's conclusions about the American frontier in the closing years of the eighteenth century, and about the motivating force behind the realization of America's promise, form a hymn to the way of life which Belknap, Brissot, and Dwight had documented, and in which Hall Jackson worked for his entire life:

> A person who had extensively seen the efforts of the New England people in colonizing new countries cannot fail of being forcibly struck by their enterprise, industry, and perseverance...I have passed the dwellings of several hundred thousands of these people, erected on grounds which in 1760 were an absolute wilderness. A large part of these tracts they have already converted into fruitful fields, covered it with productive farms, surrounded it with enclosures, planted on it orchards, and beautified it with comfortable and in many places with handsome houses. Considerable tracts I have traced through their whole progress from a desert to a garden, and have literally beheld the wilderness blossom as the rose.
>
> ...To me there is something far more delightful in contemplating the diffusion of enterprise and industry over an immense forest, where no oppression gives birth to the efforts of man, no sufferings have preceded the splendor, and no sacrifice of life, or even of comfort, is necessary to the existence of the triumph. The process is here all voluntary and free...Poverty is here commuted for competence, and competence for wealth. Towns and villages in vast multitudes rise up in the retreats of bears and wolves, and churches assemble for the worship of God the numerous inhabitants to whom he has given so goodly a heritage...Thus rational and virtuous man sees his race multiplying beyond all customary calculation, in the midst of blessings equally and universally diffused, and obtained without fraud, without oppression, and without blood.[57]

The medical implications of Dwight's testimony were clearly reflected in contemporary health and mortality statistics for the New World democracy. Jackson's patients came from a similar population—indeed, it had been described by Dwight and the other journalistic travelers to New Hampshire. Jackson clearly considered dropsy as one of his patients' most pressing problems, one that he thought should be amenable to treatment. To explore the physiological origins of dropsy, however, we must be able to trace the evolution of the medical profession's concepts of the disease. Although each generation was satisfied with its own explanation, succeeding generations were able to shed a little new light on the subject. Hall Jackson was primarily concerned with doing something that no previous generation of physicians had been able to do: providing an effective method of treatment.

CHAPTER FOUR

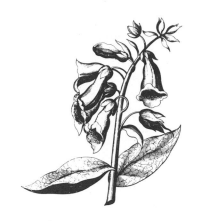

# 'A Weakness and Laxity of the Fibers'

## CHANGING FASHIONS IN

## HEART DISEASE

THE ENLIGHTENMENT was an era distinguished by careful observation, critical examination, classification, the emergence of the experimental method, and, above all, rationalism. As expected in such a milieu, new systematic approaches to medicine gained prominence, and the concept of a unifying hypothesis to explain all the varied manifestations of human disease attracted many medical rationalizers in the eighteenth century, including men who would arbitrate the acceptance of digitalis among the therapies available for dropsy and other diseases.

The stories of the evolution of concepts of dropsy, and of the introduction of its best treatment, will exemplify at least two operational facets of science that appear in widespread and generally accepted form for the first time during the Enlightenment. These facets help to characterize the historical science of that period, and to distinguish it from that of previous times. They have not disappeared; they were also among the essential preconditions for the subsequent development of science to that which we recognize, perhaps too intuitively, as science today.

First, in a conceptual context, we recognize the emergence of an increasing reliance on observed evidence to support scientific interpretations and conclusions. Even more specifically, that evidence came to be expressed as numerical data more and more often during the Enlightenment. Modern science's insistence on quantification could not come to its present flowering until after the nineteenth century's discovery (or invention) of the series of relationships we now employ in biostatistics, but its seeds were sown in the eighteenth century.

The reason for their germination at that time is clear. The emergence of the European nations as colonizing mercantile powers necessitated an increasing reliance on hard data, particularly numbers, for recording not only sums of money, but also amounts of imports and exports in board feet, pounds, barrels, bolts, and all the other units of trade. We have already seen that potential market populations were being counted. Dr. Johnson summarized the Enlightened attitude to numerical data when he told Boswell, on April 20, 1783, "That, Sir, is the good of counting. It brings everything to a certainty, which before floated in the mind indefinitely." [1]

The problems of eighteenth-century science were not new. The expansion of European populations to other continents stimulated a numerical way of thinking which found ready applicability to ancient problems, including those of health. It is no surprise that the English, in the throes of gaining and losing one empire and beginning to win a second, began to apply numbers to science long before it was universally fashionable to do so. The same reasoning applies to American science (which was, of course, English), both under the British flag, when the colonists' economic responsibilities to their homeland required the utilization of numbers, and under the new American flag, when economic survival was even more essential for maintaining political independence than it had been for satisfying colonial proprietors.

The other emerging characteristic of the science of the Enlightenment has a more social context, comprising both the new sense of scientific community and its corollary, scientific dialogue. The first foundings of learned societies in the seventeenth century led not only to more and bigger formal associations of men with common interests, but also to less formally structured organizations. The latter may, in fact, have been more productive because they were more flexible, less restricted and restraining, and even willing to let themselves die as their members moved on or died, as happened to the Lunar Society in Birmingham, composed of that town's leading scientists, including William Withering (see Chapters 5 and 6). At the far end of the spectrum were those scientists who indeed may have been on the rolls of the major societies in London, Philadelphia, or Boston, but whose real community was composed of their peers, including their out-of-town correspondents, wherever they lived and whatever their titles or job descriptions. These men recognized that their intellectual pursuits could be distinguished from those of other men, and it was the commonality of those pursuits that gave focus to their sense of identity of interests. They developed a sense of professional community which had no geographical boundaries, and which sustained them intellectually through their correspondence and publications.

These written dialogues were essential to the functioning of scientists. Correspondence was used to collect data and ideas and to transmit them, so that scientific knowledge could be acted upon, or challenged. This activity, too, may have had its roots largely in the relatively peaceful colonialism of the eighteenth century (although colonial wars were long, battles were few, and, even from 1775 to 1781, they seldom affected major American seaboard cities); there were roots also in the associated need or desire to communicate rapidly the expanding knowledge of a suddenly expanding world, knowledge that would lead to some consequent action. Although their shared language has helped maintain the transatlantic community of scientists until the present day, the Americans also sensed that their own community was unlike that of the British, and that, especially after Independence, it had its own needs and required its own propagandists.

In the circumscribed but illustrative story of the introduction of foxglove to American medicine will be found the major ingredients of Enlightenment science. Both the efficacy and the safety of the foxglove in the treatment of dropsy, and its mode of action, were "proved" by recourse to numerical data. And the transmission of the data and their interpretations were facilitated by the continuing dialogue within the newly self-conscious community of scientists.

Table 23 shows that death has been attributed to dropsy, or congestive heart failure, with consistent frequency in about 2 to 5 percent of the population for the last 400 years. The principal criterion for making the diagnosis, until the advent of such more sophisticated diagnostic tools as auscultation (1808), the stethoscope (1819), and the electrocardiograph (after 1900), was the obvious accumulation of fluid in the legs and abdomen, which gave dropsy its name (from *hydrops*, "water"). (Dropsy does not often progress to such an extent now, precisely because these same tools permit us to make the diagnosis of heart failure and to provide adequate treatment much earlier in the natural history of the condition than could Hall Jackson and his contemporaries.) The consistency of the data suggests that the criteria for diagnosing dropsy were relatively easy to identify, and were applied equally well by both physicians and non-physicians who certified causes of death (as in the London bills of mortality) over long periods of time. Although eighteenth-century concepts of the pathophysiology of dropsy were changing, all available data suggest that Hall Jackson in America, like William Withering in England, had as many patients with congestive heart failure as did practitioners of any century, even when we recognize that not all cases of dropsy were associated with heart failure alone.

It was probably the very lack of ambiguity in the signs of dropsy as well as its prominence among diseases that gave it some interest even for colonial newspaper readers. For instance, a 1736 item datelined from Bristol, Pennsylvania, describes how Mrs. Anthony Williams, who had suffered from the disease for five years, was tapped four times during her pregnancy; her physician withdrew six, five, ten, and thirteen gallons of dropsical fluid on those occasions. And thirty years later, Mrs. Sarah Davis of Portsmouth is reported to have died of dropsy in spite of twenty-eight tappings.[2]

Table 23.
Frequencies with Which Dropsy Was Diagnosed Among Both Surviving
and Dying Patients in Several American and English Populations through
1849, and the Frequencies with Which Congestive Heart Failure Is
Diagnosed in Twentieth-Century America

| HALL JACKSON'S PATIENTS, 1775–1794 | *in* 4.85% of | 247 deaths |
|---|---|---|
| Hampton, N.H., 1735–91 | in 1.24% of | 884 deaths |
| Dover, N.H., 1767–86 | in 5.31% of | 377 deaths |
| Conway, N.H., 1778–90 | in 3.64% of | 55 deaths |
| Mason, N.H., 1798–1805 | in 2.45% of | 122 deaths |
| PORTSMOUTH, N.H., 1801–20* | in 3.45% of | 1,596 deaths |
| Exeter, N.H., ca. 1805 | in 3.97% of | 126 deaths |
| Exeter, N.H., 1823 | in 4.26% of | 42 deaths |
| Concord, N.H., 1819–21 | in 4.62% of | 108 deaths |
| Salem, Mass., 1786 | in 2.87% of | 139 deaths |
| Twenty towns in New England, 1806 | in 4.91% of | 244 deaths attributed to specific causes |
| Boston, 1811–20 | in 2.40% of | 8,134 deaths |
| Boston, 1811–39* | in 2.15% of | 34,177 deaths |
| New York, 1804–19 | in 3.74% of | 37,425 deaths |
| Philadelphia, Christ Church Parish, 1746–75 | in 3.11% of | 1,798 deaths |
| Pennsylvania Hospital, Philadelphia, 1763–64 | in 4.50% of | 400 admissions, and |
|  | in 10.26% of | 39 deaths |
| Philadelphia, 1816–30* | in 6.47% of | 50,173 deaths |
| Philadelphia, 1827 | in 1.84% of | 708 deaths of blacks |
| Philadelphia, 1831 | in 3.44% of | 4,623 deaths |
| Baltimore Almshouse, 1830–31 | in 1.52% of | 2,429 admissions, and |
|  | in 5.59% of | 286 deaths |
| London, St. Botolph Parish, 1583–99 | in 1.29% of | 3,085 deaths not caused by plague |
| London, 1629–1758* | in 4.02% of | 2,439,626 deaths not caused by plague |
| London, 1770 | in 4.93% of | 20,767 deaths |
| London, St. Bride's Parish, 1820–49 | in 3.83% of | 4,513 deaths |
| Dr. Robert Willan's patients, London, 1769 and 1797–1800 | in 5.58% of | 394 deaths, and |
|  | in 2.15% of | 12,571 office and clinic patients |
| Westminster Hospital, London, 1799 | in 0.14% of | 734 admissions |
| A private practice in East London, 1799 | in 1.00% of | 1,993 patients |
| A private practice in West London, 1799 | in 2.27% of | 2,030 patients |
| London, 1799 | in 5.30% of | 8,648 deaths |

| | | |
|---|---|---|
| Baltimore, 1969–70 | in 7 % of | 403 patients discharged from a hospital medical service |
| San Francisco, 1971 | in 2.31% of | 28,996 outpatients having prescriptions filled |
| Framingham, Mass., 1971 | in 3.05% of | 5,209 persons aged over 30 years |

Stillbirths have been excluded from the bills of mortality before determining the frequency of diagnosing dropsy as a cause of death.

* There was no statistically significant constant change in the frequency with which dropsy was diagnosed over the years included in these data.

SOURCES: Hall Jackson, "Meteorological Register...," manuscript journal (1775–94). Lyman Spalding and Richard Thurston, *Bills of Mortality for Portsmouth, New Hampshire* (1801–11, 1818–20). Lemuel Shattuck, *The Vital Statistics of Boston* (Philadelphia, Lea and Blanchard, 1841), pp. xix, xl–xli. William Barton, "Observations of the Probabilities of the Duration of Human Life...," *Transactions of the American Philosophical Society*, 3 (1793), 25–62. E. B. Krumbhaar, "The State of Pathology in the British Colonies of North America," *Yale Journal of Biology and Medicine*, 19 (1947), 801–815. Roger Hart, *English Life in the Eighteenth Century* (New York, G. P. Putnam's, 1970), p. 76. Thomas R. Forbes, *Chronicle from Aldgate: Life and Death in Shakespeare's London* (New Haven, Yale University Press, 1971), pp. 103–104. Thomas R. Forbes, "Mortality Books from 1820 to 1849 from the Parish of St. Bride, Fleet Street, London," *Journal of the History of Medicine and Allied Sciences*, 27 (1972), 15–29. *A Collection of the Yearly Bills of Mortality for 1657 to 1758* (London, A. Millar, 1759), passim. Robert Willan, *Reports on the Diseases in London ...* (London, R. Phillips, 1801), passim. J. Farmer and J. B. Moore, eds., *Collections, Topographical, Historical ...* , 3 vols. (Concord, N.H., Hill and Moore, 1822), Vol. 1, pp. 82–83; Vol. 3, p. 232. *American Journal of Medical Sciences*, 10 (1832), 26, 88–89, 265–266. Jeremy Belknap, *History of New Hampshire*, 2nd ed., 3 vols. (Boston, Bradford and Read, 1813), Vol. 3, pp. 181–188. John Duffy, *A History of Public Health in New York City 1625–1866* (New York, Russell Sage Foundation, 1968), pp. 575–578, 583–584. *Pennsylvania Journal, or Weekly Advertiser* (Philadelphia), July 5, 1764. *Medical and Physical Journal* (London), 1 and 2 (1799), passim. Patrick A. McKee, William P. Castelli, Patricia M. McNamara, and William B. Kennel, "The Natural History of Congestive Heart Failure: the Framingham Heart Study," *New England Journal of Medicine*, 285 (1971), 1441–46. Robert H. Brook, Francis A. Appel, Charles Avery, Morton Orman, and Robert L. Stevenson, "Effectiveness of In-patient Follow-Up Care," *New England Journal of Medicine*, 285 (1971), 1509–14. Gary D. Friedman, Morris F. Collen, Leon E. Harris, Edmund E. Van Brunt, and Lou S. Davis, "Experience in Monitoring Drug Reactions in Outpatients: The Kaiser-Permanente Drug Monitoring System," *Journal of the American Medical Association*, 217 (1971), 567–572.

We have seen evidence in Chapter 3 that Hall Jackson had a special interest in dropsy throughout his career. He has also left us a detailed analysis of his post-mortem findings on one of his most distinguished patients with dropsy. His report on the autopsy of General William Whipple (1730–1785), a prominent patriot, judge, and signer of the Declaration of Independence, is a revealing exercise in clinicopathological correlation. It suggests that the Portsmouth surgeon was thoroughly familiar with current thinking about the dynamics of the cardiovascular system and its clinical implications:

Portsmouth February 20th 1786

Sir,

Enclosed is a rough sketch of General Whipple's very remarkable case. I have not time or patience to transcribe it. You have it with all its imperfections & inaccuracies, which I doubt not your (as well as every other gentleman who may see it) goodness & candour will overlook. I have no copy, & when you have used it as you may think proper, you will be so obliging as to return it.

Your most humble servant
Hall Jackson

William Plumer Esqr
Epping [New Hampshire]


William Whipple Esqr having for several years laboured under a disorder, the symptoms of which were of a peculiar nature, & such as to lead the Faculty in general to conclude that some material defection in or near the heart, had taken place. They were much divided in their opinions, some concluded a Polypus had formed, others that an aneurism of the aorta, or pulmonary artery's.

The general or most prevailing symptoms that attended the disorder, were, that the least encreased exercise of body or mind, or whatever in the smallest degree accelerated the motion of the blood, an uncommon palpitation of the heart, dyspena, & swooning, took place.

The fatigues of the last Superior Court circuit, so agravated these alarming symptoms as to deprive him of every expectation or hope of surviving; he gave directions that after his death his body should be opened, that the nature of his disorder if possible might be ascertained. The melancholly event took place on the 28th instant: & the following day agreeable to his request, the body was inspected, & the following appearances & observations made.

On raising the sternum the pericardium first presented, so much enlarged as to pressure the lungs much higher than in a natural situation; there appeared to be a larger proportion of fat on the pericardium than on the other viscera; in the cavity of the thorax was about one half pound of water, on opening the pericardium little or no water was found within it. The right auricle of the heart was enlarged to a surprising degree, so as closely to fill up, & greatly enlarge the pericardium. On the superior & anterior part of the auricle a little inclined to the right side was an appendage nearly the bigness of a hen's-egg, irregular, of a livid color, & appeared like a large glandular tubercle, approaching to a state of putrefaction, but on pressing it gently it lessened by discharging part of its contents into the cavity of the auricle; on opening the auricle, which by its distention had become less than half its natural thickness, & the cavity so much enlarged as to be capable of containing three times the natural quantity at the least computation. On examining the internal surface of the auricle, the before-mentioned appeared to be the internal coat of the auricle, abraded through in a great number of holes, which gave it the appearance of net work, the external coat of the auricle was pushed out, & formed this appendage, or rupture, which contained a considerable quantity of a grumous substance, of a consistence rather firmer than coagulated blood, & not altogether unlike what by some might be termed a polypus. On endeavoring to pass the finger from the auricle to the ventricle the entrance was found to be closed up with a firm ossification. The valvule tricuspides had become a solid bone & wholly closed the passage from the auricle to the ventricle excepting two small perforations that might admit a large sized probe; not a single drop of blood could pass from the auricle to the ventricle but what passed through these two apertures: Just above or rather thro' the upper edge of the ossification was an opening that passed downward in an oblique direction from the right auricle to the left ventricle, immediately under the valvule mistrales. This opening would admit the little finger. The foramentrale was not open; the walls of the left auricle, as well as those of the pulmonary arteries, were in perfect sound & natural state; the heart in every other respect had a healthy appearance, not the least preternatural adhesion or a single tubercle was found in the whole viscera, but exhibited a remarkable appearance of sound health and longevity.

When it is considered how irregularly & sparingly the lungs must have been supplied with blood, & consequently the left ventricle of the heart by the pulmonary veins, it must be concluded that unless the preternatural opening from the right auricle to the left ventricle had been formed, the ventricle could not have been supplied with a quantity of blood sufficient to have filled it immediately, & thereby excited a force necessary to propel the blood through all the remote ramifications of the arteries, even as it was, the circulation was so languid that no pulsation could be perceived in the radical artery, or any other equally large or remote from the heart, for a long time before his death.

When it is considered how small a proportion of blood could be circulated through the lungs to receive the benefit of air, & when also it is considered that so remarkable an obstruction should so long subsist in the very fountain and source of life, it must be a matter of wonder & astonishment that life could be so far prolonged, and with no more inconvenience. He appeared to enjoy a tolerable state of health, unless interrupted by encreased exercise, & at his death he was far from being an emaciated subject.

Portsmouth Nov 30th 1785

P.S. On since examining the ossification (*en situ*) it was found that a small fissure running transversely from the sides of the ossification about half an inch in length, & somewhat more than a line in breadth, terminating at each extremity in the two small perforations before mentioned. This fissure & opening appeared at the edges and points of valves not fully ossified. The papillae & upper extremities of the fleshy columns of the right ventricle were formed into numberless bony concretions. On raising the ossified valves the fleshy & tendenous columns could be drawn up, but in no situation would close the fissure, or perforations, to prevent the refluxe of blood into the auricle, a freer exit into the pulmonary arteries might prevent a return, the other way.

It is conjectured the right auricle was always filled, that by the great distention it had lost its contractile power; that the blood flowed in a slow, but a continued stream into the left ventricle through the preternatural opening from the right auricle; what could prevent the refluxe of blood from the ventricle into the auricle, through this opening, could not be ascertained. The finger would pass readily each way, without the least appearance of a valve.

On the least increased exercise the muscular motions of the heart was en-creased, little or no blood being returned from the lungs, & the preternatural opening from the right auricle, to the left ventricle, being insufficient to replace the blood thrown into the aorta, the heart from being suddenly emptied lost its action, an immediate syncope took place, which would deprive him of all motion and sensation, in less than a minute the ventricle being filled, excited the heart to renew its action, when he would recover, from his faintness and state of in-sensibility.

He complained before his death of pain in his breast, immediately over the diseased part of the right auricle, & it's very probable had he survived a short time, the auricle would have been compleatly ruptured, instantaneous death would have been the consequence.

The circulation of blood was so languid in the extremities, that he would complain of his hands & feet being cold, in the hottest day of summer.[3]

Portsmouth chronicler Nathaniel Adams felt that the facts of General Whipple's clinical course and autopsy had sufficient general interest to warrant their inclusion in his history of the town:

> About this time [1778] the General began to be troubled with stric-tures in the breast, which were at times very painful to him. A little exercise would bring on violent palpitations of the heart, which were very distressing. Riding on horseback often produced this effect, and sometimes caused him to faint. This complaint prevented his en-gaging in the active scenes of life, and induced him to resign his military command....He continued on the bench about three years, but his disorder become more painful to him; and in the fall of [1785], he was obliged to leave the Court before the Circuit was completed...By his special direction to his brother [-in-law], Doctor [Joshua] Brackett, his body was opened, and it was found that an ossification had taken place in his heart; the valve was united to the aorta, only a small aperture, the size of a large knitting needle, was open, through which all the blood flowed in its circulation; and when any sudden motion gave it a new impulse, it produced the pal-pitation and faintness, to which he was liable.[4]

Although Whipple's instructions that an autopsy be performed had been given to his brother-in-law, Jackson seems to have performed that office himself, although he does not explicitly say that he had done so. It is curious to find such complete clinical details in a book of local history, much less Adams' apparent implicit assumption that his readers would understand the physiological implications of the autopsy findings. Prob-ably Whipple's status as a local celebrity earned him this unusual wealth of post-mortem detail, a phenomenon also familiar in late twentieth-century America.

Appreciation of the role of the heart in health and disease has increased only slowly since medicine first began to emerge from its ancient confu-sion with the supernatural, although Jackson's understanding of cardio-vascular pathophysiology seems almost modern. Cotton Mather reasoned, as did most physicians until the early nineteenth century, that the heart could not be subject to disease because it "is concerned most immediately with the Praeservation of Life." [5] Because the concept of "heart disease" as a separate entity had only just begun to develop in Hall Jackson's lifetime, we should not be surprised at the uses to which digitalis was later to be put. In fact, as we shall see, there was absolutely no good reason for Hall Jackson or William Withering to think that the drug's site of action *could* be the heart.

In the late eighteenth century the pulse was still the only clue to heart action, and its implications as a clue were not well understood. The Egyptians of two millennia before Christ had conceived of the heart as the center of the body's distributing vessels, and thought that the pulse rate reflects something about heart action. Hippocrates and other physicians of the fourth century B.C. seem to have counted the pulse, but they did not associate it with the circulation of the blood, much less with the rate of cardiac contraction. Contemporary Chinese, on the other hand, had so codified pulse rates and the sites at which they were measured that they could use the pulse to diagnose disease in any given organ of the body. At least one Roman physician, Ruphos of Ephesus, appears to have realized that the pulse reflects the systolic activity (contraction) of the heart rather than its diastolic action (relaxation). He also recognized that the pulse rate reflects heart rate, as well as the force exerted by the heart. Other ancient and medieval physicians made occasional similar comments, but none was reinforced with experimental evidence. Celsus and his first-century contemporaries regarded dropsy not as a result of cardiac disease, but as a nonspecific accumulation of fluid secondary to diseases of other organs.[6]

In the late sixteenth century, Ambroise Paré (1510–1590) could differentiate between ascites, which sounds dull when the distended abdomen is percussed, and tympany, which sounds resonant, on the basis of physical examination. Paré, however, like his ancient predecessors, called them collectively dropsy. He associated dropsy with kidney and liver disease, but not with heart disease, while noting that in dropsy "The pulse is little, quicke, and hard a tention" in the 1634 English translation of his *Workes*. The treatments that Paré recommended were standard practice for two more centuries: a "drying diet, and such medicines as carry away water, both by stools and urine," including, for example, medicated baths, ointments, plasters, and cantharides. He approved the use of paracentesis, or tapping, as a last resort. For that purpose he designed a pipe with the diameter of a quill, perforated with two small holes in the tip, which was to be inserted into the body cavity to be drained of fluid.[7]

Not until after William Harvey had demonstrated that the blood circulates in one direction within a closed system of vessels (1628) could further progress be made in either the diagnosis or treatment of heart disease. His discovery that "The passing of blood through the artery upon the contraction of the heart is the cause of the pulse" was revolutionary to those who had followed Galen's teaching through the centuries. Galen had taught that the blood forms in the liver, from which it passes, by way of the vena cava, to the rest of the body for nutritive purposes, and that the right side of the heart accomplishes the same purpose for the lungs. He regarded the left side of the heart not as another sequence in the propulsion of blood to the nonpulmonary part of the body, but as the source of innate heat and vital spirits, attributes which, when distributed to the rest of the body via the arteries, sustained life. In Galenic physiology, the arterial pulse was an active function of the arteries themselves, transmitted by the heart. Even after Harvey's demonstration that the blood circulates, it was to be a long time before it could be put to real use at the patient's bedside. In fact, the concept of the motion of the blood within a closed system became obscured by other concepts which, at the time, were thought to be related but are now known not to be.[8]

One of the first developments to come from Harvey's work was the concept of fever that was to delay the appropriate therapeutic application of digitalis. For instance, Thomas Willis (1621–1675) defined fever as an "intestine motion or commotion of the blood," specifically of the blood's active chemical components, Paracelsus' triad of mercury, sulfur, and salt. Willis said that intestine motion, induced by the introduction of foreign substances into the body, occurs under normal circumstances, but that when it occurs to an excessive degree, fever is the natural and expected result. The proof that blood circulates within the body permitted Willis to postulate that the cause of fever is in the blood itself; otherwise, the offending foreign substance would be washed out of other body tissues by the blood as it circulates through them.[9]

Other seventeenth-century physicians took this reasoning the next step further, postulating that the primary seat of all disease is the blood, and that the viscera are attacked only secondarily as the blood flows through them. The proper approach to therapy, therefore, was to treat the blood itself, with a view toward mitigating the effects of the cause of whatever disease happened to afflict the patient. Willis, for instance, recommended removing fluid from the chest of a dropsical patient, as well as the use of cathartics and diuretics.[10]

John Locke (1632–1704), who is more widely remembered now for his efforts in fields other than medicine, was a physician, having studied at Oxford and with Boyle and Sydenham. He usually treated his dropsical patients with purges and diuretics, such as powdered crab's eyes. He has left us one case report, dated 1679, that illustrates common concepts of the pathophysiology of dropsy in seventeenth-century England:

> Dr. Jacob cured a young man of a dropsy only by making him lye in bed for about 14 days or 20 days. For judgeing that it proceeded from the indigested serum of his bloud which by being uprooted out of the vessells into the habit of the body which increasing every day did cool and destroy the concoction of the blood and so by degrees grew into a dangerous load. He therefore concluded that if he could

keep it within the veines it would there be concocted and to this purpose with success ordered the patient to keep to his bed and eat drying meals.

Locke did recognize that this method of cure was not infallible; he goes on to say that "In an old man [Dr. Jacob] tried this it succeeded not." [11]

Perhaps the first step toward modern concepts of dropsy was taken by Richard Lower (1631–1690). In 1669 he demonstrated in a dog that venous obstruction leads to extravasation of fluid from the veins, although he does not himself appear to have made the connection between his experiment and dropsy or heart failure. [12]

Hermann Boerhaave (1668–1738), the great teacher at Leyden whose influence was to carry on well into the nineteenth century, thought that dropsy results from a weakness of the blood vessels. He postulated that weak blood vessels release more excess fluid into body cavities than the "resorbing veins" can take up, and that dropsy, therefore, can be cured only by removing its underlying cause, laxity of the vascular fibers. Boerhaave recognized that drawing off the accumulated fluid was only symptomatic therapy. This approach was correct but ahead of its time, for in Hall Jackson's day fifty years later, dropsy was still regarded as a disease entity in itself and not as a consequence of some underlying disease. [13]

To Boerhaave a rapid pulse was the only and sufficient sign of the presence of fever. He knew that a rapid pulse indicates rapid heart action, but in his nosology the heat commonly associated with fever results from increased vascular resistance to blood flow and from increased cardiac work—that is, from friction. He saw no contradiction in the simultaneous occurrence of weak vessels and increased vascular resistance in the same patient's cardiovascular system. He thus conceived of dropsy as but one kind of fever, because the pulse is rapid. In this he labored under the disadvantage of not being able to *measure* his patients' fevers. The normal temperature had been established as early as 1740, but it was not until after 1870 that the short clinical thermometer became available. [14]

In Boerhaave's otherwise logical but experimentally unsupported concept of disease, the ultimate cause of any form of fever is the retention of some unnatural substance in the body, or the continuing presence of some excessive activity within the body. He reasoned that the best treatment for dropsy consisted of ridding the body of the obstruction responsible for the weakness of the vascular fibers, and concluded that bleeding or otherwise evacuating a dropsical patient decreases the force of the heart and the pulse by removing the offending impediment to free blood flow so that the accumulated body fluids can disappear. We have already seen that this was also Boerhaave's approach to the treatment of smallpox. As Withering was to note, Boerhaave rejected the use of digitalis for any medical purpose at all because of its toxicity. [15]

The first book on dropsy as a distinct clinical entity appeared in 1706, just midway between the appearance of Harvey's and Withering's books. Written by members of the Leopoldine Academy of Scientists at Breslau to commemorate the reign of Leopold I, Holy Roman Emperor and King of Bohemia and Hungary, who had died of dropsy in the preceding year, most of the volume is thought to be the work of Christianus Helwich (1666–1740).[16] The most important thing about the book is that its authors did not—indeed, could not—recognize that heart disease is responsible for dropsy of the chest, which is known as hydrothorax. The symptomatology and differential diagnosis of hydrothorax were understood in 1706 much as they are today even though its pathogenesis and natural history were not. The Leopoldine authors recognized that the feeling of oppression and discomfort that accompanies dropsy is not merely the result of the accumulation of fluid in the chest. They expected dropsical patients to have severe respiratory difficulty, a dry cough, and hemoptysis (spitting of blood from the lungs), but not rales (abnormal respiratory sounds) or hoarseness. A frequent symptom was awakening in the middle of the night, after only a few hours of sleep (orthopnea). The pulse was described as intermittent, and palpitations as frequent, sometimes accompanied by fainting. The patient might feel the fluid move about within his chest, which could help differentiate dropsy from empyema (pus in a body cavity), in the absence of any history of infection. Edema of the feet and scrotum might also occur. Fever occasionally occurred in dropsy, as well as pain. The patient might be extraordinarily sensitive to cold, and his fingernails might lose their normal contours.[17]

In speculating upon the cause of dropsy, the Academicians suggested that "it must be that the serous fluid is poured out into the cavity of the chest either from the blood vessels, the lymphatics, or both." They reasoned that weak and watery blood exudes its excess serum from the vessels into the thoracic cavity, but, like their contemporary Boerhaave, they had no anatomical or experimental observations to justify their thesis. They did cite Harvey several times, calling upon his demonstration of the circulation of the blood to support their concept that the basic cause of the serous effusion is a sluggish circulation. In evidence of this, they also cited Richard Lower's experiment. But the committee had no concept of defective heart function. The reason the blood did not reabsorb the effusion, they said, was that the fluid became thickened, by cold air, hot water, or alcohol. We will see that alcohol's role as a supposed cause of dropsy remained current for another century or so, probably stemming from Robert Boyle's (1627–1691) demonstration that alcohol can coagulate blood.[18]

The escape of fluid from the vessels was thought to be governed by two factors, the viscosity of the blood and the presence of disease of the blood vessels and lymphatics. The irregular and intermittent pulse in dropsy was attributed to disturbances in blood flow, not to disturbances in cardiac rhythm. Venous blood was thought to be ten times as concentrated as arterial blood, precluding its redilution to its normal, less viscous state if lymph flow is impeded or delayed. Both alteration of the physical properties of the effused lymph and narrowness or laxity of the vessels were thought to reduce lymph flow. Blood viscosity could also be increased in other, unrelated, ways, for instance by bad cooking; this resulted in what was called dyspepsia.[19]

Like Boerhaave, the Leopoldine Academicians recognized that the chest fluid must be removed and its reaccumulation prevented in order to treat hydrothorax. Contrary to their expectation, they had found that bleeding from an arm vein gave the patient no relief, and that removal of fluid directly from the chest by tapping (thoracentesis) provided only temporary relief. The principal drugs they used for dropsy were diuretics and purges. They thought that diuretics enlarged the pores of the kidney, permitting the mucous components of body fluids to escape, and that purges had to be given at the same time, to keep unclean material out of the kidneys. They also reasoned that diaphoretics (drugs that induce sweating) would help to decrease the viscosity of the blood. However reasonable this sort of approach to the therapy of dropsy seemed to its advocates, they reluctantly admitted that the disease was virtually incurable.[20]

A year later, quantitative techniques were first applied to the diagnosis of vascular diseases, including dropsy. In 1707 Sir John Floyer (1649–1734) published *The Physician's Pulse-Watch* in which he described the clinical applications of a watch that ran for just one minute. The pulse had been counted earlier, by such noted experimenters as Sanctorius (1561–1636), but his watch had no second hand, and he had to use a pendulum to gauge the time interval over which he counted pulse beats. Floyer set down his observations because "our Life consists in the Circulation of the blood, and that running too fast or slow, produces most of our Diseases. The Physician's Business is to regulate the Circulation, and to keep it in a moderate degree." This was essentially Boerhaave's concept as well. Floyer must have understood cardiovascular physiology and hemodynamics somewhat as we do now, but his clinical interpretations were markedly influenced by the general state of medical knowledge in the early eighteenth century. For instance, in writing of fevers, which were, and are, usually associated with a fast pulse, Floyer says: "By curing [them], I mean by reducing the Pulse to its natural numbers." He regarded the pulse as a property of blood passing through arteries, not as an index of the rate and force of contraction of the heart.[21]

Sir John recognized that the "natural number" of the pulse is 70 to 75 a minute. He rarely found any less than 60 a minute, and 55 a minute was the lowest he had ever observed; he wondered how much lower it could drop in the living organism. The lower limit was to be further expanded about a century later, in an experiment with the foxglove. But in spite of Floyer's work, which was more than customarily embellished with tables of numerical data, the pulse was not generally taken in medical consultations until the nineteenth century.[22]

At the same time, in Italy, Giovanni Maria Lancisi (1654–1720) published his book on the causes of sudden death, with anatomical evidence to support his conjectures. In one such case, that of the Most Reverend Bartolomeus Spada, Lancisi apparently connected the patient's heart disease (which was probably subacute bacterial endocarditis) with dropsy, but he thought that the heart disease was analogous to hemorrhoids—that is, chiefly a vascular condition. In another case, that of

Antonius Maria Brilli, Lancisi provides a good clinical description of dropsy which responded favorably, though temporarily, to a known diuretic, squill. In this instance, he postulated that the underlying defect was in the brain. In a third case he associated cardiac enlargement with dropsy, an association now well documented. Lancisi was probably unable to connect heart disease with dropsy not only because he, like his contemporaries, thought dropsy was a vascular disease, but also because he associated heart disease itself with debauchery and drunkenness, characteristics which he was unlikely to attribute to the Most Reverend Bartolomeus Spada.[23]

Some twenty years later Lancisi's second great work, on aneurysms, which were obviously diseases of the blood vessels, was published posthumously. In the two books taken together, Lancisi displays some knowledge of congestive heart failure as we now understand it, but he was not able to understand fully the pathogenesis of dropsy. He described for the first time the engorgement and pulsation of the jugular vein that may occur in right heart failure, correctly attributing it to increased retrograde pressure. In support of this conclusion he cited Lower's experiment in which ligation of the vena cava of a dog had resulted in the accumulation of fluid in the abdomen, which is called ascites. From this laboratory evidence he extrapolated to explain the effects of obstruction of blood vessels on the heart. He also recognized that heart disease may be associated with respiratory symptoms, even in the absence of any primary lung disease. His suggestions for treating the diseased heart illustrate the handicaps of an early eighteenth-century pathologist, who had to rely on contemporary physiology and pharmacology. A reasonable part of the therapy of dropsy is still restriction of water intake, but surely not snake venom, mummy dust, and myrrh.[24]

At about the same time, Raymond Vieussens (1641–1716) at Montpellier in France showed that stenosis of the mitral valve results in an apparently primary pulmonary symptom—shortness of breath—because of the retrograde congestion that results when outflow from the left auricle is obstructed. Vieussens also understood the interdependence of time, force, and resistance in explaining the hydraulic principles involved in blood flow.[25]

In his pioneering study of occupational health and medicine, Bernardino Ramazzini (1633–1714) of Modena, in Italy, regarded dropsy as a final, terminal stage of illness, and not necessarily a separate disease in itself. It would be another two centuries before this notion was confirmed. Ramazzini could find no single occupational predisposition to dropsy, which appeared in tanners, oil-pressers, corpse-bearers, millers, sifters of grain, laundresses, hunters, bathmen, salt workers (because salt makes their blood acid, he said), gardeners (because they absorb moisture from the ground), and brickmakers (because they are continually exposed to changing weather). Ramazzini observed that sedentary workers "suffer from general ill-health and an excessive accumulation of unwholesome humors caused by their sedentary life." That idea was still current in Hall Jackson's day; he blamed the sedentary life enforced by New England winters for the occurrence of dropsy there.[26]

Cotton Mather, although not a physician himself, still reflects for us today, in *The Angel of Bethesda*, much early eighteenth-century medical literature and thought about dropsy. In Mather's theologically oriented medical nosology, dropsy, like smallpox, was among the wages of sin. The associated sin in this instance was pride, because dropsy swells parts of the body out of proportion to the true whole. He even compares the thirst of dropsical patients with the insatiable and iniquitous thirst for satisfaction in the things of this life. Mather followed current medical thinking, however, in ascribing the disease to "Depauperated Blood, which having lost its due Texture, breeds a Lympha that by Stagnation or Acrimony swells or breaks the vessels." Again, appropriate treatment of dropsy properly includes abstinence from fluids, gentle laxatives, emetics (which "may not be amiss"), diuretics, and "Whey wherein a Red Hott Iron has been often quenched" to strengthen the lymphatics.[27]

In 1749 Jean-Baptiste de Senac (1693–1770) compiled then current understanding of heart disease in a text that has not yet, unfortunately, been translated into English. He described edema of the foot and dropsy in some cases of heart disease but apparently failed to recognize their association.[28] Perhaps he would have made the association had he read Stephen Hales's (1677–1761) *Statical Essays* of 1733, in which for the first time Hales made approximate estimates of cardiac output (in terms of left ventricular systolic output), of venous blood pressure and the influence of venous return on cardiac output, and of the differences between the pulmonary and peripheral circulations, all of which are now routinely considered in the diagnosis and treatment of patients with heart failure. Hales himself could not formulate general laws involving the measures, because of his own lack of mathematical expertise. His studies led him (like Mather, also a wide-ranging minister of his church), to postulate that dropsy was caused by deficits in the number of red blood cells. Dropsy may indeed occur in persons with severe anemia, but Hales's reasoning depended on Galenic concepts of heat and cold:

> In dropsical Cases when the Blood is poor and watery the Patient complains of great Degrees of Cold, the Blood being very defective in a sufficient Quantity of red Globules to give it warmth. Which yet at Intervals will be raised to a feverish Heat, for want of a due Quantity of this serum, and by the Return of some of the rancid extravasated Humours into the Course of Circulation.

He also reasoned, erroneously, that "great Compression of dropsical Humours on the Blood-vessels and secretory Ducts" would explain the "constant thirst of the Hydropic."[29]

Hales was, however, among the first to understand the reason for the abnormalities of the pulse observed in certain diseases, including dropsy: "the Pulse is weak and quick, when the Heart is supplied with little Blood; which is the Case in the Hectick Fevers, &c." Hectic fevers were generally observed in patients with consumption. (This apparent confusion will be reflected in Chapter 5, where we consider the long-lived attempts to use digitalis in consumption as well as dropsy.) Hales was unusual among his contemporaries in suggesting, on the basis of experimental evidence, that removal of blood from a dropsical patient might be deleterious to his health. He had not discovered, however, that bleeding the supposed causative agent of dropsy from the body could not possibly lead to a cure; he merely took his hypothesis about the cause of the disease one step further, reasoning (correctly) that the removal of red blood cells from the body would lead to further accumulation of water.[30]

A few years later, in 1755, Donald Monro (1727–1802), son of Alexander Monro primus, the famous professor of Anatomy at Edinburgh, wrote the second book specifically about dropsy. Monro, following Boerhaave, postulated that the cause of dropsy was "a weakness and laxity of the fibers...when the vessels do not act with sufficient force, the fluids become of a watery consistence; and the orifices of the exhaling arteries being weaker, allow a greater quantity of liquors to pass thro' them, while the veins being weakened in at least an equal proportion, do not absorb as much as they were wont to do." The Leopoldine Academicians' hypothesis that some physical alteration of the properties of blood itself was responsible for dropsy seems to have gone out of fashion —why is not known. It is not impossible that Monro had taken Hales's experiments into account in his thinking.[31]

Among the factors that would tend to weaken the blood vessels, which he thought of as the seat of the disease, Monro listed "any great evacuation," a thin watery diet, any disease that would result in the diminution of the strength of the body, kidney disease, and obstruction of small or large blood vessels (the Leopoldine authors' "dyspepsia"). To treat dropsy, then, Monro recommended the use of any drugs "which by their stimulus force the sensible organs into contraction," apparently regardless of their sites and mechanisms of action. This is now, of course, the basis for the use of digitalis in heart failure.[32]

It is somewhat surprising that Giovanni Baptista Morgagni (1682–1771), the great pathologist of Padua, failed to recognize any more anatomic correlations with dropsy than he did in his monumental 1761 masterwork *On the Seats and Causes of Disease*. He did associate disease of the liver and spleen with dropsy and ascites, but he thought that the fluid had accumulated because the motion of the blood was retarded, a conclusion not completely unwarranted for his time. He overlooked the heart as a possible cause of dropsy, even in his dissections of patients whose clinical histories strongly suggest that they had congestive heart failure. This is the more surprising because he does refer to pertinent passages by Lancisi and Vieussens. Morgagni also appears not to have associated valvular disease with the well-known signs and symptoms of dropsy; he seems to have dissected only the organs he considered a priori to be responsible for the patients' deaths. Although he knew that Lancisi had associated dropsy with venous engorgement, Morgagni did not apply that knowledge in his discussion of a patient in whom he found both right atrial enlargement and hydrothorax.[33]

In the same year, 1761, Leopold Auenbrugger (1722–1809) of Vienna first published his diagnostic innovation, percussing various areas of the body to determine, by their resonance, the condition of the organs within the body cavities. Although percussion of the chest wall provides valuable information about the amount and nature of fluids in the chest cavity and lungs, the technique was not popularized until Jean-Nicholas Corvisart (1755–1821) translated and republished Auenbrugger's book in 1808. Hall Jackson could not have known Auenbrugger's technique, but the clinical picture drawn by the Viennese physician portrays what Jackson would have expected to find in any of his patients with dropsy:

> When water is collected in the cavity of the chest, between the pleura...and the lungs, the disease is called dropsy of the chest; and this is said to be of two kinds, namely, according as the fluid occupies one or both sides.
>
> This is ascertained by percussion in the living subject; and is demonstrated by anatomical examination after death. The general symptoms of the disease are chiefly the following:
>
> 1. Difficult and laborious respiration.
> 2. A cough at intervals, which is dry, or only attended by sputa of the thin, watery nature, or occasionally somewhat viscid.
> 3. A pulse contracted, somewhat hard, frequent, unequal, and often intermitting.
> 4. A sense of breathlessness and suffocation on the slightest motion.
> 5. An incipient dislike of warm food.
> 6. Perpetual anxiety about the scrobiculus cordis [the point of the chest wall just below the lower end of the sternum].
> 7. Great pressure on the chest, and distention of the stomach during the period of digestion.
> 8. A murmuring noise about the hypochondres [the upper portion of the abdomen, just under the lowest ribs], and frequent eructation of flatus [belching], with momentary relief.
> 9. Scarcely any thirst.
> 10. Urine very scanty, and rarely made, red, with lateritious [like brick dust] sediment.
> 11. Swelling of the abdomen, more especially in the epigastrium, and particularly in that point on which the incumbent water gravitates.
> 12. A sub-livid swelling of the extremities, especially of the feet, which are, moreover, cold to the touch.
> 13. Oedematous tumescence [swelling] of the inferior palpebrae [lower eyelids].
> 14. A pallid, or, according to the nature of the affection a sub-livid, discoloration of the cheeks, lips, and tongue.

15. Inability to lie down; anxious, distressing nights, with heaviness, yet frequently sleepless.

All these symptoms vary in a wonderful manner according to the disease.

Auenbrugger's picture of dropsy is about what is found in modern textbooks of medicine. He did not mention hemoptysis among the symptoms he catalogued, but otherwise he expanded considerably on those listed by the Leopoldine Academicians some fifty-five years earlier.[34]

The importance of Auenbrugger's discovery of the value of percussion of the chest wall in the diagnosis of dropsy is apparent in William Heberden's (1710–1801) complaint that it is difficult to ascertain the presence of water in the chest cavity. Heberden was, in any event, pessimistic about the prognosis in dropsy. He regarded it as but a symptom of some underlying uncurable condition. In this he was correct, but only because he inferred correctly, not because he had any data to support his theory.[35]

Perhaps one of the most scholarly pathologists of the eighteenth century was Samuel Clossey (1724–1786). Born in Dublin, he emigrated to New York in 1763, where he was professor of anatomy at King's College until he returned to England, and then to Ireland, in 1780. His book of *Observations on Some of the Diseases of the Parts of the Human Body*, published in 1763, contains—among a number of conclusions that are erroneous but by the standards of his time reasonable—some that are remarkably perceptive.

For instance, Clossey probably drew directly on Daniel Bernouilli's discovery of the relationship between the pressure and the velocity of a fluid when he drew an analogy between the behavior of blood in the vessels and that of water in a pipe. Because the velocity of blood in an artery should be directly proportional to the force propelling the blood, and indirectly proportional to both the length of the artery and its diameter, Clossey could explain why the velocity of blood in the carotid arteries is greater in persons with short necks than in persons with long necks.[36]

He calculated the rate at which fluid would be expected to accumulate in the chest in people with dropsy. Because it would take about two years for three pints to accumulate, he reasoned that the development of hydrothorax must be a very slowly progressive process. Experiments of which he had read, in which it had been demonstrated that water injected into the chest of a dog gradually disappeared over some three months, led Clossey to postulate that some defect of resorbing membranes is responsible for the accumulation of water in the chest.[37]

Although he probably knew the works of Lancisi and Vieussens, at least at second hand, Clossey connected shortness of breath in dropsical patients not with venous congestion but with bronchial constriction. He did recognize, however, that stenosis of the heart valves would result in hydrothorax, because the lymph would leak out of the abnormally distended vessels, especially when the lungs contracted. Thus he could differentiate between dropsy associated with heart disease and that associated with ovarian or liver disease. In addition, he suggested that hepatic congestion and right ventricular failure might be associated, as had Morgagni.[38]

Among the functional defects in various organs of the body to which Clossey ascribed responsibility for the effusion of fluid from the blood vessels in dropsy, he included "want of motion in the Heart to throw it round by the veins." This is as close to what we now understand as any eighteenth-century medical writer was to come, but Clossey's understanding appears to wane when he writes: "for when the vessels are filled with healthy Blood, enriched with Spirits, the motion of the Heart, Vessels and Secretions will be much more vivid, and the Tunics of the Vessels denser; for the Heart and Fibres owe not only their nourishment but their motion to the Blood."[39]

Thus Clossey, like his contemporaries, laid the blame for dropsy on the blood vessels and not the heart. It was this conclusion that led him to recommend, for treatment, the fortification of the body as a whole, so that the heart can pump blood through the vessels at an adequate rate and with sufficient force. That was Donald Monro's concept of an appropriate basis for the treatment of dropsy. After that had been accomplished, by whatever means, Clossey recommended the use of diuretics, removal of fluid from any affected body cavities, or small punctures in the swollen tissues through which the fluid could drain away.[40]

The great classifiers and systematists of eighteenth-century medicine were the professors of medicine. Their need to present unifying hypotheses to their students probably stimulated their efforts to simplify current concepts of disease, as Hermann Boerhaave did early in the century.

Boerhaave's teachings were perpetuated in the English-speaking world by his student William Cullen (1712–1790), who, as Professor of Physic at Edinburgh, taught some of America's leading physicians. Cullen taught that all disease results from either excessive stimulation or excessive weakness of the nervous system. His thesis was that generalized debility, especially of the brain, induces arterial spasms which, in turn, irritate the heart and arteries, producing fever. Although this resembles Boerhaave's teaching, Cullen did not include dropsy among the fevers. Rather, he considered that one cause of dropsy may be an "interruption of the free return of the venous blood from the extreme vessels [including] certain conditions in the right ventricle of the heart itself, preventing it from receiving its usual quantity of blood from the vena cava; or to obstructions in the vessels of the lungs preventing the entire evacuation of the right ventricle." Among the possible obstructions to be found in the heart Cullen included "ossification of its valves." Although a few eighteenth-century physicians understood a few aspects of the pathophysiology of dropsy, no widely held unifying hypothesis involving the heart had yet gained respectability.[41]

The last great systematist of the period was Benjamin Rush (1745–1813) of Philadelphia. Although he wrote at the more enlightened end of the century, Rush's thinking resembles that of Boerhaave more than might have been expected. Like Withering, he had studied under Cullen at Edinburgh, and received his M.D. just two years after Withering received his; but the English student seems to have retained his professor's lessons better than the American was able to do.[42]

Rush started with the premise that there is a single cause of all disease—namely debility—which results from either increased or decreased stimulation of the body's excitability (more or less following Cullen's basic teaching). Rush expanded the thesis by regarding all fevers as the end result of excessive stimuli acting on the excitable function of the body to produce irregular convulsive activity of the blood vessels. In his oversimplification, dropsy was still considered a fever. To cure any fever, including dropsy, Rush reasoned that the physician must remove the responsible hyperactive stimuli from the body, with purging and bleeding. This concept follows logically from Harvey's demonstration that the blood flows within a closed system, through Willis and Boerhaave, to Rush's concept that the only way to relieve the body of the offending substance is to open up the vasculature so that it can escape. He never realized that a treatment that generally produces debility itself is unlikely to remove what he thought was the chief cause of disease— a fallacy that Hall Jackson did recognize when he discussed the therapy of diphtheria. Rush's reasoning was not homeopathic; it was merely fallacious.[43]

These closely related theories of dropsy as a consequence of "a weakness and laxity of the fibers," although none had been confirmed experimentally, dominated American and English medical approaches to the problem in Jackson's day. It is against this background that the study of digitalis must be considered in the years following Withering's publication in 1785. No further improvements in the medical profession's understanding of dropsy were made for another forty years, a period marked by an intense proliferation of textbooks of general medicine— that is, of further classification and explication—but still without further experimentation. We cannot know the full extent of Hall Jackson's reading on dropsy, but he seems to have understood the disease much as had, say, Auenbrugger, Clossey, Boerhaave, and, especially, Cullen.

The first decades of the nineteenth century began to provide a more explicit focus on the role of the diseased heart in the production of dropsy, but too late to be of use to Withering or Jackson. Although the new focus was not too late to be of use to doctors prescribing digitalis therapy, it could not be taken into consideration in explaining the *action* of digitalis. As a result, the modern concept of the effect of digitalis on the heart itself did not develop until well into the twentieth century.

In 1806 Corvisart's text on diseases of the heart made it clear that heart disease would result in the accumulation of fluid when the return of blood to the heart was impeded by disease of the heart itself. He used the same reasoning to explain shortness of breath and orthopnea, the inability to breathe comfortably when lying down, in dropsy. He relied chiefly on diuretics and tissue punctures to assist the removal of excess fluid, as had Clossey, admitting that such procedures provided only short-term relief to the patient. His book must have been known in America; it was reprinted in Boston in 1812.[44]

Allan Burns (1781–1813) of Glasgow, who also discovered endocarditis (inflammation of the heart's lining), demonstrated in 1809 that ossification of the mitral and pulmonary valves would lead to right-heart dilatation and dropsy. He used both digitalis and squill as diuretics for the treatment of such conditions. Six years later Joseph Hodgson (1788–1869) of Birmingham associated valvular disease and congestive failure. Like Rush, Hodgson favored treatment by bleeding, but for a different reason: to reduce the blood volume and, in turn, the abnormally large heart. James Hope (1801–1841) of Cheshire published his important work on diseases of the cardiovascular system in 1835. Contributing little more to our knowledge of dropsy, he used digitalis in only a few of his cases; and when he did, the patients generally failed to respond. In retrospect, Hope appears to have used too little drug, too late.[45]

In the following chapters the earliest ideas about how digitalis produces its therapeutic effects in dropsy and other diseases are presented almost entirely in the context of what was known about the pathophysiology of the cardiovascular system in the eighteenth and early nineteenth centuries, as outlined in the present chapter. Such contemporary understanding must be taken into account if one is to evaluate steps in the evolution of scientific thought with only the factitious advantage of modern knowledge and the hindsight it affords. But we can prepare ourselves further by considering, very briefly, what is now known about the way in which digitalis affects the failing heart. The experimental and clinical evidence for these conclusions, gathered and synthesized over the past sixty years, may be summarized as follows.

As heart failure develops, no matter what its cause (and there are many, primarily prolonged hypertension as well as cardiac valve disease), the heart works progressively harder to pump blood sufficient for the rest of the body. In accomplishing this task, it beats more and more rapidly and eventually becomes weak and flabby. The fluid that normally escapes from blood vessels into the body's tissues is not reabsorbed into the circulation as the blood flow becomes increasingly sluggish. As a result, this fluid accumulates in various parts of the body, especially the chest, lungs, legs, abdomen, and liver, which then are said to be congested. Such abnormal collections of fluid in tissues, which were called dropsy in the eighteenth century, are now called edema. It is true, as many eighteenth-century physicians thought, that such fluids are not resorbed well—not because of a defect in the blood vessels but because the weakened heart cannot keep the blood flowing at its usual rate.

It should be noted, however, that at least some eighteenth-century physicians whose work was, by and large, out of the main stream of the developing medical thought of which we are the direct heirs held concepts of the causes of dropsy that are remarkably like the one just outlined. Robert James (1705–1776) of London, for instance, found it "remarkable, that, in a Dropsy, whether of the Thorax or Abdomen, the Heart, and, especially, its Right Ventricle, is often distended to a surprising Bulk; so that, in two Subjects, I found it as large as the Heart of an Ox." James also pointed out that "we must observe, that where the Vessels of the Heart are full of polypous Concretions, there is, generally, a large Quantity of serum found in the Cavity of the Thorax."[46]

He goes on to advance his opinion that "a more satisfactory Reason can hardly be advanced for a dropsical Swelling, than the difficult, slow, and obstructed Circulation of the Blood thro' the Vessels," supporting his hypothesis with Lower's experiment:

> From these Experiments it is, if I mistake not, sufficiently obvious, that the true Cause of the Swelling of the Body in a Dropsy, of the Secretion of the Serum from the Blood, and of its Stagnation in the Cavities, is a too slow and languid Circulation of the Blood, especially through the Veins... From this languid Circulation of the Blood we deduce the genuine Cause and Reason, not only of the preternatural Swelling, but, also, of the other Symptoms which accompany a Dropsy; such as Weariness, Heaviness of the Body, Littleness, and a Diminution of the salutary Excretions by Sweat, Urine, and Stool. Besides these, an insupportable Difficulty of Breathing is almost a perpetual Symptom of every Dropsy, and, sometimes, rises to such a Height, as to endanger a Suffocation: This formidable Symptom can hardly have any other Cause assigned for it, than a too weak systolic Force of the Heart and Arteries; in consequence of which, the Blood, abounding with a viscid Serum, cannot pass sufficiently freely through the minute Ramifications of the Pulmonary Artery and Vein; hence it stagnates in these Ramifications, and regurgitating to the Right Ventricle of the Heart, produces a strange Uneasiness.[47]

It is probably not very surprising, however, that Dr. James's understanding of dropsy, so much like our own, did not gain prominence by Hall Jackson's time. London, where James practiced, was not then a major center of medical research, and his description is buried in James's medical dictionary of 1745, a source not likely to have been widely consulted by professional men among even his own contemporaries.

The principal direct effect of the several slightly different chemical compounds that are known collectively as the digitalis glycosides is to increase the force of contraction of both normal and failing heart muscle fibers. This effect is accomplished by facilitating the process that couples the mechanical aspects of heart muscle contraction with the electrical impulses transmitted to and through the heart along several specialized pathways.[48]

Digitalis increases the concentration of calcium ions within heart muscle cells. Because these cells function more efficiently as their intracellular calcium content increases, the net effect of digitalis is to strengthen the heart muscle, so that it contracts more forcefully. This results in an increased cardiac output, measured as the volume of blood ejected from the heart into the general circulation each minute.

In persons with congestive heart failure, digitalis exerts its principal therapeutic benefits by stimulating the weakened and flabby heart muscle so that it can operate more efficiently, allowing it to pump more blood at each beat. This, in turn, means that blood is pumped through the body with greater force, and the body receives more oxygen because of the improved cardiac output.

At the same time, more blood flows through the kidneys, so that more urine is formed and excreted. As a result, any fluid that has accumulated within the chest or elsewhere is drawn by osmotic forces back into the circulation, from which it is readily removed by the kidneys, and diuresis (increased discharge of urine) follows. It is now clear that diuresis, which Withering thought was the chief effect of digitalis, in fact occurs only secondarily to the improvement of the entire circulation brought about by the drug. Digitalis does not act on the kidneys, nor does it produce diuresis or provide any other clinical benefit for patients with forms of edema that are not caused by heart failure.

Digitalis also produces a moderate degree of constriction of both arteries and veins. In the absence of any other physiological or pharmacological influences, this effect of digitalis would result in an increased blood pressure. In people with healthy hearts, however, various reflex mechanisms that normally help to maintain the body's usual balance of heart rate and blood pressure at optimum levels, almost always mask or reverse the potential hypertensive action of digitalis, as well as its pulse-lowering action. The drug's strengthening effect on the normal heart can be detected only with special laboratory techniques that are not in common clinical use.

The drug may affect two other sites, but generally only when it is administered in excessive amounts. It acts on a portion of the brain—not on the stomach—to produce nausea and vomiting. In larger doses it may produce blurring of vision, and even make all that the patient sees appear yellow. The most dangerous side effects of digitalis occur when large amounts reach the heart itself. These complex effects, which may not even be noticeable to the patient, can be regularly expected as logical extensions of the effects that occur when only usual therapeutic doses are administered.

Digitalis has a relatively narrow margin of safety. That is, doses commonly used to achieve relief of the patient's symptoms are only slightly smaller than doses that may be harmful. For this reason, as well as the vast range of possible cardiovascular derangements encountered among cardiac patients, each patient's dose of digitalis must be carefully tailored to his special needs and limitations of tolerance for the drug.

In the chapter that follows, we turn briefly from Jackson to order to place his work in the perspective of contemporary research in England and America and to round out the account of dropsy as the case history of a disease.

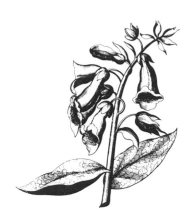

# CHAPTER FIVE

# 'The Great Abstractor of Arterial Action'

## CLINICAL RESEARCH IN THE

## EIGHTEENTH CENTURY—AND BEYOND

DROPSY'S CONTRIBUTION to overall mortality rates has been a relatively constant 2 to 5 percent for the past four centuries (Table 23), as we have seen. Until Withering discovered how to treat it, dropsy had been regarded generally, and justifiably, as inevitably fatal (see Chapter 4). It would be hazardous to regard the data in Table 24, for the one year 1799 in London, fourteen years after the publication of Withering's *Account*, as representative of the English experience with the disease, much less the American, but the data are instructive. That dropsy was diagnosed most infrequently among hospital admissions suggests that usually it was treated on an out-patient basis; hospitalization was reserved chiefly for infectious disease and for surgical cases. The two London practitioners who made the diagnosis in, respectively, one fifth and one half as many patients as were reported to have died of dropsy, may or may not have differed in their abilities to diagnose it, or in their respective patient populations. The apparent difference might have balanced out over a longer period. And if their patients with dropsy survived for at least two to five years with digitalis therapy, the incidence of deaths attributable to dropsy among those two practices would have been consistent with the overall cause-specific death rate for dropsy in London.

Withering's report of his clinical trials with digitalis had, by 1799, the year of his death, firmly secured its place in therapeutics, although without the benefit of even the simplest statistical analysis of his data. He had no mathematical skills himself, but he provided data, perhaps intuitively, with which we can study his results in the same ways we now use for data collected in the twentieth century. Mathematics, including the application of mortality statistics to social problems, had already begun to play an important role in "the propaganda of reason," but it had not yet been discovered to be useful to medicine.[1]

Re-study of the *Account* permits us to make certain characterizations of the drug that Withering apparently made without applying quantitative analytical techniques to his data. Of all the patients to whom he administered digitalis, 64 percent were relieved of their symptoms, and of those who were not relieved, at least 62 percent appear, in the light of present medical knowledge, not to have had congestive heart failure. Withering found that dried and powdered foxglove leaf was more potent than water extracts of the leaf for the relief of symptoms. Figure 3 shows, in summary form, the data that led him to reason that the dried leaf and the infusion (prepared by pouring boiled water over pieces of dried leaf, as is done in making a cup of tea) were no less successful for treating dropsy than the decoction (prepared by boiling the dried leaf fragments in water), while they were much less toxic than the decoction.

Table 24.
Incidences of the Diagnosis of Dropsy in 1799 in London: at a Hospital, in Two Private Practices, and among All Deaths in the Entire City

|  | Admissions to Westminster Hospital | New Patients in Private Practices in | | Concurrent Deaths in All London |
|---|---|---|---|---|
|  |  | East London | West London |  |
| Mean Monthly Totals | 92 | 181 | 290 | 1441 |
| Per Cent with Dropsy | 0.15% | 1.01% | 2.62% | 5.30% |
| Relative Frequencies of Diagnosing Dropsy | 1 | 7 | 17 | 35 |

SOURCE: *Medical and Physical Journal* (London) (1799), Vol. 1, pp. 110–112, 334–336; Vol. 2, pp. 318–320, 408–411.

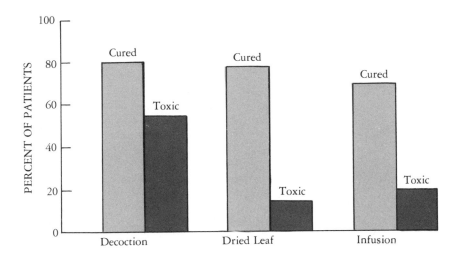

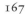

FIG. 3. *Rates of therapeutic success among Dr. Withering's patients treated with three digitalis preparations (left-hand bars), and incidence of side effects among those patients (right-hand bars).*
SOURCE: William Withering, *An Account of the Foxglove* (Birmingham, M. Swinney, 1785).

Chi-square analysis of the raw data confirms that toxicity occurred remarkably more frequently in patients treated with the decoction than with either the infusion or the dried leaf.

Figure 4 demonstrates Withering's increasing clinical skill over the ten years during which he continued to study digitalis. The incidence of side effects decreased to that which is observed today, about 25 percent, regardless of the criteria used in the diagnosis of toxicity. Although part of the decrease may be ascribed to his introduction of new dosage forms of the drug, at least part of the reduction in the incidence of side effects resulted from his increasing skill in the day-to-day, dose-to-dose management of each patient.[2]

Edward W. Pelikan, of the Department of Pharmacology of the Boston University School of Medicine, has calculated, applying current methods to data contained in the *Account*, that the therapeutic index* of Withering's usual initial dose of infusion of digitalis is close to 1.0, while that of the dried leaf is about 1.5, confirming the greater relative safety of the latter dosage form, although both are less safe, in general, than might be desirable under the best of circumstances. The therapeutic indices of the maintenance doses are in similar proportions, 4 for the infusion and 5 or more for the dried leaf.[3]

We have already seen that Withering inferred that digitalis "has a

---

* The therapeutic index is the ratio of the median of doses which produce death to the median of doses which produce a given therapeutic effect.

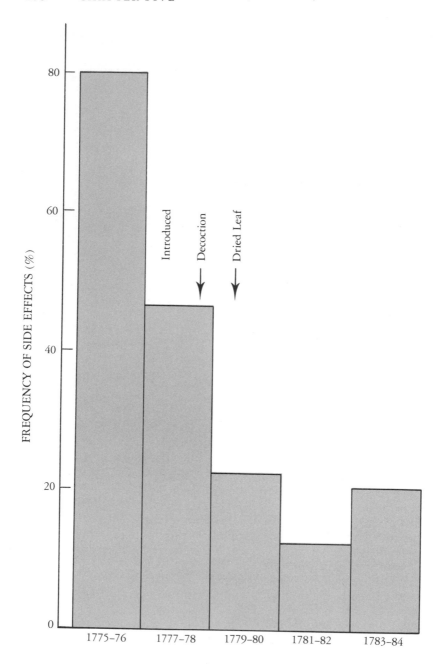

FIG. 4. *Incidence of side effects among Dr. Withering's patients treated with digitalis from 1775 to 1784.*
SOURCE: William Withering, *An Account of the Foxglove* (Birmingham, M. Swinney, 1785).

power over the motion of the heart, to a degree yet unobserved in any other medicine." He must have based this conclusion on the 9 percent of his own patients, and the 25 percent of those reported to him, on whom observations as to the frequency and the quality of the pulse were made. He thought that slowing of the heart was as much a side effect of digitalis as nausea, vomiting, and confused vision (because he considered the kidneys to be the drug's site of action), and that "if the [patient's] pulse be feeble or intermitting," the drug will effectively relieve dropsical symptoms.[4]

But Withering thought that digitalis operated chiefly on the kidneys, as a diuretic. We may never know whether he ever came to think of the heart as the true site of action of digitalis, although his letter to Hall Jackson (see Chapter 6) hints that he might have started to do so.

Several twentieth-century writers have attributed a little poem extolling the foxglove to Dr. Withering:

> The Foxglove's leaves, with caution given,
> Another proof of favouring Heav'n
> > Will happily display;
> The rapid pulse it can abate;
> The hectic flush can moderate;
> And blest by Him whose will is fate,
> > May give a lengthened day.

This slight eulogy would have suggested that perhaps Withering had come to think of digitalis as operating on the heart, or at least on the circulation. The poem was written not by Withering, however, but by Miss Sarah Hoare (1767–1855), in about 1818. Her clinical observations may have been her own; she had ample opportunity to observe the improvement the drug brought about in her father, who was treated for many years for symptoms of congestive heart failure by the famous Drs. Fothergill and Potts. Her mother was a friend of Mary Ann Schimmelpenninck, who had been present at many meetings of the Lunar Society, and the Hoare ladies may also have learned something of Withering, or at least of the properties of the foxglove, from her. The erroneous attribution to Withering probably originated from the poem's inclusion in the seventh edition of his *Botanical Arrangement*, which appeared in 1830, long after his death.[5]

Erasmus Darwin (1731–1802) attempted to discredit Withering's undoubtedly genuine claim to have first discovered—and proved—the efficacy of digitalis in the treatment of dropsy, although Darwin never provided any new information about the drug. Darwin's most strident claim of priority of discovery was in behalf of his late son Charles, whose dissertation, published in 1780, included nine case histories. Eight of the nine patients were treated with digitalis; the five who appear to have had dropsy were relieved or cured, and, of the rest, one with apparent coronary artery disease died, as did two without dropsy. The ninth patient was relieved with opium only. All eight who received digitalis vomited within two days of beginning therapy, suggesting that they had received

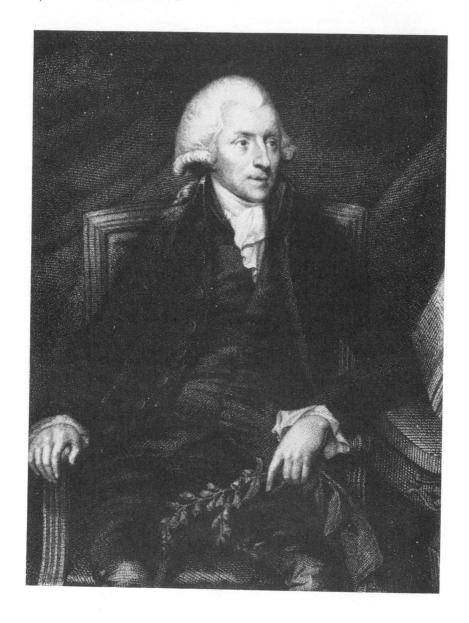

VI. *Dr. William Withering. Engraving after the portrait by Carl von Breda.*
*(Courtesy of the Countway Library of Medicine)*

overdoses of the drug. Although one might be tempted to award priority to young Darwin, as his father did, his report is more one of a few incidents than of a systematic investigation.[6]

The senior Darwin rushed his own paper into print just as Withering's book was about to appear in 1785. Darwin's paper was another attempt to preempt Withering, but Withering, one step ahead of him, included a rebuttal to Darwin in his description of Case IV in his *Account of the Foxglove*. Darwin maintained that hydrothorax results from a depressed activity of the absorbent system, but he did not adduce even anecdotal data in support of this hypothesis. He was parroting chiefly what he had learned from Cullen at Edinburgh.[7]

The chief indications for digitalis, Darwin wrote later, are dropsies and consumption. He admitted that his results were not striking in scrofulous (i.e., tuberculous) ulcers and melancholia, and that digitalis was totally ineffective in asthma. The dropsies he considered most likely to respond were those with "unequal pulse." In the next paper in the same issue of the journal to which Darwin had contributed his 1785 study, Sir George Baker (1722–1809), physician to Their Majesties the King and Queen, discussed the successful use of digitalis in a case of what appears to have been congestive heart failure.[8]

Erasmus Darwin's poems were as widely read as his medical works, but with less reason; his eulogy to the foxglove speaks for itself to this point:

> Bolster'd with down, amid a thousand wants,
> Pale Dropsy rears his bloated form, and pants;
> "Quench me, ye cool pellucid rills!" he cries,
> Wets his parched tongue, and rolls his hollow eyes.
> So bends tormented Tantalus to drink,
> While from his lips the refluent waters shrink;
> Again the rising stream his bosom laves
> And thirst consumes him mid circumfluent waves.
>
> Divine Hygeia, from the bending sky
> Descending, listens to his piercing cry;
> Assumes bright Digitalis' dress and air;
> Her ruby cheek, white neck and raven hair;
> Four youths protect her from the circling throng,
> And like the Nymph the Goddess steps along.
> O'er him She waves her serpent wreathed wand,
> Cheers with her voice, and raises with her hand,
> Warms with rekindling bloom his visage wan,
> And charms the shapeless monster into man.[9]

Following the publication of Withering's *Account*, more clinical trials were reported, but they can hardly be regarded as clinical studies in the same sense. His local influence is reflected in the case reported by Birmingham surgeon William Jones, who had contributed a similar report to the *Account*. He noted that foxglove reduced the pulse in his subsequent patient. In fact, he wrote that he had given the drug to his patient with hemoptysis on the advice of Mr. Mynors, another Birmingham surgeon, who "recommended [it] with a view to diminish the increased action of the heart, and of the whole vascular system." Although Mynors may have conceived of dropsy in the same way as Cullen had taught about it, it is possible that at least some Birmingham doctors were beginning to think of the heart as the foxglove's site of action. If so, Withering would surely have been aware of their thinking, if not partly responsible for it himself.[10]

William Cullen, in 1789, considered digitalis to be a diuretic, "but upon what sort of operation these powers depend, I am at a loss to explain." While he doubted that the drug directly affected the kidney, he admitted that he had no conclusive data on this point. Cullen, who was acquainted with Withering, speculated that, "as besides the increased quantity of water in the mass of the blood, or a stimulus particularly applied to the kidneys, there may be a medicine [digitalis] which, by a general operation of the system, may promote the secretion of urine." He felt that the foxglove's effect on the pulse is certain proof of its "general operation upon the system," that is, as a "sedative," which is how it would have to work to fit Cullen's concept of the etiology of dropsy.[11]

In 1794 John Coakley Lettsom (1744–1815) published eight cases in which he had used digitalis from 1785 to 1788, to rectify an earlier adverse report he had made. He cited another London physician who had used the drug successfully as early as 1760 or 1766, before Withering had even finished medical school. Lettsom himself had graduated in medicine in 1769 from Leyden, where Boerhaave had taught, and was a founder of the Medical Society of London. Although Lettsom noted that digitalis slowed the pulse, the drug had produced equivocal or unfavorable clinical results in all eight of his patients. It appears, in retrospect, that most of them may not have had congestive failure, and would not have been expected to respond favorably to digitalis. However, Lettsom was convinced that the drug is an important diuretic for patients with dropsy.[12]

In 1794 Thomas Beddoes (1760–1808) published a case report demonstrating that the sedative effect of opium was not additive to that of digitalis, and, in fact, that it counteracted digitalis toxicity. Because of the lack of appropriate quantitative data in his paper, however, it is not possible to determine whether Beddoes really did have data sufficient to suggest that the drugs might be antagonists, although Withering had used opium to counteract the irritant effects of digitalis on the intestinal tract.[13]

Beddoes is one of the very few principal participants in the early history of digitalis who did not attend Edinburgh. After obtaining his M.D. at Oxford in 1788, he set up practice in Clifton in Derbyshire. He was a business and professional colleague of many members of the Lunar Society in Birmingham, although not a member himself, and so must have known Withering.

Even if he was not the first to experiment with digitalis in animals, Beddoes was the first to use animals to try to ascertain the site and mode of action of the drug in animals, as well as to use negative controls in its study. His only predecessor in the laboratory investigation of digitalis had been Dr. François Salerne of Orleans, in France. In his introduction to Withering's *Account*, Jonathan Stokes cited Salerne's experiments, which had been reported in 1748.[14]

Salerne had undertaken his experiments merely to determine whether foxglove leaves could, in fact, poison turkeys, as he had heard. To this end he fed foxglove leaves to two birds. A turkey, fed one dose, recovered from its gastrointestinal effects in eight days; a rooster, given digitalis leaves daily for four days, died after another fourteen days, and at autopsy was found to be severely dehydrated. Dr. Salerne drew no conclusions from his experiments about the effects on man of "la grande digitale à fleurs rouges." He stated only:

> On voit par ces expériences le dérangement que l'usage de cette plante peut causer dans les organes de ces animaux, & combien on doit être attentif à la détruire dans les endroits où on les élève.[15]
> [These experiments illustrate the disorder which the use of this plant can cause in these animals' organs, and how one should be alert to destroy the plant in places where animals are raised.]

Beddoes tried to ascertain the way in which digitalis affects the body so that he could use it to better effect in the treatment of his patients. He wrote: "The most profitable course...would be to settle in what a knowledge of the operation of any medicine may consist; and then to compare this idea with our actual attainments." In the case of digitalis, his supposition was that because it "very regularly increases the momentum of the blood...it is the contrary of a sedative," but he thought that digitalis shared some other pharmacological properties with opium. To investigate the similarities common to the two drugs, Beddoes designed a series of experiments. He asked one of his surgical colleagues, a Mr. King, to perform the experiments and record the appropriate observations, in order to avoid the bias that Beddoes felt he might bring to the study because of his preconceived hypothesis.[16]

They performed experiments with six frogs; two were untreated controls, and two each were treated with aquaeous solutions of opium and digitalis applied to the skin. The experiments involved at least three replications at different time intervals between doses. Beddoes and King observed that both drugs produced an initial excitement, followed by a period of inactivity and unresponsiveness to external stimuli. In a second series of experiments they treated five toads with digitalis, opium, wine, laurel extract, and water, respectively. Because all five toads, including the untreated negative control toad, died, the investigators concluded that all of the animals were ill and therefore discounted their results. They did not, apparently, try to repeat the toad experiment.[17]

Beddoes then considered the effects of digitalis that he had observed in patients in conjunction with his experimental data, and concluded:

1. That digitalis, in a certain dose, will increase the action of the arterial system [i.e., is a stimulant].
2. That it will increase the digestive power of the stomach, when that is impaired [i.e., is a stimulant].
3. That it will often induce sleep, like opium [i.e., is a sedative].
4. That, like opium, in an over dose it occasions languor and excessive sensibility, head-ache, dimness of vision, nausea and bilious vomiting.
5. That it almost immediately produces great excitement in frogs, somewhat as opium does; and produces certain other effects similar to those of opium [i.e., is a stimulant as well as a sedative].

[Finally, that digitalis:] increases the organic action of the contractile fibers as much, or more, than opium; but that it does not so much, or so immediately, increase the organic action of the nerves...I hope I have brought together facts enough to induce those to pause who may be tempted to argue from a decreased number of pulsations to a decrease of living action, and from this to the propriety of employing digitalis, in the height of inflammatory orgasm.[18]

In other words, Beddoes differentiated between digitalis' effects on the pulse and on the "system"—its opium-like effect—conceiving of the effect on the pulse as a predictable but therapeutically unnecessary side effect.

One fallacy in Beddoes' reasoning is apparent when we consider some of his own clinical data. For instance, one of his dropsical patients, a Dr. Briggs, recorded his own pulse rate before and after Beddoes gave him digitalis. The pulse data are summarized in Figure 5. Even without making a graph, Beddoes should have been able to conclude that digitalis lowered Dr. Briggs's pulse. In fact, when it reached a low on the nineteenth day of treatment, Beddoes omitted that day's medication. Perhaps Beddoes forgot these data, misunderstood them, or perhaps chose to ignore them because they did not fit his hypothesis. The eighteenth-century propensity to simplify its classification schemes led to great difficulties in understanding how digitalis works. The apparent distinction between "sedatives" and "stimulants" became disorganized and ineffective when it was applied to contemporary indistinct concepts of the components of the cardiovascular and nervous systems. As we will see, the confusion was compounded by differences in outlook between physicians in England and in America, as could be recognized even at the time.

Beddoes, then, regarded digitalis as a drug that would stimulate the body generally, to remove unwanted fluids or other substances, a sort of Boerhaavian thesis. He did not realize that consumption is an inflammatory condition, for he continued to wonder how digitalis exerted its beneficial effects in that disease. He supposed only that the drug stimulated the lymphatics to remove more diseased material from the lungs, in the same way as digitalis was thought to remove water in patients with dropsy.

Others were studying, or at least pondering, the obvious effect of foxglove on the circulatory system. William Currie had written in 1789 that the drug was a general sedative, "diminishing the irritability of the brain and nervous system, and...inducing sleep," not to mention "diminishing the irritability of the heart, and...weakening the force of the circulation." Currie apparently lumped together effects that are secondary to the symptomatic relief of heart failure to digitalis (such as relief of the wakefulness that is commonly caused by fluid in the chest) as a single drug effect. To this single conglomerate effect he attached the designation of one of the few drug classes recognized at the time, seda-

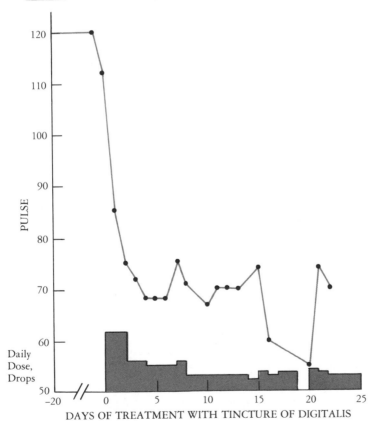

FIG. 5. *Daily dose of digitalis administered to Dr. Briggs in 1799, and his pulse rate during therapy.*
SOURCE: Thomas Beddoes, *Observations on the Medical and Domestic Management of the Consumption* (Troy, N.Y., O. Penniman, 1803), pp. 78–89.

tives. Although Currie was enthusiastic about the use of digitalis in the therapy of hemorrhage, he readily admitted that "It is extremely difficult to distinguish between the spontaneous cessation of the disease, and the operation of the medicine," a rather advanced conclusion for the eighteenth century, and even, sometimes, for the twentieth.[19]

John Ferriar (1761–1815) has been credited with being the first to publish his realization that the site of digitalis' action is the heart. After receiving his M.D. from Edinburgh in 1781, he settled in Manchester, where he practiced medicine and wrote papers on the theater, philosophy, and archaeology, among other subjects. His little book on the foxglove, the culmination of nine years' observations, was published in 1799. In it Ferriar wrote:

> The effect of Foxglove, in retarding the velocity of the pulse, as a direct sedative, was too striking to be long over-looked; and when its application, to diminish morbid irritation in the vascular system, was once pointed out, the consequences of the idea were easily comprehended.[20]

Ferriar was fully aware of the existence of dose-effect relationships for digitalis, at least for each patient, as well as of biological variation among the responses of individuals in a population, although he could not differentiate the effects of foxglove in normal persons from those in congestive heart failure:

> [It is] capable of reducing the pulse, without danger, from 120 in a minute to 75 or 80, at the will of the Practitioner... Let me observe, once for all, that nothing is less accurately fixed in medicine, than one of its most important objects, the doses of remedies. The proper dose of a medicine, is undoubtedly that which produces the effect required, whatever be its numerical denomination. A full dose of Foxglove is, therefore, merely a relative term. To one patient, half a grain may be a full dose; to another, six or eight grains may be given, not only without inconvenience, but without producing any sensible effect.
>
> These varieties of sensibility and habit can only be ascertained, by beginning with the lowest dose, and encreasing it with the most scrupulous care.[21]

Ferriar had trouble interpreting the data available to him in his efforts to ascertain the true site and mode of action of the foxglove:

> A great difficulty, respecting the theory of the action of Digitalis, has often occurred to me, on this subject. While it lessens the frequency and quickness of arterial contraction, it often encreases, at the same time, the secretion in the kidnies... I feel it impossible to explain this phenomenon, at present. The diuretic power of Digitalis, does not appear to me a constant and essential quality of the plant; the power of reducing the pulse is its true characteristic.[22]

Many medical historians have taken this last sentence to indicate that John Ferriar was, in 1799, the first to suggest that digitalis exerts its chief effect on the heart itself. It is clear from the previous sentences, however, that he regarded it as acting on the "arterial system" and not on the heart. He went on to amplify this theory:

> To say that the action of the arterial system is retarded, and that of the absorbents stimulated, by the same remedy, is rather stating the fact in different terms, than explaining it. The secreting vessels of the kidnies are, in general, affected by stimulants, which act upon the whole of the blood-vessels; but it is conceivable, that a spasmodic state of the vessels secreting urine, or a diseased action in them, may be overcome by a remedy, which lessens the force of the general circulation, as, in either of the cases which I have supposed, the *vis a tergo* (as the physiologists of the last age termed it) must act as an irritating cause, constantly supporting the disease.[23]

Ferriar can be credited with some recognition of the foxglove's direct action on the heart, although he seems to have thought that it suppresses the entire vascular system:

> I have had occasion to mention, formerly, the utility of Digitalis in palpitations of the heart. As the direct action of the medicine, is the salutary power required, in these cases, it is strongly indicated, and is indeed eminently serviceable. I have known it to remove the complaint entirely, where it had risen to an alarming degree, in consequence of terror, and intemperance; and even in cases depending on organic laesions of the heart, or great blood vessels, it has relieved the symptoms, and rendered life not only longer, but more supportable...I have seen all the symptoms of general dropsy, attended with a fluttering, feeble pulse, removed by small doses of Digitalis, in the course of a week; and in one remarkable case...the vigour and steadiness of the pulse encreased, exactly in proportion as the water was withdrawn from the cellular membrane.[24]

However, neither the cellular basis of disease nor the principles governing the passage of water and electrolytes across biological membranes were known to Ferriar; they had not yet been discovered. Understanding these factors would be prerequisite to ascertaining the way in which digitalis is now known to operate.

On the contrary, Ferriar used the drug to treat his patients with consumption, clearly following Cullen's concepts of the etiology of dropsy and inflammatory diseases:

> I hoped, by diminishing the velocity of the pulse, to lessen one cause of irritation to the lungs; and it appeared possible, that the abatement of the impetus of circulation might lead to a suspension of the diseased action, subsisting in them...I believe that Digitalis, properly administered at the beginning of Phthisical affections, may

suspend the morbid action of the lungs, by which tubercles are formed; that by its continued exhibition, after haemoptysis, it may be possible to procure the cicatrization of the ruptured vessels, and thus present the formation of ulcers; and I am even disposed to hope, that its power of soothing irritation may extend so far, as sometimes to heal ulcerations of the lungs, in the advanced stage of consumption.[25]

When Ferriar gave digitalis leaf or infusion to patients with dropsy and not consumption, however, he achieved about what his contemporary investigators had accomplished. About 45 percent of his patients responded favorably to digitalis and 21 percent displayed side effects.[26]

Volume 3 of the *Medical and Physical Journal of London*, published in 1800, contains nine papers on digitalis, from all parts of England; the volume is almost a symposium on the foxglove. In one paper, Robert Kinglake (1765–1842) of Bristol, who had taken his M.D. at Göttingen and studied at Edinburgh, described the successful use of digitalis in consumption. Kinglake has been called the first to have shown that "the force of the pulse was increased by the drug—the first clinical recognition of the increased stroke volume [the volume of blood expelled at each contraction] of a digitalized heart." This interpretation was probably based on Kinglake's recognition that "With reduced frequency of pulse ...are necessarily associated proportionate fullness and swiftness, conditions less separable from the beneficial agency of digitalis than increased slowness." It is more likely that Kinglake was able to differentiate the effects of digitalis seen in his patients than that he understood the physiological changes brought about by the drug as we do today.[27]

John Bailey of St. Thomas' Hospital in London presented a novel concept of the mode of action of digitalis: "Like opium, it restrains the action of the heart and arteries, through the medium of the stomach; i.e., by the harmony that subsists between those organs; consequently the blood is propelled with less energy to the pulmonic system." Bailey's rationale for using digitalis in consumption was like that of Beddoes; both thought it would remove the pathological substances causing the disease.[28] Other aspects of the preparation of digitalis and its clinical use in consumption were discussed in the "symposium" by Nathan Drake (1766–1836), a 1789 Edinburgh graduate living in Suffolk; John Sherwen (1749–1826), a 1798 Aberdeen graduate who practiced surgery at Bath; Thomas Harrington of Piccadilly; and William Carson, an obstetrician of Birmingham.[29]

John Penkivil of Plymouth Dock tried to relate his patient's pulse rate to the dose of digitalis administered each day; his data are summarized in Figure 6. Because Penkivil found that a dose of 90 drops of tincture of digitalis daily did not reduce the pulse to less than 90 or 100, he considered the case to be "proof that the good effects of this medicine does not depend upon the retardation of the circulation." The Figure shows, however, that he could have achieved slowing of the pulse without giving doses large enough to induce vomiting in his patient; the maximum effect on heart rate occurred at doses of about 50 to 60 drops daily, whereas vomiting did not occur until the dose had been increased to eighty drops a day.[30]

George Mossman (fl. 1788–1800) of Bradford, in Yorkshire, presented data on two patients with respiratory disease, possibly tuberculosis, whose symptoms and pulse rates lessened during the administration of digitalis. He argued that its clinical utility depended on its effects on the cardiovascular system, and on achieving a sufficient dose of drug in the body. Mossman attempted to set a standard for evaluating the foxglove's clinical effects:

> I have, however, met with none who did eventually resist its influence; and I think, that unless it obtain dominion over vascular action, it will never produce any curative effect. It is therefore incumbent on every practitioner, who details failures, to state with precision, whether the Digitalis did or did not retard the motion of the heart; for without this information we are not certain that their patients were charged with the plant; and the cases are good for nothing.[31]

The most detailed observations presented in the 1800 "symposium" on digitalis were those of James Magennis, surgeon at the Royal Naval Hospital at Plymouth. He studied the effects of digitalis in a 27-year-old Dutch prisoner who had been hospitalized for consumption, in compliance with a 1798 directive from the Sick and Hurt Office for Prisoners of War that foxglove be used in the treatment of prisoners with pulmonary

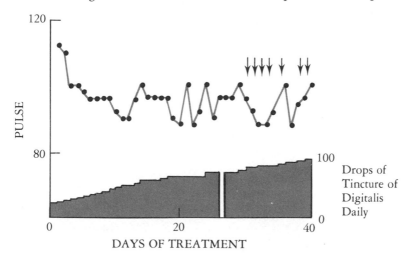

FIG. 6. *Daily dose of digitalis administered by Dr. Penkivil in 1800 to his patient, and the patient's pulse and episodes of nausea and vomiting (indicated by arrows).*
SOURCE: John Penkivil, "On Digitalis," *Medical and Physical Journal of London*, 3 (1800), 315–321.

diseases. In his paper Magennis listed the dose of digitalis administered to the patient each day, three times a day, whether the patient vomited the dose, his pulse every morning, afternoon, and evening, and the occurrence of side effects, all over a period of 108 days. These data, which he presented in paragraph form, are summarized graphically in Figure 7.[32]

Magennis wrote that the "pulse was examined systematically," that is, at the same time each day, by himself or a trusted associate, "from an anxious desire of becoming acquainted with the exact properties of the digitalis." The drug was successful in "curing" the patient's respiratory disease, and had the expected effect on the pulse: "The power of the

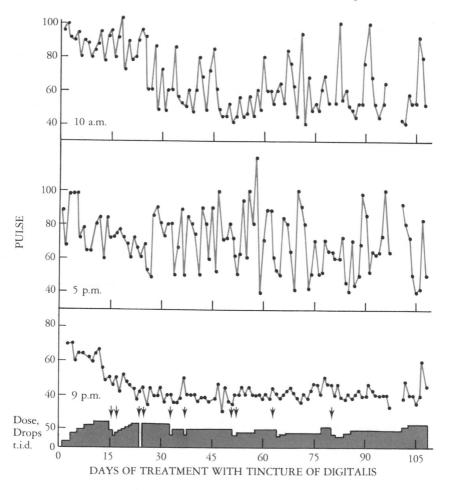

FIG. 7. *Dose of digitalis administered at 8 A.M., 1 P.M., and 7 P.M. by Dr. Magennis in 1800 to his patient, and the patient's pulse at 10 A.M., 5 P.M., and 9 P.M. Episodes of nausea and vomiting are indicated by arrows.*
SOURCE: James Magennis, "On the Effects of Digitalis," *Medical and Physical Journal of London*, 3 (1800), 128–135.

medicine was most conspicuous in diminishing the quantity, changing the quality, and removing the factor of expectoration, as well as in lessening the force of the vascular system." Magennis realized, as had Kinglake, that the pulse was always more regular, and generally fuller, when digitalis had reduced it to less than forty, even when diuresis did not occur. Charles Aldis (?1775–1863), who, like Magennis, was a physician to prisoners of war, found foxglove to be completely ineffective in his patients at Norman Cross Barracks.[33]

Figure 7 shows that the patient's morning and afternoon pulses fluctuated to a greater extent than his evening pulse, when, presumably, he was resting in bed. Statistical analysis of the raw data shows that the three pulses are correlated ($P < 0.01$) only over the first five weeks, reflecting the drug's gradually increasing effect, regardless of the patient's daily activity, while he was being digitalized to the maximum extent achieved. The pulses were not correlated during the last ten weeks of the study. Although Dr. Magennis could not know about statistical measures of association, any more than he could draw graphs, he could still conclude, in reference to the daily variation in heart rate:

> After a certain length of time, when the system is charged, and completely under [the foxglove's] influence, it possesses a power of arresting the motion of the heart and arteries in a surprising manner; but . . . under such influence, they are exquisitely susceptible of being roused into action on the slightest bodily exertion.[34]

He was astonished at the extent of the foxglove's effect on the pulse: "The pulse may be brought to a degree of reduction [i.e., to less than 40 beats per minute] hitherto thought incompatible with the existence of animal life, for any considerable time, without danger to, or even any material derangement of, the animal oeconomy."[35] He concluded, then, after considering all his data:

> That the criterion by which we are to be guided in regulating the increase, diminution, or total omission of the medicine, depends on the phenomena arising from its action on the sensorium and stomach, and not on the quantum of reduction in the pulse.

In his paper Magennis has provided extensive data that confirm Withering's admonition that digitalis should be given until either beneficial or side effects occur, because the two are separable, but he, too, considered slowing of the pulse to be a side effect.[36]

Textbook writers of the time took all these and other writings into account in their summaries of the effects of digitalis. For instance, John Murray (d. 1820), an apothecary who late in life obtained the M.D. degree from St. Andrews in 1814, wrote in his 1804 text of materia medica:

> Of all narcotics, Digitalis is that which diminishes most powerfully the action of the system; and it does so without occasioning any previous excitement. Even in the most moderate dose it diminishes the force and frequency of the pulse, and in a large dose reduces it

to a great extent, occasioning, at the same time, vertigo, indistinct vision, violent and durable sickness, with vomiting... [It is] one of the most certain diuretics in dropsy apparently from its power of promoting absorption.

Murray, then, like his contemporaries in England, ascribed the pharmacologic and therapeutic properties of digitalis to its ability to suppress the hyperactive "system" which they thought characterized dropsy.[37]

Charles William Quin of Dublin was a medical student at Edinburgh in 1779 when he heard a paper presented at the Royal Medical Society which referred to Withering's continuing successful trials of digitalis. Quin administered the new drug to one of his patients, but without success, and he did not repeat the experiment until he read Withering's book seven years later, with its clear directions for the drug's clinical use. Quin then gave digitalis to at least eleven patients with ascites or anasarca. Only five of these patients responded favorably to the drug, but the case histories also indicate that the other six did not, in fact, have congestive heart failure. The two patients who developed side effects had not responded to the drug's diuretic effect.[38]

The report of the largest clinical trial of digitalis in patients with dropsy, after Withering's pioneering study, appeared in England in 1810 and was republished in the United States four years later. Dr. L. Maclean of Sudbury, in Suffolk, reported on seventy-two patients with hydrothorax associated with congestive heart failure. Of the sixty-four whom he treated with digitalis, 83 percent recovered. Of thirteen who were not treated, including three who had been treated successfully on previous occasions but who would not or could not take the drug later, only 8 percent recovered.[39] Table 25 shows that Maclean's overall therapeutic success rate, and the incidence of side effects among his patients, were like those found by Withering and others, including Jackson (see Chapter 6). Even with improved methods of detecting the presence of side effects, such as the electrocardiograph, the reported incidence of digitalis toxicity has not changed appreciably over the past 180 years.

By the time he compiled his data, Maclean must have learned in what circumstances digitalis would be most likely to be clinically effective. Eleven years earlier, in 1799, he had written of its use in cases of consumption: "My own experience in upwards of twenty cases, will not suffer me to speak in such high terms of it [as Beddoes does]."[40]

The next entire book to be devoted exclusively to the medicinal properties of the foxglove was by William Hamilton, a physician of Bury St. Edmunds. Dr. Hamilton's 1807 treatise was largely a review of the literature, focusing on Withering's *Account*. Hamilton reported only six cases of his own, plus four additional cases reported to him by Maclean. Hamilton thought that reduction of the pulse need not, in itself, reduce fever and its associated symptoms, and he agreed that the foxglove's efficacy in patients with hydrothorax was the result of its diuretic properties. He concluded that digitalis caused recovery from consumption because, as his predecessors had reasoned, the drug provided either:

Table 25.
Incidences of Therapeutic Success and Side Effects Attributable to
Digitalis in Earliest Clinical Studies of Its Efficacy, 1785–1818, and
in 1971

| | *Digitalis Preparation* | *Number of Patients* | *Therapeutic Success Rate* | *Incidence of Side Effects* |
|---|---|---|---|---|
| WITHERING (1785) | Decoction | 15 | 80% | 55% |
| | Dried Leaf | 35 | 77% | 14% |
| | Infusion | 78 | 69% | 19% |
| JACKSON (1790) | Infusion | 11 | 73% | 9% |
| QUIN (1790) | Infusion | 11 | 46% | 18% |
| MACLEAN (1810) | Infusion | 94 | 83% | 16% |
| FERRIAR (1816) | Not specified | 29 | 45% | 21% |
| BLACKALL (1818) | Infusion and Tincture | 35 | 71% | 17% |
| BELLER, et al. (1971) | Leaf and pure Glycosides | 135 | 100% | 23–29% |

SOURCES: J. Worth Estes and Paul Dudley White, "William Withering and the Purple Foxglove," *Scientific American*, 212 (June 1965), 110–119. George A. Beller, Thomas W. Smith, Walter H. Abelmann, Edgar Haber, and William B. Hood, Jr., "Digitalis Intoxication," *New England Journal of Medicine*, 284 (1971), 989–997. John Ferriar, *Medical Histories and Reflections*, 1st American ed. (Philadelphia, Thomas Dobson, 1816), pp. 18–30, 212. Charles William Quin, *A Treatise on the Dropsy of the Brain* . . . (London, J. Murray and W. Jones, 1790). John Blackall, *Observations on the Nature and Cure of Dropsies* (London, Longman, Hurst, Rees, Orme, and Brown, 1818). L. Maclean, *An Inquiry into the Nature, Causes, and Cure of Hydrothorax* (Hartford, 1814). Hall Jackson, "Some Cases of the Administration of the Foxglove," unpublished manuscript, 1790 (see below, p. 214, for the complete text).

a means of exciting the absorption of matter from ulcers in the lungs as rapidly as it became secreted, [or] the power of retarding the velocity of the pulse; and consequently, of preventing the growth of new and morbid parts, and restraining the secretion of Pus by diminishing the supply of arterial blood—at the same time that absorption was increased.[41]

In 1813 John Blackall (1771–1860), who also discovered that dropsy is often associated with the presence of albumin in the urine, published

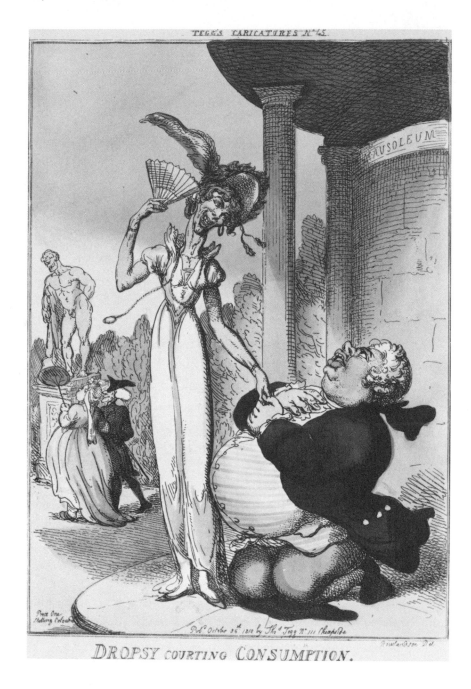

VII. *"Dropsy Courting Consumption" by Thomas Rowlandson, 1810. (Yale Medical Library)*

his observations on 73 patients with dropsy. Explicitly citing and confirming Maclean's results, he found that the foxglove provided effective therapy in virtually all patients who developed dropsy following attacks of scarlet fever (Withering had recommended digitalis for patients with scarlet fever only if they were resistant to rhubarb, squills, or other drugs; he may have been reluctant to use the more potent digitalis in children, who are the most likely to have scarlet fever). From his perspective of almost thirty years since the publication of the *Account of the Foxglove*, Blackall summed up Withering's contribution to medicine as it was commonly perceived at the time:

> This plant has certainly made a great addition of late years to our means of cure. For although before the time of Dr. Withering's publication on that subject it had been employed very frequently, both in this and other countries, as a domestic [i.e., household] drug, yet its exhibition was regulated by no sort of principle or distinction; and accuracy, as to dose, was wholly out of the question. Even lately, the common people of this neighborhood have been in the habit of throwing boiling water on the leaves, stem, and root, without any measure or weight. The results have been unexpected recoveries much talked of, and more failures, which tell no tales.
>
> Dr. Withering, by showing its safety as well as its efficacy, and by greatly diminishing the dose, has taken the only means of rendering it applicable to common use... It is not too much to say, that lives are prolonged for many years by the discreet management of this remedy alone... Our first object, undoubtedly, should be to choose such doses of it, as will cure; our second, carefully to avoid such as may act with violence or offence.

But the drug's action on the heart remained tantalizingly elusive, even if it was *almost* evident to Blackall: "Digitalis greatly depresses the action of the heart and arteries, and controuls the circulation; and it seems not unreasonable to believe, that its curative powers can be independent of such an effect, or at least in contradiction to it." [42]

Virtually all the published medical literature of England was available to American physicians in the years following the Revolution, either imported directly or republished in American editions. We have seen that English medical periodicals were cited by American physicians. In fact, during the early years of the new republic Europe remained the chief source of formal medical training and literature. By 1800 four medical schools had appeared in the United States, and by the end of our story, 1820, there were nine. These schools were designed originally to supplement, rather than replace, apprenticeship training, although their mission had changed to that of the best European schools by the end of the period. [43]

The cultural nationalism that belatedly arose after the Revolution began to stimulate some research. Shryock has observed that "It is surprising how few professional leaders of that time rushed into print," but they had only a few outlets for their research for some years to come. The first medical periodical in the United States was the *Medical Repertory*, founded in 1797. Between 1804 and 1820 the *Philadelphia Medical Museum*, the *American Medical and Philosophical Register*, the *Eclectic Repertory*, the *New England Journal of Medicine and Surgery*, and the *Philadelphia Journal of Medical and Physical Science* (later the *American Journal of Medical Sciences*) were established. The advent of these native publications probably did stimulate American practitioners to contribute papers, at least on their own interesting cases, and to read them, more often than they could have done as colonists.[44]

Professional journals published at home and abroad began to replace the popular lay press as the usual forum for medical data and opinions. Most of the new journals were edited in Philadelphia, which had long superseded Boston as the nation's intellectual capital. Before the Revolution much medical writing was intended to influence the public rather than the profession,[45] as, for instance, we noted while following Hall Jackson's involvement with smallpox inoculation. The same situation is recurring in late twentieth-century America, unlikely as it may seem, largely because of the rediscovery of the political implications of health care.

Medical books for home use were included in the advertisements of eighteenth-century bookshops. For instance, Charles Pierce's Book and Stationery Shop in Portsmouth advertised the *Afflicted Man's Companion or a Directory for Persons and Families Afflicted with Sickness or Any Other Distress, with Directions to the Sick, &c.* The 1794 catalog for Lamson and Odiorne's at Exeter, New Hampshire, included Bell's books on surgery and ulcers, Cullen's *Materia Medica*, and Hamilton's *Midwifery*. Some of these were suitable for do-it-yourself-at-home medicine, but others were not. Most medical books came from England, and many were reprinted here. William Buchan's *Domestic Medicine* went through some twenty-one American editions in the thirty years before the turn of the century, attesting to its popularity on the home bookshelf.[46]

In 1790 Dr. John Warren (1753–1815) of Boston lamented to John Coakley Lettsom in London the absence of native medical publications in America:

> The poverty of this country, with respect to literary productions, is such, that I am not enabled, by any means, to make that return which your notices to me in this way, merit. We are, however, making some advances, I trust, in the paths of science, and we shall think it no dishonour to imitate the means by which the enlightened nations of Europe, and particularly England, have become so celebrated for their cultivation of the arts. At a humble distance, we shall indeed long remain, but from the labours of the industrious, something advantageous may, in all countries, be derived.[47]

Native publications were, however, a luxury that the young country could ill afford at the time.

Billings has tabulated the extent of the country's meager output of strictly medical works, excluding pamphlets and broadsheets, from 1776 through 1799:

| American-authored medical books: | First editions | 39 |
| | Later editions | 9 |
| | Total volumes | 51 |
| Foreign-authored medical books: | First editions | 28 |
| | Later editions | 11 |
| | Total volumes | 49 |
| American medical journals: | | 1 |
| | Volumes completed | 1 |
| Transactions of medical societies: | | — |
| | Volumes completed | 7 |

The total medical output of the young country was, of course, much greater than this list might indicate. For instance, abundant material related to health and disease can be found in transactions of general scientific and "philosophic" societies, even in agricultural volumes.[48]

Precious little original research was accomplished in America before 1820. Save for the development of smallpox inoculation, the few important discoveries made between 1720 and 1820 were not the result of organized investigation, as Withering's had been. For instance, Ephraim McDowell's performance of the first planned abdominal surgery in 1809 resulted not from an investigative approach, but from the pragmatic necessity of removing a tumor from his patient's abdomen. Furthermore, McDowell was not a backwoods practitioner in a small Kentucky town, but the possessor of an Edinburgh M.D. degree who knew enough anatomy to realize that the operation was feasible.[49]

Shryock points out that American physicians, even in the best medical centers, did not appreciate the significance of scientific investigation. He also quotes Alexis de Tocqueville's 1835 observation that "theoretical science" has been neglected in America because access to the European literature is so easy, and because the ideology of the republic placed more emphasis on the practicality of application of new discoveries than on satisfaction of intellectual curiosity. The few scientists of Jefferson's America urged chauvinism and utilitarianism as sufficient reasons for support of the sciences, arguments that are still being employed. Less philosophically, Spector has ascribed the lack of original publications in young America to the American physicians' greater need to make a living. It is telling, perhaps, that the foxglove was never discussed formally at meetings of the American Philosophical Society, at least through 1838, although in his prospectus for the Society, Benjamin Franklin had stipulated that its members should discuss "new methods of curing or preventing disease." Even the theses submitted for the M.D. degree at American medical schools were prepared more to satisfy academic degree requirements than for the sake of investigation. Many—but, as we will see, not all—medical theses were merely regurgitated digests of published literature.[50]

It is not possible to be truly astonished, or ashamed by implication, at the apparent paucity of American medical research during George III's sixty-year reign. The reason is that a young and impoverished country with no developed resources cannot be expected to have competed with the then richest nations as a substantial producer of research, any more than today's poorest nations can be. Even John Warren's fervent familial patriotism should not have kept him from recognizing that factor almost two centuries ago. Nor, as these chapters show, can it be confirmed that the year 1850 is "the approximate date of the end of the empiric and the beginning of scientific American medicine," even if for "scientific" we substitute the word "experimental." [51] American medicine has had its scientific component all along, although occasionally it has been camouflaged by twentieth-century concepts, mitigated by financial constraints, or rendered ineffective by the absence of appropriate methods of measurement.

We have seen that Benjamin Rush regarded all disease as the result of a generalized "debility" of the body, a concept he is said to have developed in order to help consolidate his position in the principal chair of the University of Pennsylvania School of Medicine. His majestic self-confidence in his own reasoning and research is demonstrated by his exultation, almost surprise, at finding that bleeding and purging "cured" yellow fever:

> Never before did I experience such sublime joy as I now felt in contemplating the success of my remedies. It repaid me for all the toils and studies of my life. The conquest of this formidable disease, was not the effect of an accident, nor of the application of a single medicine; but, it was the triumph of a principle in medicine. [52]

In his *Medical Inquiries and Observations*, Rush displays a reasonably accurate grasp of the pathophysiology of dropsy, and of the mechanism of action of digitalis, although he follows his colleagues at Philadelphia and in England in regarding the drug as a sedative to the arterial system. Rush described dropsies as being characterized by a hard, rapid pulse, but laments that "Many physicians visit and examine patients in these disorders, without feeling the pulse." Of appropriate drug therapy for dropsy he wrote:

> Certain medicines, which by lessening the *action of the arterial system*, favor the absorption of and evacuation of water. The only medicines of this class which I shall name are *nitre, cream of tartar*, and *foxglove* ... [Foxglove] has been supposed to exert a specific action on the kidneys as a diuretic; but I am rather disposed to believe, that it acts only by lessening the action of the arterial system by a sedative quality which appears to reside with in it.

Rush did not close his mind to new developments in digitalis therapy; in 1809 he wrote in his *Commonplace Book* for his son who was about to go to Europe: "Converse on medicine with physicians. Ask what new medicines or new forms of old medicines &c they are in the habit of giving, e.g. digitalis, &c." [53]

The first publication specifically about digitalis by an American was a paper published in 1797, ten years after Jackson received Withering's foxglove shipment, by Dr. James Mease (1771–1846), Resident Physician of the Port of Philadelphia. Mease, who had obtained his M.D. from the University of Pennsylvania in 1792, was also a noted antiquarian and philanthropist. In his paper he pointed out that lack of success with digitalis probably does not result from any inactivity of the drug, but from other factors, such as its faulty preparation or its administration to patients who are not likely to respond. He recommended that Withering's directions for the administration of digitalis be followed, but, emulating his former professor, Benjamin Rush, with something bordering on adoration, Mease disagreed with Withering as to what kind of patients would be most likely to respond favorably. In this respect, Mease was unable to differentiate congestive heart failure from other wasting disease of the elderly. Like Hall Jackson he feared that digitalis would fall into undeserved disrepute if more was expected of it than it could deliver. [54]

Dr. James S. Stringham (1775–1817) of Columbia University, the first professor of medical jurisprudence in the United States, had just obtained his M.D. from Edinburgh when he wrote about the effects of digitalis on the vasculature in 1801. After presenting two case reports, he wrote, almost as if presenting a new discovery: "I have often thought, that a medicine which would diminish the action of the vascular system, without previously occasioning an increased excitement, was a great desideratum amongst physicians," and that foxglove is probably that medicine. Stringham's concept of dropsy was derived ultimately from Boerhaave. Although he regarded the pharmacological reduction of the pulse in his patients as beneficial, because he assumed that a slower blood flow would permit the blood to enter the smallest vessels more easily, he felt that diuresis was the best way to encourage the discharge of fluids from the body and therefore was the true mode of action of digitalis. [55]

Ferriar's 1799 book was reviewed in an editorial accompanying Stringham's paper in the same issue of the *Medical Repository*. The editorial probably was written by either Dr. Samuel I. Mitchill (1764–1831) or Dr. Edward Miller (1760–1812), the editors of that journal, which was published in New York. The writer also mentioned letters the editors had received about cases in which digitalis had been used in Wilmington, North Carolina, and Dumfries, Virginia. He reviewed the current conflict over the foxglove's mode of action: to some it was a sedative, "rendering the heart and arteries less susceptible of the stimulus of the blood and other agents," while others thought it had a stimulant effect on the absorbents, or lymphatics, as we now know them, "speedily evacuating watery accumulations in many cases of dropsy." American physicians could still not recognize that the heart is the foxglove's target organ. [56]

Dr. Mahlon Gregg of Attleboro, Pennsylvania, wrote a paper in 1801 that appeared three years later in the first issue of the *Philadelphia Medical and Physical Journal*. Gregg reported on two patients with phthisis pulmonale who developed excessive salivation upon exposure to, and later re-challenge with, digitalis. In a note to Gregg's paper, the editor, Benjamin Smith Barton, noted that Withering, too, had observed that digitalis sometimes may "excite a copious flow of saliva." [57]

Barton (1766–1815) was professor of materia medica at the University of Pennsylvania; he received his M.D. from Göttingen in 1789, having previously studied at Edinburgh and London. In 1798 he wrote that digitalis was "so much and so justly celebrated at present." Later he almost rhapsodized in his textbook of botany: "Every physician now acknowledges the highly valuable powers of the Digitalis purpurea, or Purple Foxglove: one of the most inestimable articles in the Materia Medica." [58]

In 1804 Dr. Isaac Rand of Boston delivered a paper on the use of digitalis in phthisis pulmonale to the Massachusetts Medical Society. After acknowledging the "experiments" of Drs. Darwin and Baker, he discussed his concept of the foxglove's mode of action in phthisis, which was much like that of Beddoes, Ferriar, and Hamilton:

> The digitalis...promotes two important processes; it promotes the absorption of the pus before it is converted into an ichorous poison by the air, and by lessening the irritability of the heart and arteries, prevents the profuse secretion of pus...The pulse is retarded in consequence of nausea; and as subsequent to the retardation of the action of the heart, absorption [of pus, not of edema fluid] frequently occurs.

To illustrate this point, Rand presented the case of Mr. Crocker, noting that "The digitalis rendered his body soluble." [59]

The first civilian pharmacopoeia published in the new republic was the work of John Redman Coxe (1773–1864), professor of chemistry and later of materia medica, at the University of Pennsylvania, where he obtained his medical degree in 1794. He had also been apprenticed to Rush for a time. Coxe listed the effects of digitalis in *The American Dispensary*:

> Its effects when swallowed are,
> 1. To diminish the frequency of the pulse [i.e., as a sedative].
> 2. To diminish the irritability of the system [i.e., as a sedative].
> 3. To increase the action of the absorbents [i.e., as a stimulant].
> 4. To increase the discharge by urine.

In this terse outline Coxe summarized all the thinking about both dropsy and digitalis over the past 20 years, although he could not yet synthesize it into a unifying hypothesis. He went on to recommend the use of digitalis:

> 1. In inflammatory diseases, for its very remarkable power of diminishing the activity of the circulation.
> 2. In active hemorrhagies, in phthisis.
> 3. In some spasmodic affections, as in spasmodic asthma, palpitations, etc.

4. In mania from effusion on the brain [because hydrocephalus and other kinds of mental disease were sometimes regarded as forms of dropsy].
5. In anasarcous and dropsical effusions.
6. In scrofulous tumours.
7. In aneurism of the aorta, it has alleviated the most distressing symptoms.

Coxe relegated dropsy only to fifth place among his indications for the use of digitalis, while first place went to consumption and other respiratory infections, as his former professors had taught. It must be remembered, in Coxe's defense, that at the time it was often difficult or impossible to make the differential diagnosis that would now help distinguish certain respiratory and cardiac diseases that have similar symptoms.[60]

There are other possible reasons for the order in which Coxe listed the clinical indications for digitalis. The specific order of the list may reflect only the relative incidences of the diseases. For instance, consumption was the leading cause of death at the turn of the eighteenth century. Hemorrhage and "spasmodic affections" were, as we have seen, attributed to hyperactive disorders of the blood vessels, so it was to be expected that a "sedative" drug which "diminished the irritability of the system" would counteract such disease.

Other reports of the usefulness of the foxglove in the treatment of various diseases are all but lost in papers with omnibus or otherwise misleading titles that may camouflage any mention of digitalis. For instance, in his paper on "Organic diseases of the heart," Dr. John Collins Warren (1778–1856), professor of anatomy and surgery at the Harvard Medical School and a graduate of that school, noted in passing only that "The digitalis seems to be a medicine well adapted to the alleviation of symptoms [of heart disease], not only by diminishing the impetus of the heart, but by lessening the quantity of circulating fluids."[61]

It is probable that the first experimental observations of the effects of single doses of digitalis on the pulse rate in man were those reported by John Moore in his M.D. thesis for the University of Pennsylvania. Moore (1778–1836) was born in Upper Merion Township (now in Haverford) in Montgomery County, Pennsylvania, and began to study medicine with Dr. John Wilson in Bucks County. In 1797 he became a private student of Caspar Wistar in Philadelphia, and the following year was appointed apothecary to the Philadelphia Hospital, resigning that position after a year for reasons of poor health. Moore dedicated his dissertation to his two principal medical mentors, Drs. Wilson and Wistar. He received his degree in 1800 and returned to Montgomery County to practice. From 1818 to 1820 he was a member of the obstetrical staff of the Pennsylvania Hospital in Philadelphia.[62]

In the introduction to this thesis Moore quoted one of Withering's cautions about medical research:

"It is much easier to write upon a disease than upon a remedy. The former is in the hands of nature, and a faithful observer, with an eye of tolerable judgment, cannot fail to delineate a disease. The latter will ever be subject to the whims, the inaccuracies and the blunders of mankind." [63]

We will see that Moore himself fell into some of these traps in his thinking about digitalis. Withering had demonstrated in his own M.D. thesis of 1766, on scarlet fever, that it was easy to write about a disease, although twenty years later he also managed to write accurately and systematically about the foxglove as a remedy. [64]

Moore went on to explain why he decided to perform his experiments with the foxglove:

> As its effects can be more clearly ascertained in a state of health, than when complicated with the symptoms of disease; and as its operation in morbid affections will be more properly considered after its mode of action has undergone examination, I shall here confine myself to an enumeration of its effects on the body in a state of health, and particularly of its primary effects on the arterial system. [65]

Under many circumstances it is appropriate to investigate the effects of a new drug in healthy persons before administering it to sick patients. The situation is somewhat different with digitalis, however. Although it can at least temporarily and to a slight degree lower the pulse of healthy persons, it does not produce diuresis in persons who are not in congestive heart failure. (The reasons for the unequal effect in normal and ill subjects are discussed above in Chapter 4.)

Figure 8 shows in graphic form the data reported by Moore in tabular form. Unfortunately, he reported only these eight experiments in detail, because he felt that all his other experiments had produced such similar results that no loss would be suffered if he omitted them for the sake of brevity of his thesis. Moore then summarized, explained, and justified his conclusions.

> [Digitalis] was considered as a sedative medicine, from the time of its first introduction into the materia medica, until the winter 1798–9, when Dr. Barton taught, in his lectures, that notwithstanding all that had been said in proof of its lowering or diminishing of the pulse, he was induced to believe that it was a stimulant. My experiments, or at least, the first, second, fourth, fifth, seventh and eighth, lead to a very similar conclusion, and seem sufficient to establish the opinion above stated. If we mean by a stimulant, a medicine which will always increase the force and frequency of the pulse, digitalis may not be entitled to that appellation, but, if I mistake not, there are medicines denominated stimulants, or incitants, which will not, on every constitution and habit, produce the same effect of accelerating the pulse. [66]

Although he tried to avoid the power of suggestion on his experimental subjects, Moore fell victim to the power of Benjamin Smith Barton's suggestion, in that he took account solely of the initial increase of the

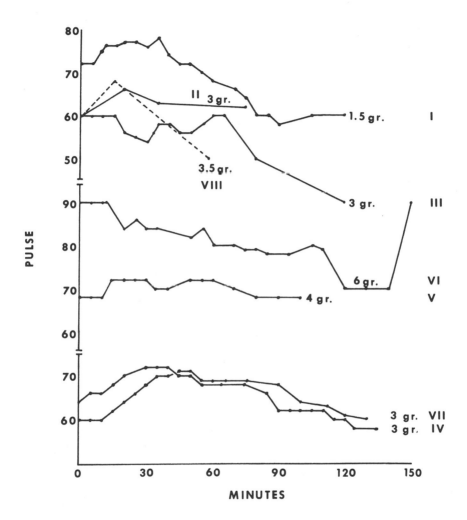

FIG. 8. *Effects of digitalis on the pulse in eight experiments by medical student John Moore, in 1800. Moore performed experiments I, II, III, and VIII on himself, experiment VI on Thomas Maborough, "a black man aged 48," experiment V on George Taverner, "aged 40, a robust healthy man, who had been accustomed to drink freely of ardent spirits," and experiments IV and VII on his "worthy friend and colleague, Dr. Enoch Wilson."*
SOURCE: John Moore, *Inaugural Dissertation on Digitalis Purpurea* (Philadelphia, Way and Groff, 1800), pp. 11–16.

pulse in seeking to describe the mode of action of foxglove. Perhaps if he had known about graphing his data, a tool that was not yet used in medicine, he would have seen that after the initial increase in pulse rate, digitalis in fact *decreased* the pulse in most of his experiments. He surely had not seen such papers as those of Penkivil and Magennis, which probably had not arrived in Philadelphia by then. (Seven years later an anonymous letter to the editor of the *Philadelphia Medical Museum* would note that the *London Medical and Physical Journal* "is in the hands of but few practitioners in this country.")[67]

Like Beddoes, who was performing his frog experiments at about the same time, Moore thought that digitalis and opium had several properties in common, because both drugs had been observed to increase the frequency and fullness of the pulse, and to increase the flow of saliva, sweat, and urine. But unlike Beddoes and his English colleagues, and unlike Rush and others at Philadelphia, Moore postulated that digitalis stimulates the arterial system via the nerves. In other words, he used his experimental results to justify Professor Barton's hypothesis, which dates from at least 1798 and which had already caused confusion by 1801.[68]

The next thesis on digitalis appeared in 1805, again at the University of Pennsylvania. Its author, Lewis Burwell (1783–1826), was born on a still magnificent James River plantation, "Carter's Grove," near Williamsburg. After graduating in medicine at Philadelphia in 1805, he visited and studied at hospitals in Paris and elsewhere in Europe. Upon his return to America he built "Prospect Hill" in Clarke County, Virginia, and having come into an inheritance, never practiced medicine.[69]

Burwell appears to have been a wealthy student who barely managed to get by scholastically, at least by modern standards. Apparently attempting to curry favor all around, he dedicated his dissertation to the entire University of Pennsylvania faculty. His paper is a blustering corroboration of what he had been taught by Benjamin Smith Barton. It leans heavily on Moore's experiments and presents new data for only two subjects, shown in Figure 9. Because of the small doses administered, as well as the drug's usual lack of observable effect in normal subjects and the fact that we now know that digitalis could not have been absorbed from the gastrointestinal tract to its maximum extent during the sixty-minute experiments (nor in Moore's 120- to 150-minute experiments, for that matter), we are not surprised at the apparent absence of effect. He quoted his notes from Barton's lectures, who thought foxglove "more properly classed amongst the more powerful Stimuli." With sarcasm Burwell reported that the drug had been called "the Sampson of the Materia Medica" because of its stimulant effects on the stomach and the salivary glands, and condescendingly asserted that Withering praised digitalis all too much.[70]

Combining Rush's theory of tonic and atonic dropsies and Barton's theory of the stimulant nature of digitalis, Burwell proposed his own synopsis of how the drug affects patients with dropsy, following current theory:

The cure of Tonic Dropsy, should be attempted by all those means which tend to lessen the inflammatory action of the system; as Blood-letting, Cathartics, &c. with the Anti-phlogistic regimen. Here it might be said the Digitalis would be a very proper remedy, from its remarkable effect of lowering the Pulse. To this, I answer; that this is a secondary effect, and the consequence of a primary stimulant operation on the system; which is not peculiar to the Digitalis, but common, more or less, with all Stimuli. And as stimulants are certainly injurious in this state of the system, I think we should loose more, by the primary stimulant operation; than we should gain by the secondary effect of this medicine.

This being the case I think we may fairly conclude, that the Digitalis cannot be advantageously administered in tonic Dropsy, which is frequently the state of that disease.

If then our medicine cannot be advantageously used in tonic Dropsy, and as it certainly has been so used in this disease, it must be adapted to the atonic stage of it, or that species which is attended with feeble morbid action...I believe, the experience of all authors unite in telling us, to expect very little or no benefit from the exhi-

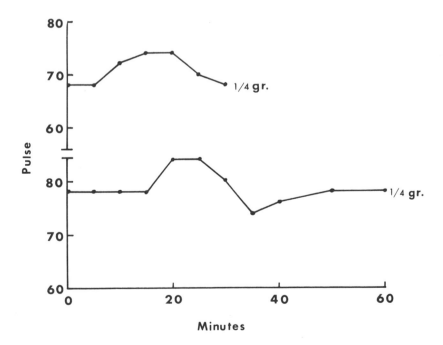

FIG. 9. *Effects of digitalis on the pulse in two experiments by medical student Lewis Burwell on himself, in 1805.*
SOURCE: Lewis Burwell, *Observations on the Digitalis Purpurea* (Philadelphia, printed for the author by Hugh Maxwell, 1805), pp. 10–11.

bition of the Digitalis in those cases of Dropsy, where there is great Debility...

I shall conclude my observations on the use of Digitalis in this disease by observing: that I would always use it when other medicines have failed; but would not in the first instance prefer it to some other Hydragogues [diuretics].[71]

In contrast to Burwell's very logical but dogmatic treatise is Thomas Edward Steell's 1811 M.D. thesis for the College of Physicians at New York. Steell (ca. 1785–1818), a native of New Jersey, must have had his first and most influential exposure to medicine at home, because the dissertation is respectfully and devotedly dedicated to his father, Dr. Thomas Steell. The younger Steell attended Columbia College before he entered the medical school, but nothing more is known of him before his death. From the quality of his thesis one suspects, or perhaps hopes, that more might be known of him today had he not died only seven years after completing his medical education.[72]

Steell began his thesis with a discussion of national peculiarities of medical practice:

The wide difference in the treatment of similar diseases in this country and Great-Britain, is surprising, and in some cases almost unaccountable.

The same circumstance occurs in the employment of particular remedies in certain classes of disease. This observation applies with great force to the employment of the digitalis purpurea. This great abstractor of arterial action is employed with most advantage in acute diseases of high excitement in the United States... while its exhibition in Europe has been confined to dropsy, pulmonary consumption, and other diseases of debility...

Climate, soil, government, and other causes operate in producing a difference in the symptoms of diseases and their consequent treatment. These no doubt have their full operation. But there is another cause that affects nations as opinions do individuals. Hence arises a national practical prejudice, if we may so call it. Dr. Rush observes, that "whole nations are as much distinguished by it as they are by language and manners"...

Universities tend to establish such opinions and practice when they do not allow that liberal discussion and expression of sentiment which is peculiar to the government and medical institutions of the United States. National ideas may thus contribute to the adoption of digitalis in opposite diseases.[73]

In the last paragraph Steell apparently differentiated between the concepts of digitalis as a sedative, then current in England and among some of the Pennsylvania faculty, and as a stimulant, the concept then being promoted by Barton and his students. When Steell, in New York, differentiated among the diseases for which digitalis was used in America and Europe, however, he further confused the concepts and theories of disease in the two areas, concepts that bore little relationship to modern ideas of pathology, with the differing political philosophies of the mother country and her former colonies. He concluded that the liberal politics of America is more likely to be associated with proper experimentation than in the more tradition-oriented society associated with the ancient universities of Britain—especially because Cambridge and Oxford had a monopoly on medical licensing.

Boorstin has suggested that eighteenth-century American physicians practiced better medicine than did their European colleagues; at least, they "interfered less with the patient's recovery." He attributes this not only to the Americans' emphasis on practical ways of treating disease, but also to their appeal to evidence, regardless of prevailing academic theory. Such thinking inevitably would have been linked with the colonial situation, far removed from the mother country, and with the Americans' long-ingrained sense of democracy. The same message, we have seen, is implicit in the Americans' enthusiasm for rural life and for the long life. Their confidence that the will can master circumstances is rare among the "historical flourishings" of creativity.[74]

Steell went on to discuss Moore's conclusion that digitalis shares some stimulant properties with opium: "Of late years... [digitalis] has been considered as an excitor, and applied accordingly. I am in hopes to show this to be a fallacious result of partial observation and experiment." He differentiated clearly between opium's specific soporific effect, which occurs at lower doses than those required to produce sedation with digitalis, and the foxglove's specific effect on the pulse: "for though it at first increases the number of arterial pulsations, it afterwards diminishes them in a greater ratio than the increase, according to the time."[75]

Using John Redman Coxe's list of pharmacological properties of digitalis, Steell commented on the known characteristics of the drug. He considered its effect on the pulse to be its most important action, and concluded that it should be most efficacious in inflammatory diseases and hemorrhage, to slow down the flow of blood. He was not so impressed by its efficacy in dropsy, because he considered dropsy to be a disease of the lymphatics, and he knew that the effects of digitalis on the lymphatics were not constant. Steell felt the foxglove's effects on diuresis to be "trifling and precarious," in spite of Withering's conclusions.[76]

Steell believed that digitalis operates primarily on the vascular system, and based his opinion on experimental observations, although he could not have known that the drug directly affects the heart and not the arteries:

> My opinions of the operation of digitalis are deduced from its effects on the pulse. I was about to institute a set of experiments for the purpose of ascertaining this point, when some already made occurred to me, which will verify my ideas on the subject, though they were made, and have been used [by John Moore] to substantiate an opposite opinion, viz. that digitalis is a stimulus. These experiments, when *properly analyzed* [italics mine]... will, it is hoped,

place the operation of this medicine in a clear point of view, and remove every objection to its employment in diseases of excitement.[77]

In his reanalysis of Moore's eight experiments, Steell noted the number of pulses per minute below the baseline pulse that was produced on each occasion (see above, Figure 8). He then concluded:

First, that digitalis, in many instances, increases the number of pulsations for a limited time; and second, that a depression then takes place to a greater degree. Without further observation we are immediately led to this conclusion, that the sedative effect of digitalis is greater than its stimulant, since the latter is limited, less, and not so permanent...

Here then, we find, that by a partial view of the subject Dr. Moore has been led into an error, in order to confirm the opinion of his professor (Dr. Barton) that digitalis is a stimulant.[78]

Finally, Steell enumerated diseases in which he thought digitalis could properly be used. They are those that we now know are often associated with fever and, consequently, a rapid pulse, such as pneumonia, rheumatism, certain kinds of hemoptysis, and consumption in its early stages.[79]

A major problem in extrapolating from the data collected by Moore and Burwell to the patient in congestive heart failure is that the data show no statistically remarkable elevation or depression of the heart rate in any subject. We now expect digitalis to induce no remarkable change in normal subjects with intact compensatory reflex mechanisms. However, the average time to achieve half the actually achieved maximum slowing of the heart observed by Moore (in his cases I, III, IV, VI, and VII) was about 1½ hours, which is like that found in patients treated with oral doses of digoxin—two hours.[80]

Rush's concept of dropsy as a form of debility led Steell to advocate that digitalis not be used in that disease:

According to nosological arrangement digitalis would be rejected in the cure of [dropsy], for though it sometimes has a diuretic effect, its powerful sedative operation would counteract its other qualities in these cases of debility. Were it not that [dropsies] sometimes take on a febrile appearance, digitalis would perhaps be totally inadmissable.[81]

It appears that Benjamin Rush had so thoroughly convinced his contemporaries of the value of his own unifying concept of disease that they could not make appropriate use of experimental data at the bedside, despite what Withering and Ferriar had written.

Steell's thesis was summarized in a review in the *Medical Repertory* a year later. The reviewer concluded that the use of digitalis may be extended to diseases other than those Steell had listed, those in which there is "strong febrile excitement" and "where the pulse requires reduction in the number of its pulsations, or in tension or hardness." Such a comment naturally led to the use of digitalis in many situations in which we now know it to be ineffective.[82]

William Currie (1754–1828) was an eminent Philadelphia surgeon who kept up with current developments in medicine and wrote extensively on the diseases of America. In 1792 he cited physicians in New Jersey and Maryland who had used digitalis successfully in the treatment of dropsy by at least the previous year. One, however, had learned of the new drug not via a route that began with Withering's book, much less with Jackson, but directly from Erasmus Darwin's 1785 paper.[83]

Currie may be the first to have recognized that digitalis accumulates in the body, although the phenomenon he describes may almost be taken for what we now call tachyphylaxis:

> when a sufficient dose of the Foxglove Decoction is given at first to produce the effect desired, a much less quantity will have the same effect afterwards. This I suppose is owing to the facility our Constitutions possess of acquiring habits of action after having been excited by adapted stimuli.

Currie goes on to use this model to explain the effects of alcohol in alcoholics.[84]

James Ewell (1773–1832) of Savannah, Georgia, published, in 1807, a popular home medicine text called *The Planter's and Mariner's Medical Companion*. The section on dropsy is very much like Donald Monro's book on the subject (see above, Chapter 4), but Ewell's remedies are new: blood letting (straight from Rush), cream of tartar (for purging) and foxglove, "for lessening the action of the pulse, and thereby increasing absorption."[85]

Nathan Smith (1762–1829) included digitalis in his lectures on the theory and practice of physic at the Medical Institution of Yale College in 1814–15. He recommended it for anasarca and pneumonia but was unsure of its usefulness in consumption. However, he also recommended cantharides (Spanish flies), cream of tartar, dwarf elder, juniper, olive oil, squills, and uva ursi for anasarca, antimony for pneumonia, and bloodroot for consumption.[86]

Solomon Drowne included the foxglove in his lectures on materia medica at Brown University in Rhode Island after 1811. The following notes, which he scribbled on a scrap of paper, appear to be his own observations, because nothing similar appears from any other author:

> Consumptions are cured infallibly by weak decoctions of Foxglove leaves in water, or wine and water, and drank for constant drink. Or take the juice of the herb and flowers, clarify it, and make a fine syrup with honey, of which take three spoonfuls thrice in a day, at physical hours... But be cautious of its use, for it is of a vomiting nature. In these things begin sparingly, and increase the dose as the patient's strength will bear, lest instead of a sovereign medicine, you do real damage by this infusion or syrup.[87]

The question of how digitalis affects the body remained unanswered for almost a century. Not until the twentieth century was the mechanism of dropsy finally ascertained, along with the proof that digitalis stimulates the weak heart. It is not possible to trace the impact of Thomas Steell's reasoned deductions that digitalis is a sedative on subsequent practitioners or researchers, but by 1820 Barton's theory that the drug is a stimulant was dead. The chain of reasoning set in motion by William Harvey two hundred years before remained yet unbroken.[88]

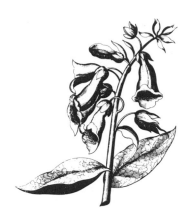

# CHAPTER SIX

# The Purple Foxglove

## A NEW DRUG IN EIGHTEENTH-

## CENTURY AMERICA

THE BACKDROP against which digitalis was introduced into American—and English—medicine was an animated panorama of Western experience. The one continuing actor in the scene was King George III of England, who reigned, however fitfully, during our entire period, from 1760, when Hall Jackson was just starting his practice, until 1820, the year in which digitalis gained official sanction in America.

During George's reign, and in spite of him, a number of new social principles that would later influence the development of American medical practice were established. The Americans gave experimental proof to the hypothesis that in order to alter an unpopular form of government a revolution may be justified. Hall Jackson's countrymen had gone even further when they introduced the concept of a government that is responsible to the wishes of the people, an idea that was unthinkable even to the elected Parliament at the time. Jackson's New England was a principal origin of these social and political changes.

The ideas generated by the American Revolution gained momentum in that of the French, but Napoleon's retrogressive Roman imperialism left only America to carry on the experiment in practical democracy after 1800. For England, the great victories at Trafalgar and Waterloo more than made up for the losses written off at Yorktown, and the British navy was freed to consolidate the growing British Empire for a second time around, with India, Australia, and Canada as its nuclei.

George III also saw the beginnings of another great social upheaval, the Industrial Revolution. It was Withering's circle in Birmingham, the Lunar Society, that provided the tools for this longer-lasting innovation —James Watt's steam engine, the manufacturing methods introduced by Matthew Boulton and Josiah Wedgwood, and the chemistry of Joseph Priestley.

Both the establishment and the radical left of George's reign had their own leaders and chroniclers. Catherine the Great of Russia, Louis XVI of France, Maria Theresa and Joseph II of Austria, as well as George and Napoleon, could conceive of no government other than by personal rule. This autocratic concept brought down the French radical left— Marat, Danton, and Robespierre. Only Adams, Jefferson, and Washington saw the idea of republicanism in permanent form.

It was also a period of ferment in nonpolitical arenas, but often with political and social results. Edward Gibbon was demonstrating the lessons to be learned from the precise study of historical records, while Lavoisier and Jenner, as well as the Lunar Society, were demonstrating the value of careful observation and experimentation. Scientific exploration, in contrast to far-flung economic expansion, was being practiced by Baron von Humboldt. John Wesley was establishing new articles of faith. While Haydn was composing for the court, Mozart was writing operas of revolution, and Sheridan was mocking the manners of all social groups. Johann Wolfgang von Goethe, William Blake, and J.M.W. Turner were developing new views of the world around them, portraits that, in their final development, would leave no room for the principles of scientific investigation to which members of the Lunar Society applied themselves.

In the closing years of the eighteenth century the humanities and the sciences went arm in arm. Physicians could be as conversant in literature and art as in medicine. They formed learned societies, both formal and informal, dedicated to discussions of interesting subjects. Among the most distinguished in England were the Lunar Society, which included two of the country's most famous physicians, Drs. Withering and Erasmus Darwin, and the Manchester Literary and Philosophical Society, founded by two physicians. Although neither English society outlived its charter members, their contemporary American counterparts still engage in scholarly activities: the American Philosophical Society, in Philadelphia, and the American Academy of Arts and Sciences, in Boston. Members of the cast of the story of the foxglove in America were on the rolls of both the American and the English societies.

The members of these organizations were dedicated, like the American Philosophical Society, to "promoting useful knowledge." To promote their knowledge they wrote voluminously—books, memoirs, pamphlets, journal articles, and personal letters. They made and recorded careful observations in their notebooks, discussed their results with their colleagues, and published their data and conclusions in many forms.

Letters to their associates were the most frequently used form of communication among these philosophical scientists, or scientific philosophers. Not only did they exchange letters, they retained their own first drafts, thus preserving a number of letters that otherwise might have been lost. We wonder how men as busy as Benjamin Franklin and Thomas Jefferson, not to mention the busy medical practitioners who are the leading characters in our story, found time to continue their correspondences with men of all interests and on both sides of the Atlantic, without the aid of carbon paper. They must have relied on their letters, perhaps only intuitively, as an essential cement for their new worldwide scientific community.

The letters of such men are microcosms of intellectual activity. Not content merely to request some foxglove seeds from Withering, Hall Jackson also discussed the etiology of dropsy, and those meteorological characteristics of Portsmouth which might be applicable to the growth requirements of the plant. Withering himself was a recognized authority on botany and geology, and became an informed dabbler in archaeology. He did not hesitate to outline in detail for Jackson his thoughts on the etiology of dropsy.

Withering's *Account of the Foxglove* went to press sometime after July 1785, and had reached Portsmouth by the end of the year. The exciting new clinical study immediately convinced Jackson that digitalis was a new therapeutic tool in which he could place complete confidence. He considered it so important that for the next several years he tried to encourage its use among his colleagues. But first, to obtain a continuing supply, he wrote to his new intellectual hero in Birmingham.

TO: Doctor William Withering

Portsmouth, New Hampshire
North America, February 9th 1786

Sir:

Your inestimable treatise or account of the Foxglove and its medical uses, with practical remarks on dropsy, and other diseases, has found its way to this remote part of the globe. It must greatly add to the satisfaction that daily arises in your mind, on seeing so many distressed fellow-mortals relieved by your personal advice and administrations, to reflect that thousands at the most distant ends of the earth are wishing to offer their tribute of gratitude for your indefatigable endeavours for the good of mankind.

The Gentlemen of the Society of medical observations, and enquiries, in London, the ingenious and worthy Doctors, Percival, and White, of Manchester, with many others, of this day in England, will never know how much the world is indebted to them for their publications; not only the present age, but generations yet unborn will bless their memory.

There is no disorder more prevalent in this country than dropsy, our summers are extremely hot, our winters intensely cold; only two of the spring and fall months may be called temperate; our days in the winter are short; consequently our labouring people work but a few hours, the remainder of the time is spent in a sedentary, idle manner, and too often in an immoderate use of spirituous liquors. Our lumber trade to the West Indica Islands returns us large quantities of rum, and Molasses; of the latter is distilled amongst us an inferior, cheap kind of rum, which is evidently unwholsome, it is generally used immediately from the still, it has an empyreumatic taste, and is wholly destitute of the mildness of rum that has undergone agitation at sea, and a few months age; a common labourer may receive five quarts of this new, strong, and fiery spirit, for a short day's work from this plenty and cheapness. The use is too general and immoderate, and it is a just observation that those who indulge too freely in the use of spirit are least anxious for substantial food, their appetites are palled, the solids weakened, the fluids vitiated, and increased obstructions formed, and dropsies become frequent. As yet no specific has been found, but in most cases after a longer, or shorter time, the disease has proved mortal. Life in many cases has been prolonged to a considerable length of time by repeated tapings [tappings], but this has generally been with female subjects, where the disorder was of the encysted kind. Our remedies in general have been such as are used in Europe, in like cases; the squills have been considered as the most powerful diuretic, and mostly depended upon, and some few have been relieved by their use, where resolution has been strong enough to persevere against the nauseating effects thereof.

I have taken your treatise in my pocket for six weeks. I have shown it with the incomparable, accurate, and elegant drawing, to all my acquaintance within twenty miles, but no one can recollect of ever seeing any of its kind in America. I am perswaded, however, that it would arrive in sufficient maturity in this country, by attentive cultivation as our natural productions in general are much the same as those of England, with this difference, the wood of our large trees is not so compact and hard, our fruit trees, nor the fruits, so large, smooth, and succulent, as those of the same kind in Great Britain, our plants and herbage in general are a degree, or two, inferior to those in England, planted in equal good soil, and cultivated with equal attention. Chamomile will not flower in this country, tho I have seen, in a very favorable season, a few scattered single flowers in a large bed. These remarks are from my own observations, having spent the year 1762 in England for the advantage of medical improvements.

I have the honor of being acquainted with John Lane Esq., Mercht, in London. To him I have sent for a small invoice of medicines; I have directed a small quantity of Fol. Digitalis purp; siccat., also some of the powder, and seeds, but I greatly fear they have not as yet become articles of the shops in London. Could I be so fortunate as to obtain (to the care of Mr. Lane), thro' your influence, and direction, a small quantity of the genuine seed, the plant should be most attentively cultivated, most carefully prepared; and as opportunities will not be wanting to administer it, the most accurate observations and remarks on its operation, and effects, shall be noted, and if you will permit me the honor, shall be communicated to you, for any further satisfaction, or remarks, you may wish to make on this truly valuable discovery.

And now, Sir, I should be most painfully embarrassed for an apology in troubling a Gentleman of your character with so lengthy, and uninteresting a letter, without the least personal knowledge, or the remotest introduction, was I not assured that where so much merit, and goodness obtains, an indulgent candour will not be wanting towards one who is sincerely desireous of doing all the possible good, in the narrow sphere in which providence has placed him, and hopes not altogether from those motives that too often actuate the generality of mankind.

> I am, Sir (tho' unknown)
> with the utmost veneration
> and respect, your most
> obliged most obedient
> humb: serv:
> Hall Jackson

P.S. I have directed to be sent me two or three sets of your account of the Fox-glove for the purpose of dispersing them. Also your Scarlatina Anginosa, outlines of Mineralogy; and anticipate with great pleasure your promised Botanical Arrangement. I hope it will be published before my directions are compleated and sent out from London.
The extreme heat and cold in this country may be judged from the following:
  The Thermometer, Fahrenheit's scale, stood as followeth:

|                          |            |   |   |          |
|--------------------------|------------|---|---|----------|
| Portsmouth 1785          | July 1st   | . | . | . 83°    |
|                          | July 15th  | . | . | . 75°    |
|                          | July 30th  | . | . | . 80°    |
| August from the 15th to 30th |        | . | . | . 80°    |
| 1786 January 15th        |            |   |   |          |
|         to 19th          |            | . | . | . 8° below 0 |

N.B. The Thermometer was placed in the open air, and the observations made at noon.[1]


It is clear from this letter that Drs. Jackson and Withering had never been acquainted personally, even during Jackson's stay in England, in spite of later reports to the contrary. It also appears that he spent not more than the one year 1762 in England. Even if Jackson had known Withering in England, Jackson could not have learned about digitalis at that time, because Withering did not begin his evaluation of the drug until 1775.[2]

Jackson's letter is a culogy of Withering, consisting largely of unmitigated adulation in conventional eighteenth-century style. It is not clear why Jackson adds the praise of Drs. Percival and White of Manchester, unless he was carried away by a burst of Anglophilic enthusiasm. Thomas Percival (1740–1804) and Charles White (1728–1813) were among the founders of the Manchester Literary and Philosophical Society, and both were frequent contributors to various medical journals.[3]

Jackson noted that the drug most likely to relieve dropsical patients is squill. Among the many medicines that were registered by the British Patent Office from 1620 to 1786, only five were claimed to be effective in the treatment of dropsy. None contained foxglove or squill, and none can now be considered to be specific, much less effective, for any known disease. Typical is the claim made in the letters patent issued to Joseph Collett and James Jackson in 1752, for:

A certain medicine called oleum anodinum, or British balsam of health, for the cure of gouty nodes and tumours, rheumatick and sciatick pains, fistulas and ulcers, the evil and leprosy, bruises, and sprains, the dropsy, stone, and gravel, sterility and impotence, consumptions, and other disorders of the breast and lungs.

This wonder drug consisted of coal and red sand distilled over a slow fire. The residue was subjected to a sand heat bath, boiled and skimmed until it became transparent, mixed with the distillate, and digested until it attained the consistency of a balsam. No wonder its proprietors claimed that the drug was efficacious in so many conditions. It was certainly equally efficacious for all of them. And there is equally little wonder that an effective antidropsy medicine was so much to be desired.[4]

The Portsmouth physician recognized the *Account* for what it is: a straightforward, unbiased clinical evaluation of a new drug. It is likely that the book's purely scientific approach to establishing guidelines for appropriate therapeutic application of digitalis—including both corroborative and noncorroborative data—influenced Hall Jackson's decision not only to try the drug himself, but also to inform other American physicians about it. Although he may have known of Withering by reputation before he read the *Account*, it was probably the excellence of the book that led him to order the Englishman's other works, on scarlet fever, mineralogy, and botany.[5]

Eight months later Withering replied to Jackson, in a letter that is here published in its entirety for the first time:

Birmingham 27th Oct: 1786

Sir—

Your letter of Febr: 9th arrived here in due time, and the Seed of the Digitalis purpurea which accompanies this, will shew that I have not been inattentive to your request. I send much more than will be necessary for your own use, in the hope that you will distribute it into other provinces, and [illegible] to transmit some to my friend Dr. Jones in Virginia for the same purpose. Mr. Cutler, in the memoirs of the American Academy of Arts and Sciences, printed in Boston 1785 & now before me, gives in his account of indigenous American vegetables page 465, the Linnean character of Digitalis purpurea and supposes it a native of that part of America; but I have reason to believe that his species is not the *purpurea*. Perhaps you may have an opportunity of sending him a few of these seeds; and please to mention my suspicion to him.

It has been remarked that in cold countries the sedentary and the intemperate are particularly the victims to disease, and the diseases which attack them are I think mostly such as arise from debility. If the kind of rum you mention be really more unwholesome than that we have from the West Indies, it must be from some combination with the ardent spirit, though I am inclined to suspect that the intemperate use of Spirits, as such, will occasion the disorders you mention. If however the new rum distilled from the Molasses be as you believe more deleterious than such as we use, and that deleterious quality abates by keeping, we must suppose its amelioration is caused by separation of the hurtful impregnation. The noxious part I believe to be sometimes Lead, and sometimes an essential Oil. The oil escapes in time, and I know the Lead will be precipitated by the astringent extract the Spirit gets from the Casks; but I never have been satisfied whether the Lead is held in solution by an Oil or an Acid; probably by the latter, for we find the corks of rum bottles soon become rotten. If you suppose with me that dropsies, either with or without glandular disease in the abdomen, may be caused by want of action in the absorbent vesicles and too great laxity in the exhalants, you will readily conceive that this inaction must follow the repeated use of strong stimulants, such as ardent Spirits, Essential oils, or both combined, nor will you be at a loss to judge why a cold climate and an inactive Life should aid the formation of the disease. I should attempt in your dropsies to evacuate the Water by the Digitalis, and to prevent its repeated aggregation by frictions, exercise, flannel Shirts and other warm clothing, and I should also call in the aid of Aromatics, Steel, & sometimes Mercury.

I am more & more convinced that the Digitalis, under a judicious management, is one of the mildest & safest medicines we have, as well as one of the most
efficacious. It is I believe *never* necessary to create nausea or any other distur-
bance in the system. I never now use more than 1 drachm fol: sicc: to one pound
of infusion, and in substance rarely 3 grains in 24 hours. An Account of your
tryals with this medicine will be highly grateful to me, and fully recompense
any trouble you have given me.

The Exp[t]s on the freezing of Quicksilver were extremely well conducted, &
correspond sufficiently with the most accurate we have had from other quarters.
I read them to a Society of Philosophic friends in this place, and they met the
approbation of all. Reason and Philosophy are making rapid strides in every
quarter of the globe to emancipate and to enlighten Mankind.

We cure our intermittents [intermittent fevers, most of which were caused by
malaria] of every kind by a solution of white Arsenic in Water, 1 grain to 1 ounce
—Dose 25 to 30 drops, 3 times a day in 6 or 8 ounces of Gruel or Barley Water.
In or out of the paroxysms we go on, until the disease is stopped. The cure is
then to be finished with the usual tonics. Under proper management it produces
no sensible effects.

I must beg you to accept my grateful thanks for the opinion you are pleased
to entertain of me, and believe me that no one is more happy to promote the
spread of Science than your obliged and very
obd[t]. serv[t].<br>W. Withering
The new Botan[l]. Arrangement will not be out sooner than the beginning of
next summer.

Digitalis has cured 2 other cases of insanity in this neighbourhood and 3 cases
of Haemoptoe. The latter were of the kind attended with a quick bounding pulse,
and I directed the Medicine from [the] quality I knew it possessed of abating the
action of the heart.[6]


Withering's "friend Dr. Jones" was Dr. Walter Jones (1745–1815),
who was born in Williamsburg, Virginia, and received his M.D. in 1770
after three years at Edinburgh. Although it has been said that Jones knew
Withering in England, and the tone of Withering's remark supports this,
it is not likely that they were fellow students at Edinburgh, because Withering had graduated in 1766. Jones was Physician General of the Middle
Military Department for three months in 1777, just prior to Benjamin
Rush's appointment to the post. After the war he practiced in North-
umberland County, Virginia and was elected to the House of Representatives (1797–1799, 1803–1811). There is no evidence to indicate whether
he did, in fact, receive any of Withering's foxglove seeds from Hall Jackson, at least as far as can be ascertained from two collections of Dr.
Jones' papers.[7]

Manasseh Cutler, in his monograph on plants indigenous to New England, mentions that many of the "medical and oeconomical uses" which
he attributes to the plants he describes have been selected "from a late
ingenious and useful publication by William Withering, M.D. entitled,
'The botanical arrangement of British plants.'" Because Cutler completed his paper on January 26, 1784 (although he did not deliver it to
the American Academy of Arts and Sciences until September 2, 1785),

he could not yet have seen Withering's *Account of the Foxglove*. As will be seen later, that volume may not have been available generally in Boston before the end of 1787. I cannot determine how Jackson happened to see it almost two years earlier.[8]

Cutler (1742–1823) was pastor in the parish of Ipswich (now called Hamilton), Massachusetts, at this time. After receiving A.B. and M.A. degrees from Yale, he practiced law and then medicine. He became an honorary member of the Massachusetts Medical Society in 1785, two years after Jackson, and in 1789 Yale awarded Cutler an LL.D. His interests and vocations were many: astronomy, meteorology, and botany, among the natural sciences, as well as teaching, merchandising, exploration (of Ohio), politics, and preaching.[9]

Undoubtedly Withering was correct in thinking that the Reverend Mr. Cutler had mistakenly identified *Digitalis purpurea* in his entry on "Digitatis." Cutler described the plant to which he applied Linnaeus' terminology for *Digitalis purpurea* as red, and as flourishing in moist soil. Perhaps Withering's clues were that the plant's flower is definitely purple, and that it thrives best in dry gravelly or sandy soil. There is no record of whether Jackson did communicate Withering's suspicion of an erroneous identification to Cutler, although he probably did. Jackson and Cutler had met at least once, on October 18, 1773, when Cutler had gone to the smallpox hospital on Cat Island at Marblehead, just after Jackson had become the hospital superintendent. However, Cutler was not inoculated at that time.[10]

Jackson's letter to Withering shows that none of his "acquaintances within twenty miles" had ever seen *Digitalis purpurea* in America, and therefore it is unlikely to have been Cutler's "Digitatis." Jackson's New England friends probably could not have overlooked a flower as showy as the foxglove. Cutler himself found a number of errors in his own paper, for on December 5, 1792, he wrote to Count Luigi Castiglioni, who was then traveling in America: "I have found many errors in my botanical Paper in the Species, which I have also corrected. I have much regretted that I communicated that Paper to the Academy so hastily."[11]

Withering's concept of the role of ardent spirits in the etiology of dropsy differed somewhat from Jackson's. The latter—in predictable early New England fashion, following the established Puritan ethic—blamed the life style of chronic drinkers as well as the biological effects of cheap rum. Jackson's attitude seems typical of the contemporary "dawning suspicion that the American appetite for strong drink might well be endangering the glorious future that was being forecast for the country," as Cassedy has summarized the then developing temperance movement. Withering, on the other hand, who suggested that certain impurities—especially lead, leached from distilling pipes, and essential oils—might be the responsible agents, must have known about the first demonstration of the connection between lead poisoning and Jamaican rum in 1745 by Dr. Thomas Cadwalader (1708–1799) of Philadelphia. To Withering, "an inactive life" in the long, cold New England winters

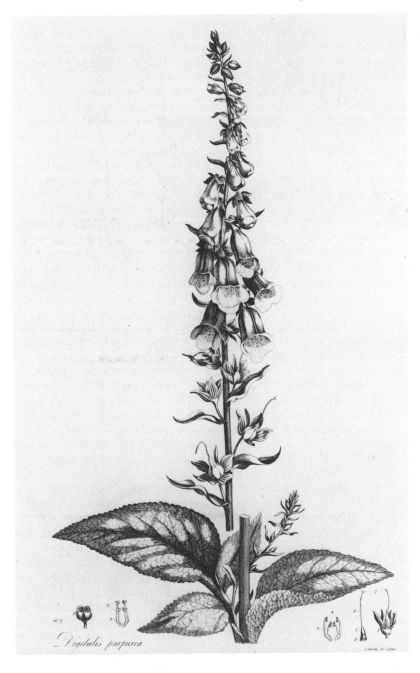

VIII. Digitalis purpurea. *Uncolored frontispiece from a presentation copy of* Withering's *Account of the Foxglove.* (*Courtesy of the Countway Library of Medicine*)

would tend to increase the likelihood of the occurrence of dropsy, but he did not consider it to be causally responsible for the disease.[12]

Although there is no evidence that Jackson ever sent an "account of [his] tryal" of digitalis to Withering, later we will examine what records he did keep of his clinical trials with the drug, perhaps following Withering's example.

The "Society of Philosophic Friends of this place" to whom Withering read Jackson's temperature data, which were abstracted from his "Meteorological Register" (see Chapter 3), was the famous Lunar Society, an informal group that consisted of fourteen Birmingham-area scientists and industrialists (although not all fourteen were members at the same time) who have been called "the harbingers of the Industrial Revolution." Among the joint studies about which they were most enthusiastic was meteorology, and it was probably during a discussion of the measurement of temperature that Withering read Jackson's data to his friends. No formal records of the proceedings of the Lunar Society were kept, but the data must have been read at one of its regular monthly meetings on the Monday nearest the full moon, between March and October 1786.[13]

It is not clear why Withering included the paragraph on the current treatment of intermittent fevers; Jackson did not mention the problem in his letter, and there is no evidence of any other correspondence between them on this or any other subject. Withering probably mentioned the arsenic treatment by way of keeping Jackson informed as to the latest thinking on an important medical problem in England, in the same spirit one always associates with Withering, that of a scientist in the newly awakening era of scientific enlightment, full of enthusiasm not only for his own work but also for publicizing important new advances in any field. His comment on "Reason and Philosophy" supports this appraisal of his thinking.

In writing of the current treatment for intermittent fevers in England, Withering clearly was referring to Thomas Fowler's newly reported arsenic solution. Fowler (1736–1801), both Withering's friend and his successor as physician at Stafford, had just published his treatment for the intermittent fevers in 1786. In his book Fowler included a letter from Withering reporting on forty-eight patients whom he had treated with arsenic. Of these, thirty-six (75 percent) were cured of their fevers, and three (6 percent) exhibited reversible side effects. Fowler, in turn, had encouraged Withering to publish his results with the foxglove.[14]

Withering's postscript suggests that during the fifteen months since the Account of the Foxglove had gone to press, he had come to realize that the drug is likely to be effective in instances of hemoptysis (spitting up blood from the lungs) accompanied by atrial fibrillation with a "quick bounding pulse" (because of a too rapid beating of the upper chambers of the heart). In the book, in reference to the foxglove's cardiac activity, he concludes only that "it has a power over the motions of the heart, to a degree yet unobserved in any other medicine, and that this power may be converted to salutary ends."[15]

That inference must have been based on the effects of digitalis on the pulse, which Withering observed in fourteen of his own 162 cases, and in thirteen of 54 cases sent to him by correspondents. He noted that digitalis provided no clinical benefit to his own patient CXXI, but he included the case "to point out the great effect the Digitalis has upon the heart; for the pulse came down [from 132] to 96." In the case of Mrs. M submitted by Dr. Jonathan Stokes (1755–1831) of Stourbridge, the autopsy and clinical evidence led Stokes to conclude: "The intermitting pulse should seem to have been owing to effusions of water in some of the cavities of the breast, as it disappeared on the removal of the waters." Withering made no comment on this case, perhaps because he continued to assume that the foxglove's principal target organ was the kidney. He had only secondarily observed, during the course of his investigations, that digitalis had an effect on the heart, regardless of whether it also produced diuresis. The letter to Jackson hints, then, that Withering was beginning to think of the heart as at least another site of action of digitalis. Unfortunately, it is not possible to study further the evolution of his thought in this direction, for no extant later Withering manuscripts mention this subject.[16]

Hall Jackson tried to comply with Withering's request that he "distribute it [the foxglove] into other provinces." We can assume that he did send some to Dr. Jones in Virginia. The story of Jackson's efforts to convince his colleagues in New England of the new drug's potential usefulness can be traced in detail among the papers of Dr. Edward Augustus Holyoke of Salem, Massachusetts.

Dr. Holyoke (1728–1829) received the first honorary medical degree awarded by Harvard. By 1786 he had been practicing in Salem for forty years, and would practice there for another forty. He was the first president of the Massachusetts Medical Society (1782–1784), and was serving a second term (1786–1787) when Jackson received the foxglove seeds from Withering. Although his correspondence shows that he became acquainted with the efficacy of digitalis for patients with dropsy, in his scrapbook of news clippings about medical and other items that interested him he included not a single reference to the foxglove, nor do the two clippings indexed under dropsy mention the drug.[17]

Holyoke's most frequent and faithful correspondent was Dr. Nathaniel Walker Appleton (1755–1795) of Boston. Appleton obtained his M.D. degree from Harvard, studied with Dr. Holyoke for a time, and established his practice in Boston in 1780. He was the first recording secretary of the Massachusetts Medical Society, and, with Holyoke, was among its founders, as well as a founder of the American Academy of Arts and Sciences. Appleton was a constant and meticulous recorder of the New England medical scene until he moved to Ohio in 1794, although he did return to Boston shortly before his death.[18]

On October 14, 1786, two weeks before Withering replied to Jackson's letter and about six months before Jackson probably received that reply, Appleton wrote to Holyoke about a patient with ascites and anasarca who was refractory to the usual forms of treatment:

About a fortnight since Dr. [Nathaniel Appleton] Haven [Dr. N. W. Appleton's cousin] of Portsmouth was in town. He mentioned that the physicians there had lately experienced very beneficial results from the use of the *Digitalis purpurea* or Foxglove. First recommended by Dr. Withring as a powerful diuretic. Yesterday I rec'd some of it and propose to give it a trial agreable to Withring's Directions.[19]

Unless Appleton erred in dating his letter (which is likely), this letter would suggest, at least circumstantially, that Jackson had already convinced his colleagues in Portsmouth of the new drug's advantages. If so, not only must he have obtained a supply of digitalis before Withering's seeds reached him, but it was also available in sufficient quantity even then for someone, perhaps Haven, to have been able to spare some for Appleton.

Jackson received Withering's letter in the spring of 1787; soon after, on April 24, he wrote to Holyoke:

from several trials made here, I am fully convinced that neither Doctor Withering or his numerous correspondents have exaggerated its salutary effects: It is perhaps the greatest diuretic in nature, and possesses in a remarkable manner, a power of abating the action of the Heart, and retarding the circulation of the blood. In the last Ship from London and last Post from Boston, I was honored with a very polite, obliging, and interesting letter from Doctor Withering, together with some of the Seeds of the Foxglove... It is with much pleasure I inclose you some of the Seeds. I am perswaded you will have equal pleasure in cultivating the Plant, which besides its utility in medicine, bears a beautiful flower, with a place in any garden...

Presumably Jackson sent the seeds to Holyoke because Holyoke, as president of the Massachusetts Medical Society, would be in a good position to recommend its use to his local colleagues. Jackson may have at least met him, because Jackson was made an honorary member of the Society during Holyoke's first term as its president. Most of Jackson's letter consists of verbatim quotations from Withering, pertaining to methods of administering the drug, and its virtues.[20]

Nine days later (May 3, 1787) Holyoke drafted a reply to Jackson thanking him for the foxglove seeds and saying that he did not understand the exact dosage schedule because "I have not had the pleasure of seeing Dr. Withering's book." Three weeks later, Jackson wrote again to Holyoke, copying out the directions Withering gave in his *Account* for compounding the infusion of digitalis.[21]

Holyoke wrote to Appleton about Jackson's letter on the same day he replied to Jackson. In a letter of May 17, 1787, Appleton refers to Holyoke's letter of two weeks earlier, and goes on:

I had before received some of the Seeds of the *Digit. purpur.* which were sown about 10 Days since in my Father's Garden. I fear that the hard rain will prove injurious to them. Tho they were covered some of the time. Those you sent, I gave to Dr. Gardner to be sown on a proper soil & properly attended. I have run over Dr. Withering's treatise on the *Foxglove* to which you allude. By his acc°. it is a very valuable Medicine. I have tried it in two Cases—to one I gave it in pills made up with Soap—& to the other I have it in Infusion agreably to Withering's Directions. It had no sensible Effect in either...[22]

The busy practitioner had, apparently, given his young former trainee and present fellow officer of the state medical society the tasks of checking out the new report from abroad and of making a clinical trial with the drug. Appleton does not mention the source of his new batch of seeds, nor where he saw the copy of Withering's book (it took him some months to find a copy for Holyoke). Up to that point Appleton was not impressed by the new drug, but we do not know whether the two patients in whom he tried it so unsuccessfully could have been expected to respond to it. He, in turn, asked his colleague Dr. Gardner to try to raise the seeds that Holyoke sent him—probably some of the batch sent by Withering to Jackson. Either Appleton had no facilities for gardening or no inclination toward horticulture. Gardner is most likely Dr. Joseph Gardner (1727–1788), another of the founders of the Massachusetts Medical Society in 1781 and one of Jackson's fellow inoculators at Boston in 1764.[23]

Five months later, on October 10, 1787, Appleton wrote to Holyoke that he had had at least some horticultural success (or his father had):

I shewed [a visitor] the FoxGlove Plants which I have come up in my Father's Garden. They are the first he had seen. They are very flourishing, he advises to gathering some of the leaves for use now, to leave out some of the Roots exposed to the weather... all which I propose to do...P.S. I shall send you some of the Leaves of the *Digitalis purpur*. for Trial.

Within the next twelve days, Appleton harvested and prepared his crop of digitalis leaves: "I now send you by Cousin Harry Appleton a number of the Leaves of the *Digitalis purpur*.: I have not yet been able to get Dr. Withering's Book for you. I am told that II Vol. of Ed: Med: Comment: contains many acc°. of its use in Haemoptoe & Ascites." The recent reference cited by Appleton is a paper by Mr. William Jones, a surgeon of Birmingham. It is written as a letter to Withering, who probably caused it to be printed in the journal. Jones had also contributed a case report to Withering's book two years earlier. Appleton appears not yet to have read the new paper at the time he wrote this letter.[24]

Jackson and Holyoke remained in correspondence during that winter. Upon a request from Holyoke on February 27, 1788, Jackson sent him two lengthy and not very perceptive reports on cases of lockjaw and ophthisthotonos that he had treated successfully. He did not mention foxglove.[25]

Into the spring of 1788 Appleton and Holyoke continued to discuss digitalis. In an undated letter, probably written during this period, Appleton indicated his awareness that the drug's margin of safety is relatively small: "I have at last procured Dr. Withering's Book for you. By what I can learn it is necessary to be very cautious as to the Dose & to attend closely to it's operation." At least the book was now available in Boston.[26]

On February 8 Appleton inquired about Holyoke's clinical success with the drug. On March 20 Appleton could at least claim that he had observed a drug effect from the administration of digitalis, confirming Withering's assertion that digitalis stimulates salivation in some persons; but he did not mention specifically whether the patient's dropsical symptoms were relieved: "I have lately tried the *Digitalis* I think with success, it appeared to bring on a ptyalism [salivation]." And a year later Appleton had a patient whose urine output did not increase after treatment with digitalis, but who suffered only nausea and vomiting.[27]

In the early summer of 1790 Holyoke must have written to Jackson requesting further information about digitalis, as well as more supplies of the drug, for on July 12, 1790, Jackson replied to Holyoke:

> I ... am happy that I have it in my power to comply with your request; have sent you some of the leaves of the Foxglove for present use, and some of the seeds for cultivation; I find no difficulty in raising it. I sow the seeds in the spring and take no further care of it until the next spring, when I transplant it, only for the sake of giving it good room and placing it in some agreable situating in the garden, for when in full bloom it has a very pleasing appearance ... I have always made a practice to keep a kind of diary or journal of particular cases that occurred in the course of my business, and have found myself fully compensated for my troubles ... I have used the Foxglove in a great number of cases, it has for the most part answered my expectations, whenever I had a plausible right to expect relief from any medication whatsoever ...

Apparently Holyoke had not yet tried to grow the plant himself, and had finally decided it might be useful to do so.[28]

Along with his letter to Holyoke, Jackson sent descriptions of his "particular cases" in which he had used digitalis. None of these cases can be identified among the deaths listed in the "Meteorological Register," but the journal is, of course, less detailed, and was kept for another purpose altogether. In his summary report Jackson describes eleven patients to whom he had administered digitalis. It is a rather formal document, consisting of two folded foolscap pages sewn in the centerfold to make an eight-page booklet, which is transcribed below:

SOME CASES OF THE ADMINISTRATION OF THE FOXGLOVE

The wife of Mr. Josiah Dow of Lee, aged 30 years, was naturally very corpulent, in the 8th month of her pregnancy, had her legs, thighs & belly enlarged to an astonishing degree, and so hard no impression could be made on them. She had taken squills, nitre, crystals of tartar & other medicines: She made but little urine. She took 1 gn: of the powder of foxglove at night, and a slight infusion of the same in the morning; after a few days she became faint, oppressed &c: her urine much increased; the medicine was discontinued hoping for a more favorable opportunity of administering it after delivery; she unexpectedly went her full time, was delivered of a dead child, and she died a few days after.

Jones of Portsmouth, a labouring man, 50 years of age, naturally of a good construction and not intemperate in his manner of living, early in the winter fell into an anasarcous dropsy; his legs, thighs, scrotum and penis greatly enlarged; he made but little urine; he took 2 gn: foxglove night and morning for 8 days, had a proper discharge of urine; in three weeks with the use of the Bark he was perfectly cured.

Zachariah Browne of Hampton, aged 70 years, in the same condition as Jones, only much worse, obtained the same relief as speedily and effectually by the use of the foxglove taken in powder; there was no visible effects of the medicine in. either of these cases, but in the profuse discharge of urine.

On the 8th day of March I was desired to visit Miss Lidia Pukernail, a maiden of about 57 years of age, who resided with her brother Mr. Nelson Pukernail, in Kittery. She had been confined with the dropsy during the winter, was given over by her physician. The application was more out of ceremony than an expectation that any relief could be afforded her: Her face, arms and hands were those of a skeleton, her countenance ghastly, her belly, thighs, and legs big to an incredible degree, and very transparent; her difficulty of breathing in a reclined posture was so great she had not laid down in her bed for a long time, nor was there the least reasonable hope for her surviving many days; some slight scarifications were made on her legs which discharged a considerable quantity of water; the scarifications soon inflamed, became very painful, with an alarming appearance; they soon, however, alter'd for the better by the application of a fermenting cataplasm; She was directed to take two grains of foxglove in powder, night and morning and to continue it until the effects of it were perceived; after six days, she became very sick, faint, giddy, and her vision confused, the medicine was omitted; her urine greatly increased, her breathing relieved; her body lessened; after the effects of the medicine were gone off she was directed to take it again, sometimes in powder, sometimes in an infusion, and she continued in a course of taking and omitting, as occasion required, until June 4th, when she had little or no appearance of the dropsy excepting in her legs, which were smaller tho' considerably ulcerated in the scarifications. Her breathing was free, and she could rest well in her bed; her countenance and appetite good, and she continued in a fair way of recovery until August 20th, when she was seized with a violent pain in her right side, fever, and great difficulty of breathing, and died the 7th day after this attack. The lung was evidently the Seat of her last complaints, and it is more than probable her liver was distressed.

Mrs. Meriam, the wife of the Revd. Mr. Meriam of Berwick, had for some time been under a dropsical habit, she had taken mercury, squills, nitre, crystals of tartar, and many other medicines to no good effect. Her legs, feet, and abdomen were much swelled, she made not more than 12 ounces of Water in 24 hours. July 21st she took 1½ gn: of foxglove in powder, and continued morning and evening for 8 days. It had no sensible operation or effect; July 31st she began on an infusion of the dried leaves, 1 dram in 8 ounces of water, and 2 ounces of geneva [gin] added to the strained liquor, [in a] dose [of] 1 ounce twice a day. After the fourth day she made three quarts of water in the night, and half that quantity in the day, and continued to do the same for eight days. When the swelling in the abdomen had decreased 11 inches, the swelling of the legs and feet nearly gone, a difficulty of breathing which had prevented her from laying down in bed for a long time was wholly relieved; a preparation of steel, and bark, with a flannel wastcoat next the skin was recommended as the weather became cool, since which time (near 12 months) she has had no occasion to apply for medicines or advice.

The wife of Mr. Joseph Marden of Portsmouth [being] under an ascites, took the foxglove. It had no effect on the disorder; she was tapped and died soon after.

A Lady in Portsmouth 40 years of age who had enjoyed a good share of health suddenly lost her appetite, complained of great oppression, difficulty of breathing —could not lay down in bed, her countenance became palid and dejected, and she emaciated very fast; the disorder was supposed to be an asthma, the more so as some of her relations had been afflicted with it. At length her feet, legs and thig[h]s became swelled and very oedematous; and she perceived herself considerably enlarged in the waist; the disorder was now pronounced dropsical, and the difficulty of breathing from an effusion in the thorax; she made but little urine; every other medicine was now laid aside and half an ounce of the infusion of foxglove evening and morning was substituted instead; it soon had the desired effect, proved sufficiently diuretic, and removed every symptom of the disorder. She has now regained her flesh, and in the course of 12 months she has had no returns of the oppression and difficulty of breathing, but has always been relieved by the foxglove; the swelling of the feet, &c. never returned.

The wife of Mr. John Tobey, aged 45 years, under an ascites, took the foxglove as freely as it could with safety be urged; it had no effect on the urine; she was tapped, a large quantity of coagulated lymph was taken away; the greatest part remained, it being too thick to pass thro' the canula of a trocar purposely made three times larger than the common size. She survived six weeks after this operation, and died wasted to a skeleton.

A negro woman near 40 years of age laboured under an asthma; and swelled legs; she took the foxglove, it was effectually diuretic, her difficulty of breathing and the swellings of her legs were entirely improved; she some months after fell into an ascites—when the foxglove had no effect, she was tapped 11 times in the course of 15 months; 9 quarts of water were taken away one time with another; she died soon after the last tapping, entirely wasted.

Capt. Samuel Shapleigh of Kittery, a Bachelor 60 years of age, who from a sedentary inactive life become exceedingly corpulent, and unhealthy, his legs and thighs were somewhat swelled; his scrotum and penis from an effusion in the cellular membranes were enlarged to an astonishing degree; the largest ox-bladder could not be blown to near the size of the scrotum. The penis was in like proportion and so distorted that the glans penis turned quite backward, the little water he made appeared to flow from a cavity at the bottom of his belly in which the penis was almost wholly buried; the scrotum was hard and so discoloured that any scarification on the part was judged unadvisable; Two grains of foxglove was directed to be taken in a pill evening and morning, and an ounce of the infusion at noon. In eight days his urine flowed involuntary in so large a quantity as in one night to run thro' a thick blanket folded under him, a pail, and stood in a pool on the floor. This profuse discharge of urine continued until he was reduced to his common size, and is at present in tolerable health; he took no other medicine excepting two purges of Jalap with cream of tartar.

Mr. Josiah Norton of Kittery had great oppression and difficulty of breathing with swelled oedematous legs and thighs, was relieved with the foxglove.

Enclosed is a letter from Doctor Barker, a gentleman of eminence in his profession in Portland [illegible], with an account of the foxglove in the case of Capt. Frickey of that Place. I have also a letter from a gentleman of Conway informing me that Thomas Merrell Esqr: of that place, who was past all hope of recovery under an anasarcous dropsy, with great oppression and difficulty of breathing [,] was effectually relieved by the foxglove when every other remedy had failed; that he continued in tolerable health for some months; being threatened with a return of the disorder, applied for another supply of the medicine; since which have not heard from him.

The foxglove cases here related were of the latter part of the year 1786, and beginning of 1787 [,] the others since that time. These cases were all minuted from time to time as they occured, that from a comparative view of the unsuccessful cases a just estimate of the virtues of a medicine so highly recommended might be obtained; and from a consideration of the foregoing facts it cannot be doubted that the foxglove is a powerful diuretic and efficacious remedy in most cases of anasarca and cellular effusions. Dropsies of the abdomen, more especially those in female subjects, are generally of the encysted kind. The absorbent vessels cannot be made to act on the fluid, consequently diuretics or other remedies are ineffectual, besides, it is probable that in most cases of ascites, there is incurable glandular disease of the abdomen. Doctor Withering and his correspondents whose veracity cannot be doubted, recite many cases of acites cured by the foxglove, but in the trials made here we have not been so fortunate.

The foxglove has been administered in several other disorders, some cases of Haemoptoe, one of insanity, one profuse and continued bleeding at the nose, but as it was accompanied by the use of other remedies it cannot with any degree of certainty be determined what share it might have in affording the relief that was obtained.[29]

Of these eleven cases, eight (73 percent) were relieved of their dropsical symptoms (although two of them died later, presumably from the underlying disease responsible for their dropsies), and only one of the eleven (9 percent) showed side effects (nausea, vomiting, and confused vision). These incidences are much like those reported by Withering (see Chapter 5 and Table 25). At the end of his report to Dr. Holyoke, Jackson shows that he is aware of the necessity of administering only one drug at a time to determine its clinical utility.[30]

In his July 12th communication to Holyoke, Jackson also included an unsolicited testimonial from the husband of one of his patients. The Reverend Matthew Merriam wrote from Berwick, Maine, a few miles upriver from Portsmouth:

After so long experience of the beneficial effects of the foxglove it is high time that I should express my gratitude for your goodness in favouring Mrs. Merriam with so efficacious a remedy for the dropsy ...It appears to be provided and designed by the great author of nature as a remedy exactly fitted for such a disease...[31]

Jackson concluded his covering letter to Holyoke with a reasonably accurate prediction of the foxglove's course over the next century or so, but it is difficult to tell whether he was being cynical or merely realistic:

I doubt not but the Foxglove will in time share the fate of many other valuable remedies. They are first used with great success in cases where they are with propriety applicable. We become too sanguine, and depend on them in cases that are incurable, out of the reach of any medicine whatever. We find ourselves sadly disappointed and forgetful of our former success, begin to look on the medicine with indifference, it grows into disrepute, and finally becomes totally neglected.[32]

Appleton and Holyoke discussed by letter what might be done with Jackson's report to Holyoke. In all likelihood Jackson had no intention other than communicating his results and recommendations to the elder statesman of New England medicine, a conclusion also reached by Appleton, to whom Holyoke had sent Jackson's correspondence: "So far as I can judge by once running over the Letter I do not see that it was his intention to have them [the letter and accompanying papers] communicated [to the Massachusetts Medical Society].[33]

It remained unclear to Appleton for the next several months whether it was Holyoke's intention that Jackson's letter be read at the April 1791 meeting of the Society. On March 11 Appleton asked Holyoke: "Is it your intention to communicate [Jackson's report] to the Soc^y, at their next meeting, which will be on 13th of next month[?]." And on April 5 Appleton replied to a conjecture by Holyoke: "as to Dr. Jackson's [paper] I have some doubts as to his intentions."[34] The matter seems to have been resolved without actually determining the wishes of either Jackson or Holyoke. In Appleton's letter of April 18 reporting to Holyoke the proceedings of the Society's meeting five days earlier, there is no mention that Jackson's cases were, in fact, communicated to the Society.[35]

In the meantime, Holyoke had been trying digitalis on some of his own patients, for on April 26, 1791, Appleton wrote to him: "[I] note that you write respecting the happy effects of the Digitalis. I wish you may continue to experience it." Perhaps Holyoke had become a convert. But because his practice is reputed to have been based largely on the use of mercury, antimony, opium, and quinine, it is unlikely that digitalis ever became a standard feature of his personal materia medica. The tenor of the latter suggests that Holyoke might have taken digitalis himself; he was 63 years old. When he died 37 years later, however, his heart was found to be in perfect condition.[36]

Holyoke may have encouraged others to use digitalis. In 1799 Dr. Jeremiah Barker (1752–1835) wrote to him from Portland, Maine, that Holyoke's directions for administering the decoction of digitalis had been successful: "Have the pleasure to inform you that Digitalis has done wonders in Cpt. J[illegible]'s case."[37]

Some years later the drug was used with good results in a member of Holyoke's own family. In 1813 Dr. Isaac Rand of Boston wrote about his treatment of Holyoke's daughter, Mrs. William Turner, who appears to have had tuberculosis:

> The digitalis produced faintness, depression of spirits & sickness of the stomach, and did not lessen the frequency of the pulse [it had ranged from 92 to 110] ... I have never observed any advantage from the digitalis purpur. unless it lessen the number of pulses in a minute, notwithstanding I have a good opinion of its effects in this disease.

It can be inferred from this, too, that digitalis was by then, twenty-seven years after Withering's letter to Jackson, well known to the doctors of Boston. Dr. Rand's appreciation of clinical indices of the drug's therapeutic effect was reasonably accurate. Two weeks later Rand wrote that Mrs. Turner had improved on a regimen of myrrh, digitalis, and quinine, and that digitalis had, after all, decreased the pulse moderately.[38]

Isaac Rand (1743–1822) had studied medicine with his father, Dr. Isaac Rand of Charlestown, and Dr. James Lloyd, Boston's first obstetrician. Rand's specialty, too, was obstetrics. He was another cofounder of the Massachusetts Medical Society and served as its president from 1798 to 1804. In 1804 he delivered the Society's annual discourse, a paper on phthisis pulmonalis (tuberculosis) and the use of digitalis in its treatment (see Chapter 5).[39]

Jackson did not limit his attempts to promote the use of the foxglove to Dr. Holyoke and his circle. He wrote to Dr. James Thacher (1754–1844) of Plymouth, the early biographer of American physicians, on April 29, 1789:

> With much pleasure I send you seeds of foxglove and some of the leaves of the same for your trial of its efficacy until you can cultivate it. It is a beautiful flower in a garden, and has arrived at full perfection in my garden from seeds sent me by Dr. Withering.[40]

Thacher may have known of Withering's book either at first hand or through previous communication with Jackson. By 1817 he considered digitalis to be the drug of choice for the treatment of dropsy.[41]

On April 30, 1787, a week after he first wrote to Holyoke, Jackson sent some of Withering's newly arrived foxglove seeds to the Reverend Ezra Stiles (1727–1795), president of Yale College from 1778 until his death, along with appropriate quotations from Withering's letter. Although Stiles was not a physician, Jackson sent the seeds to him because, as a college president in the young republic, he would have had sufficient intellectual authority among the doctors in Connecticut, none of whom

Jackson knew, to encourage trials with the drug. Jackson had known Stiles at least moderately well, for he had lived in Portsmouth about ten months before moving to New Haven, and Jackson would have been familiar with Stiles's many other scientific interests. Although no further correspondence between Stiles and Jackson has been found, Stiles at least attempted to propagate the seeds. On a margin of Jackson's letter he noted that he sowed the seed in his garden on June 6, 1787. Stiles also tried to propagate the letter's message; he probably contributed it to *The American Museum, or Repository of Ancient and Modern Fugitive Pieces* for 1788.[42]

Although the occasion of the purposeful introduction of digitalis to medical therapeutics in America can be ascribed with certainty to the Jackson-Withering correspondence of 1786, the very first arrival of the plant in the North American colonies cannot be ascertained so precisely. A considerable body of negative evidence shows that foxglove did not grow wild in the United States prior to the early nineteenth century. The earliest botanical catalogues of North America—such as John Banister's (1680) and John Clayton's (1739)—contain no reference to anything that can be substantiated as digitalis.

As late as 1781 Thomas Jefferson did not mention foxglove as being found in Virginia among "those trees, plants, fruits, etc.... which would principally attract notice as being 1. Medicinal, 2. Esculent, 3. Ornamental, or 4. Useful for fabrication." Even if Jefferson had not known of foxglove's pharmacologic properties, that astute observer of both natural and political history would have recognized such a striking plant for its ornamental properties. The earliest documented mention of its escape to the wild is from a stand originally planted in New York state in 1820.[43]

Foxglove apparently was not cultivated in seventeenth-century American gardens, but it had been introduced into a few colonial gardens by the 1740's. John Custis (1678–1749) of Williamsburg, Virginia, was among several colonists who carried on extensive correspondences with Peter Collinson (1694–1768), at the time one of England's leading botanists. His American correspondents often sent plants to Collinson for identification and propagation at his botanic garden at Mill Hill, near London, but he also sent English plants to the colonies. In 1737, probably on May 28, Custis wrote to Collinson:

> I have a plant you sent last year that bears a [flatt?] stalk full of white long hollow blossoms. I forgot the name; that and the sage tree were the only things that braved our intolerable hard frosts and do believe they would live in Greenland; should be glad to know the name of the long white hollow flower.[44]

Collinson thought that he had sent what we now know as *Digitalis lanata*; on December 5, 1737, he replied:

> The White Flower by your description I take to be the White Fox Glove. I am glad you have it, for it is a rare flower with us and in

fewe Gardens. I sent the seed without hope but on Experim't for it will not keep long unsown—but as you are so Lucky to have it make much of it—it generally sows itself which generally makes the best plants.

The following year, about the time when seeds of a biennial sown in 1736 would have been expected to flower, Custis wrote (on or before July 18, 1738): "the fox glove thrives very well, and blossoms very full..." Later that year or perhaps the next, Custis listed for his own records "What Seed I planted or sow'd." The list included the "rose colored fox glove." Perhaps he had acquired *Digitalis purpurea* by then.[45]

In 1748 the Swedish naturalist Peter Kalm (1715–1779) was traveling in North America. While visiting Philadelphia, on October 18 of that year, he recorded in his journal: "Plants in blossom. At present I did not find above ten different kinds of plants in blossom: they [included] ...the foxglove, or Digitalis purpurea..." It is unlikely that a student of Linnaeus' would have identified such an unusual plant erroneously.[46]

Three years later the most noted and influential of all the early American botanists, John Bartram (1699–1777), who lived near Philadelphia, added a preface and running commentary to an American reprint of Thomas Short's 1746 *Medicina Britannica*. In a footnote to the entry on *Digitalis purpurea* Bartram wrote: "This species of Digitalis, grows only in curious Gardens with us in America." At least we can be sure it was being cultivated in gardens of mid-eighteenth century Philadelphia. Bartram, who was another of Peter Collinson's many colonial correspondents, wrote to his English colleague and fellow Quaker on June 24, 1760: "The seed thee sent last fall was choice good and most of them came up...I hope the yellow foxglove...is come up." Perhaps Bartram was referring to what we would now call *Digitalis lutea*.[47]

In his *British Herbal* of 1756 Dr. John Hill of London (1707–1775), the first Englishman to recognize the significance of Linnaeus' work, wrote that *Digitalis perfoliata* is a "native of Virginia." However, the accompanying plate is of a plant most likely to be *Gerardia*, or *Agalinis*; it certainly is not a member of the genus *Digitalis*.[48]

Caspar Wistar (1760–1818), the distinguished anatomist at Philadelphia, wrote in 1787 to Humphrey Marshall (1722–1801), another noted Philadelphia botanist and a cousin of John Bartram, about Withering's *Account*, which must have arrived in Philadelphia not long before:

> I send a treatise on the effects of the Foxglove...Dr. M. will be pleased to find that he is in possession of a plant of such efficacy, and perhaps will cultivate a greater quantity of it...The book is in great demand...If you have any of the plant to spare, I will be much obliged for a few leaves of it, and also a few seeds...I cannot omit mentioning, that a patient in the Edinburgh Infirmary, who took the medicine as directed by Dr. Withering, vomited to death. This determined me to avoid the medicine; but dropsies are so often fatal, that we must try everything.

"Dr. M." is Dr. Moses Marshall (1758–1813), Humphrey's nephew, and himself a botanist. In the same year that Withering published his *Account*, Humphrey Marshall had published his *Arbustrum Americanum*, the first work on American plants by a native American printed in this country. It is not clear that Wistar would try the new drug on his patients, and no evidence that he or the younger Marshall did use it has been found. The plant is not included in the herbarium specimens of either Humphrey or Moses Marshall.[49]

Dr. William P. C. Barton (1786–1856) did not include it in his 1818 catalog of "indigenous and naturalized plants within ten mile radius of Philadelphia," nor did Dr. John Torrey (1796–1873) in his similar list of plants growing around New York. In his 1829 manual, Amos Eaton (1776–1842) listed *Digitalis purpurea*, but did not indicate whether it was cultivated or wild.[50]

In New England, Boston's Dr. Benjamin Waterhouse did not include a specimen of digitalis in the dried botanical collection he made around 1800, and Dr. Jacob Bigelow (1787–1879) did not list the foxglove among the plants he found growing around Boston as late as 1840. Bigelow surely would have included this striking medicinal plant had it grown in the vicinity; he, with Lyman Spalding, was among the five editors of the first *United States Pharmacopoeia* (1820).[51]

Bigelow in his 1822 *Sequel to the United States Pharmacopoeia* had noted that digitalis was not native to the United States but was easily cultivated. He remarked that the best specimens of the plant in this country were raised by the Shakers, which suggests that the drug was in large-scale commercial preparation by then, for the Shakers were the leading wholesale purveyors of medicinal plants. About thirty-five years after its introduction to American medicine, digitalis had therefore gone into wholesale production, which provides one kind of testimony to the drug's acceptance as medically valuable therapy.[52]

It appears, then, that upon receiving a supply of foxglove seeds from Withering, Hall Jackson wrote to a number of prominent physicians and scientists around the country, sending each a number of the precious seeds. He certainly sent some to Holyoke, Thacher, and Stiles, and probably to Cutler and Jones. He may have sent some to Dr. Solomon Drowne (1753–1834), who was practicing in Providence. Although there is no mention of Jackson in the extensive collection of Drowne papers at Brown University, the two surgeons very likely met during the Revolutionary War when they were both stationed in Providence. Drowne did have foxglove plants in his large botanical garden at Union, Pennsylvania, at least as early as 1792–94. Whether Jackson sent foxglove seeds to any other American physicians, especially those at the country's leading medical center, Philadelphia, is not known, but he probably did send some to other physicians, or at least drew their attention to Withering's *Account*.[53]

Some of Jackson's letters to his patients show that he administered the new wonder drug in exactly the same way and for the same clinical indications as those Withering had recommended. Jackson informed a

Boston gentleman that his wife should exploit the same supportive measures that Withering had suggested, and that she should take cream of tartar and squill rather than digitalis, because if she did not have dropsy, no benefit could be expected from digitalis. Jackson appears to have followed Withering's guidelines rather strictly.[54]

The Jackson-Holyoke-Appleton correspondence shows that Hall Jackson was the first to persevere in making known the effects of digitalis in the New England states at least. William Plumer, even if not a physician, recognized Jackson's contribution when he noted that Jackson "was one of the earliest, if not the first physician who introduced the culture and use of foxglove into New England." Although he may not have been the very first to introduce it as a drug to America, there is no conclusive evidence to support any other claim of pride of place, and he was clearly the first to take active measures to ensure its incorporation into the remedies regularly available to patients with dropsy.[55].

CHAPTER SEVEN

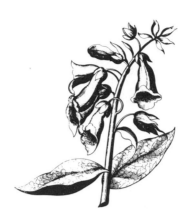

# Patterns and Conclusions

THE NINETEENTH CENTURY witnessed an insistence that digitalis should provide effective therapy for consumption—tuberculosis—in spite of the accumulation of discouraging data. Ackerknecht has ascribed the attempts to use digitalis for noncardiological diseases, during the century after Withering's book appeared, as an example of physicians' age-old and still fruitless search for a true panacea, a wonder drug that will cure every disease.[1]

Another explanation is suggested by the fact that of all those who published more than mere anecdotal case reports of the use of digitalis, about two thirds had earned their M.D. degrees at Edinburgh or at Philadelphia, the two anchors of the influential transatlantic medical axis. It is clear that physicians trained in the wake of Boerhaave, through Cullen and Rush, had good reason to think that they could use digitalis in the treatment of patients with consumption and other conditions they regarded as diseases arising from pathological weaknesses of some part of the body.[2]

We have seen that William Hamilton based his concept of the mechanism of action of digitalis in consumption on the premise that its ability to slow the heart prevents the growth of tubercles by diminishing their blood supply, while facilitating reabsorption of the morbid material at the same time. Other American inheritors of the Edinburgh tradition would have agreed with William Currie's reflection of the same concept:

> The healing of an ulcer is supposed by eminent teachers to depend on procuring an absorption on its surface greater than the secretion or deposition of purulent matter, and those medicines which induce nausea and sickness having been observed to produce this effect, and the digitalis in particular to an eminent degree . . . [digitalis is the drug of choice in consumption].[3]

Ackerknecht, noting that Thomas Beddoes, "a man of many therapeutic enthusiasms, became the main promoter of this misuse of digitalis," argues that because digitalis is now known to be a "specific for heart disease," so should it have been to eighteenth-century physicians.[4] With the advantage of hindsight it is all too easy to fault our professional predecessors. Conscientious and responsible physicians of all centuries—and we have no reason for omitting Beddoes from that group—can apply only the best physiological and therapeutic principles that they can know. Thus Beddoes, along with Currie, Ferriar, Bailey, Hamilton, Rand, and Coxe, as we have seen, all had good reason to employ digitalis in the treatment of their consumptive patients.

By 1775 American physicians had already brought English medical education to incipient fruition in the colonies, providing sufficient backlog and confidence to permit the expansion of American training facilities after the war. That many American doctors had been politically active in the drive for independence made it inevitable that nationalism would lead to some resentment toward America's intellectual dependence on England and Europe. But it was not an irrational or overly emotional resentment, and the lines of scientific communication were back in operation long before the two countries were at lasting peace with each other, as often happens within the international scientific community. This facet of international cooperation provided the essential stepping stone for the history of the foxglove in America.

It is difficult to follow all the routes by which knowledge of digitalis spread throughout the medical profession in the years following 1785. In Figure 10, however, I have tried to illustrate all the known and presumptive routes by which the drug was publicized during the forty years after Withering began his studies of its clinical efficacy. The dates given in parentheses are of the publications of the journal articles or books (the latter are underlined) written by the men listed.

Many of the pathways illustrated go on for no more than two "generations," although some can be traced for three. In only one instance was a purposeful block imposed, that which precluded the reading of Hall Jackson's case reports to the Massachusetts Medical Society in 1790. For all the rest, interest in digitalis seems to have just petered out, for reasons that will become apparent.

Because not all medical practitioners in America had academic training and degrees, it might be assumed that fewer learned about new drugs from the published literature at that time than now. Probably the same factors influenced drug acceptance from 1785 to 1820 as now, and in roughly the same order of importance: professional "opinion leaders," both those known socially and those known through their writings; verbal communication, including advertising; and personal observation of both product effectiveness and product quality.[5]

For instance, both William Withering and Hall Jackson were demonstrably opinion leaders among their colleagues in Birmingham and Portsmouth, respectively. Of the two, only Withering was an opinion leader through the medical literature, as were Maclean, Beddoes, Lettsom,

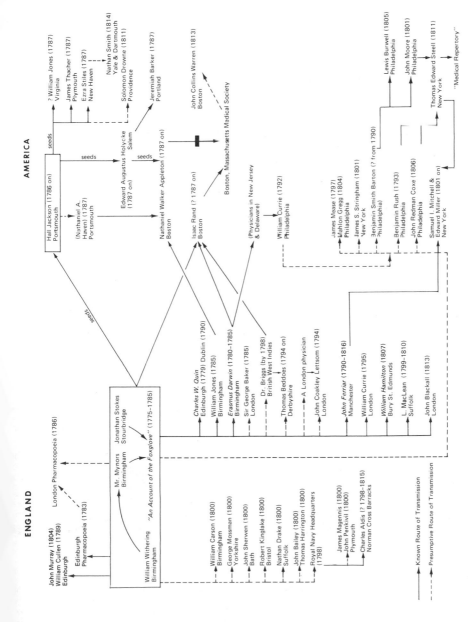

FIG. 10. *Documented routes of transmission of new knowledge about digitalis, 1775–1815. Dotted lines represent routes reconstructed on the basis of presumptive connections, and solid lines represent routes reconstructed on the basis of evidence contained in each publication. The dates in parentheses are of the publications by each physician. All are discussed in the text.*

Rand, and Rush. Drug advertising directed to physicians was not developed in the late eighteenth century to the extent that it would be in the late nineteenth and again in the mid-twentieth centuries.[6]

We cannot assume that digitalis gained official status in America, its admission to the first *United States Pharmacopoeia*, solely because of its virtues as extolled in the medical literature. Although the succession of reports asserting its efficacy may have provided confirmatory evidence to the compilers of the *U.S.P.*—and it should be remembered that proof of efficacy was not a requirement for any entry in that list—digitalis was probably included in the compendium because it was also listed in the Edinburgh and then the London *Pharmacopoeias*, as a direct result of Withering's work.

The first official drug compendium in America, the *Pharmacopoeia Simplicorum* (sometimes known as the "Lititz Pharmacopoeia"), was assembled in 1778 for the Continental Army by Dr. William Brown (d. 1792) of Virginia. Digitalis does not appear among the approximately one hundred preparations listed in the first or second (1781) editions, because at that time digitalis was not an official preparation anywhere.[7] But by 1787 the foxglove had become official in the *Pharmacopoeias* of Edinburgh and London, the pacesetters for therapeutics in the English-speaking world. In 1808, then, we are not surprised to find digitalis included in the *Pharmacopoeia of the Massachusetts Medical Society*, which was based largely on the British pharmacopoeias.[8] We cannot even hazard a guess as to what extent Hall Jackson's missionary zeal facilitated the drug's acceptance among members of the Society. Nor can we know whether the drug was included *only* because it had appeared in the earlier European pharmacopoeias, even though that is likely to have been the case. And by this time Jackson and many others had had ample opportunity to evaluate the foxglove's medical virtues in their own patients.

Eight years later digitalis appeared in the pharmacopoeia of the New York Hospital and, finally, in the 1820 *United States Pharmacopoeia*, of which Boston's Jacob Bigelow was among the editors, as well as Lyman Spalding, formerly of Portsmouth (although he lived there after Jackson's death). All three of these early pharmacopoeias gave the same directions for preparing the infusion: spirit of cinnamon was added to make the otherwise acrid medicine more palatable. Only the *U.S.P.* included the tincture (alcohol extract) of digitalis as an official drug.[9]

Jawetz has postulated that four discrete stages mark the establishment of a new drug within the profession: discovery and enthusiasm, initial stabilization, disappointment, and final stabilization.[10] In this sequence, outlined for digitalis in Figure 11, approval of a new drug first rises very rapidly to its highest peak; it then wanes to a lower plateau; next, professional approval declines precipitately but then rises to a new final plateau that is lower than the first one. Jawetz' models are the antibiotics, and the story of chloramphenicol comes first to mind as an appropriate illustration.[11]

For the antibiotics in particular, the disappointment phase may be associated with the discovery of unanticipated side effects as much as with unfulfilled therapeutic promise. Final stabilization often awaits the ascertainment of the drug's most appropriate and safest selectivity of action. For instance, disappointment in chloramphenicol, introduced in 1948, was precipitated by a series of reports, beginning in 1952, of bone marrow toxicity associated with its use; final stabilization occurred only after the drug's recommended spectrum of action had been limited to typhoid fever and the rickettsial diseases, for which other drugs are often less efficacious. The medical literature of the 1950's and 1960's reflected this pattern for chloramphenicol, in the published data as well as in the profession's almost horrified response to chloramphenicol-induced aplastic anemia. Understanding this, Jawetz cautioned that "Awareness of this pattern of response will permit the physician to evaluate a new agent according to the successive phases and to avoid unwarranted optimism or undue disappointment." [12]

Approval of digitalis in medical therapeutics followed much the same evolutionary pattern. After the first publication about the drug provided all the data necessary at the time to permit its introduction in 1785, enthusiasm for it waxed strongly to its greatest peak by about 1800, on both sides of the Atlantic. Hall Jackson was the leading American participant in this crest of enthusiasm. By 1820 the foxglove had become firmly established in the national pharmacopoeias.

The phase of disappointment had at least begun by 1832, when Sir Charles Aldis wrote in a book that had nothing to do with either dropsy or foxglove that the latter "is nearly become obsolete, though some years since nothing could be more fashionable; and miracles were almost ascribed to its potent agency." [13] In this case, however, it was not the foxglove's propensity for causing dangerous side effects that led to its

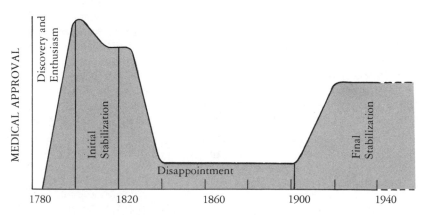

FIG. 11. *Summary of the historical fluctuations of the medical profession's collective "approval" of digitalis, based on Jawetz' model as described in the text.*

abandonment, but its apparent ineffectiveness in curing consumption, the chief public health problem of the time, as Aldis recognized.

We have noted that both Hall Jackson and James Mease feared that the foxglove would fall out of professional favor if more were expected of it than the drug could deliver. And by the 1830's their fear had begun to be realized. In 1835 A. L. J. Bayle of Paris compiled all the case reports in which digitalis had been used and reviewed the existing literature. His results (omitting Withering's data) are tabulated below:

| Diagnostic Category | Number of Cases | Cured or Helped | Not Cured |
|---|---|---|---|
| Dropsy, other forms of Edema | 144 | 91% | 9% |
| Other heart disease | 18 | 61% | 39% |
| Phthisis (consumption) | 151 | 78% | 22% |
| Scrofula | 11 | 100% | 0% |
| Other pulmonary disease | 16 | 50% | 50% |
| Central nervous system disease | 13 | 53% | 46% |
| Miscellaneous | 9 | 67% | 33% |
| (All nondropsical diseases) | (218) | (74%) | (26%) |

Bayle studied his compilation and found himself forced to ask why, if digitalis helps so many patients, is it not prescribed more often than it is? The data do show that the drug helped more patients with dropsy than with any other disease in which it had been employed, and that the treatment failure rate among dropsical patients was only one third the failure rate among patients with other diseases. Bayle's own answer was that treatment failures are not commonly reported, and that new clinical trials were not, in recent years, being reported.[14]

Even Hall Jackson came to the logical conclusion that digitalis should be effective for the treatment of consumption. He had taught his pupil Jabez Dow that digitalis is a "certain Diuretic in Dropsy," and that it "greatly reduces the force of the circulation, sometimes terminating in syncope [fainting] and convulsions." But Dow also observed that his mentor used the drug for "cases of Tubercles of the Lungs and all debilities consequent to inflammation of that organ."[15]

By mid-century, digitalis was regarded by textbook authors as a nervous sedative, and a poor one at that, following the same kind of reasoning as Thomas Edward Steell had used. George B. Wood (1797–1879), a distinguished Philadelphia physician, noted, in 1860, that:

> At one time digitalis had a high reputation in phthisis, and great success was apparently met with, in the cure of the disease, by its use. The journals teemed with favourable reports of its efficiency. It is needless to say that, with the imperfect means then existing of diagnosticating thoracic disease, chronic catarrh and other affections of the chest were not unfrequently confounded with geniune tuberculous consumption, and that the cases cured belonged in all probability to the former category. No one now expects to cure

phthisis with digitalis... although there are occasions, in the course of phthisis, in which the remedy may be advantageously resorted to as a palliative...

It would be another twenty-two years before Robert Koch in Germany would discover the bacterium that causes tuberculosis, finally proving that consumption is an infectious disease.[16]

It appears that the failure of digitalis to fulfill its earlier promise, which had been predicated on current concepts of the pathogenesis of consumption, accounts for the onset of the medical profession's sense of disappointment in the drug. If it could not provide dependable treatment for patients with the major public health problem of the nineteenth century, the reasoning seems to have been, then perhaps digitalis was not even helpful in dropsy. Despite Withering's unequivocal demonstration of the drug's efficacy in dropsy, his specific recommendations had been widely forgotten a hundred years later. Not until the early twentieth century, when new methods for studying heart disease became available, could digitalis begin its ascent into the period of final stabilization among the medical profession's tools.

Franz Ingelfinger has emphasized the medical journal editor's concern with newsworthiness as a criterion for publication.[17] We can exploit this hypothesis to explore further the implications of publishing patterns for studying the applicability of Jawetz' model to the history of digitalis.

The accumulation of books and papers mentioning digitalis in their titles from 1785 to 1820 is shown in Figure 12. Although 41 percent of the titles are British (English and Scots) and less than 10 percent American, the publications in German, French, and Italian were known to and cited by American authors. (Withering's *Account* seems to have been read in English in France, but it was translated into German in 1786.) Some important major works, however, such as Maclean's book on hydrothorax, are not included in these data because they do not have the words digitalis or foxglove in their titles. From the data in Figure 12 we can calculate that it took about nine years for the literature on digitalis to double over the first 35 years after the publication of Withering's *Account*, the years which encompass the periods of discovery and enthusiasm, and initial stabilization. Although we lack similar data for the rest of the nineteenth century, Bayle's 1835 observation that new publications pertaining to digitalis are rare seems to be a fair estimate of the situation for the next eighty years.

A graduate student in pharmacology, Andrew Katsampes, has collected data from which the doubling times of the literature pertaining to digitalis in the twentieth century can be estimated. The twenty years following 1910 were marked by the invention of the electrocardiograph and renewed clinical interest in the selectivity of digitalis for cardiac function, following studies on both sides of the Atlantic which narrowed the scope of its reasonable expectations in medical therapeutics. During this period citations to digitalis in the *Index Medicus* doubled about every twelve years, a little more slowly than during its original introduction but much more rapidly than during the last half of the nineteenth century. Once the drug had completed its reemergence from the disappointment phase to the final stabilization phase, the rate of accumulation of papers pertaining to it dropped to a doubling time of about 40 to 50 years. (During 1931–59 publications pertaining to cardiovascular drugs doubled every 4.6 years, even though that rate was only 9 years following the introduction of the first potent antihypertensive agents in 1950). If the doubling time of the literature pertaining to a drug is a valid measure of its newsworthiness, then such data can be expected to assess the profession's approval of the drug—or at least physicians' interest in it.[18]

Thus the story of the foxglove's acceptance into, and approval by the medical profession appears to fit the model which Jawetz postulated would be helpful in monitoring the development of new drugs. The overall shape of the curve in Figure 11 probably does not vary from drug to drug; only the dates placed at intervals along the horizontal axis will be

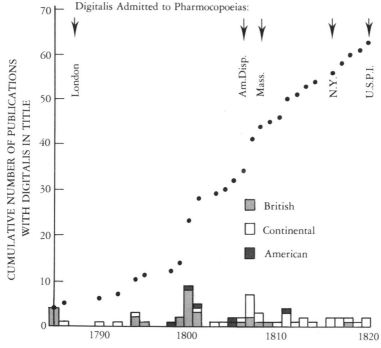

FIG. 12. *Accumulation of literature on digitalis published over the first thirty-five years after Withering's book appeared in 1785, and the years in which digitalis was admitted to the earliest American pharmacopoeias (arrows). It had been readmitted to the* Edinburgh Pharmacopoeia *in 1783, two years before Withering published his book, as a direct result of his unpublished but widely known investigations.*
SOURCE: *Index-Catalogue of the Library of the Surgeon-General's Office* (Washington, D.C., Government Printing Office, 1882), s.v. "Digitalis" and "Foxglove."

expected to differ, depending on the drug whose history is being summarized.

We still cannot ascertain why the appropriate clinical applications of the foxglove were so long delayed, why the disappointment phase in its approval lasted for almost a century. Was it because Withering had "shown" it to be a diuretic, and therefore, no more investigation was thought necessary? Was it only because the profession's concepts of the pathophysiologies of both dropsy and consumption were so similar that disappointment in the drug's efficacy in consumption became inevitable? Or, was the delay necessitated by the technological hiatus that precluded the electrophysiological studies of cardiac function necessary before digitalis could be applied to the treatment of the failing heart and its disordered rhythms, more than thirty years after the tubercle bacillus had been discovered? Presumably, all of these factors interacted within the medical profession to produce, as their net effect, a disappointment phase of such length.

According to King, "The eighteenth century physician was expected to be a keen and discriminating thinker...He must observe accurately, reflect carefully, and reason soundly." [19] We expect no more and no less today. Throughout his professional career Dr. Hall Jackson met successfully, by the standards of his own times as well as of ours, the usual medical challenges of the eighteenth century. Many of the medical problems he encountered are with us still, receiving essentially similar solutions.

We have few contemporary accounts of Hall Jackson's personality other than what can be inferred from the few newspaper accounts and correspondences already quoted. Widely respected among differing groups throughout New England, he was, for instance, one of the founders of the New Hampshire Medical Society, the second Grand Master of the Grand Masonic Lodge of New Hampshire from 1790 until his death seven years later, and one of the fifteen prominent citizens of the town who founded the Federal Fire Society of Portsmouth on March 6, 1789. Although the society was a somewhat secret social organization —its membership, limited to twenty-five, had a secret watchword—it was organized for the very serious purpose of fighting fires. Jackson's major professional accolades came when he was made an honorary member of the Massachusetts Medical Society in 1783 and when he received an honorary M.D. degree from Harvard in 1793. [20]

The colonial physician (and, presumably, his immediate post-Revolutionary successor) has been described as holding only a modest rank in early American society. Jackson's social attainments, as gauged by his known memberships, suggest, however, that in his own community at least he enjoyed the company of the "best families." His journals show that he enjoyed their patronage, although the Royal Governor employed Jackson's expertise while disdaining his democratic behavior. And, when Portsmouth paraded itself in honor of New Hampshire's having cast the ninth and deciding vote for ratification of the new federal Constitution in

June 1788, the physicians of the town, undoubtedly including Jackson, followed the clergy but preceded the representatives of the law, the legislature, and the military in the line of march. This order of precedence was not unique with Portsmouth; it was followed in Boston a year later, when President Washington paid that town a highly ceremonial visit. New Englanders, then, seem to have awarded their physicians a higher rank than was common in other colonies.[21]

The only known portrait of Hall Jackson shows him as a rather stern, perhaps even complacent, young man. The picture, which is attributed to John Singleton Copley, seems to have been painted in 1772, when Jackson was thirty-three. It shows him with a book, probably his monograph on diphtheria, and his instruments for cataract surgery.[22] (See Illustration I, p. 2.)

By the time he was thirty-nine Jackson wrote that he was plagued constantly by gout. Ten years later it had become virtually incapacitating. His letters show that his handwriting became angular and obviously tortured during attacks of the disease—which may, in fact, have been arthritis. He was not stoic: "[I am] afflicted also, with a most painful Disease that confines me near half my time, and must shortly put an end to my temporal existence."[23]

It was not gout, or arthritis, however, but an accident in which his sulky overturned, crushing his ribs, that ended Jackson's temporal existence in 1797, at the age of 58. His funeral was "the largest procession ever known in this town on such an occasion." Members of the Federal Fire Society, the St. John's Lodge of Portsmouth, and the Grand Lodge of New Hampshire made up the cortege. Although obituaries appeared in several papers throughout southern New Hampshire and northeastern Massachusetts, they were parroted largely from the original in Jackson's local paper, *The Oracle of the Day*. It emphasized his skills in surgery, obstetrics, and inoculation, embellished with the customary flourishing eulogies: "His merit alone will be his best panegyric, and will erect the most durable monument to his memory."[24]

Annalist Nathaniel Adams, who must have known Jackson, wrote, more than twenty-five years after his death:

> His sprightly talents, lively imagination, and social habits, rendered him an agreeable companion; facetious and pleasant in conversation, his friends enjoyed in his company "the feast of reason," with the flow of wit; and the several societies of which he was a member found their entertainment greatly heightened by his presence.[25]

In his *American Epitaphs and Inscriptions* the Reverend Timothy Alden, who had once lived in Portsmouth, portrays the same kind of person, although the picture could be of any well-educated man in any late eighteenth-century community: "He was a man of brilliant genius, lively fancy, extensive reading; and of such social qualities, as rendered him, at all times, a pleasing companion, particularly to those who adopt the maxim, *dum vivimus vivamus*."[26]

Although the Latin maxim scarcely requires translation, a contemporary poetic treatment of same theme provides further insight into how Alden might have applied it to Hall Jackson. The poem is by Philip Doddridge (1702–1751), a Presbyterian minister whose works were among those most widely read in the colonies:

> Live while you live, the Epicure would say,
> And seize the pleasures of the present day.
> Live while you live, the sacred Preacher cries,
> And give to God each moment as it flies.
> Lord, in *my* view, let both united be,
> I live in pleasure if I live to thee.[27]

Jackson's own manuscript "Hymn for the New Year" combines, as Doddridge urged was proper, the philosophies of the Epicureans and of Ecclesiastes:

> The lord of Earth and sky,
>     The God of ages, praise!
> Who reigns enthron'd on high,
>     Ancient of endless days.
> Who lengthens out our trials here
> And yet we see another year.
>
> Barren and wither'd Trees,
>     We've cumber'd long the ground,
> No fruit of righteousness,
>     On our dead souls was found.
> Yet did he us in mercy spare
> Another and another year.
>
> When Justice bore the sword
>     To cut the fig-tree down,
> The pity of our Lord
>     Cry'd—"let it still alone!"
> The Father mild inclin'd his Ear,
> And spares us yet another year.
>
> Then dig about our Root,
>     Dig up our fallow ground,
> And let our gracious fruit
>     To thy great praise abound.
> O! may we all thy praise declare,
> And fruit unto perfection bear.[28]

At least one other example of Jacksonian verse has come down to us, a bit of doggerel which refers to the rumor that in his controversial 1794 negotiations Chief Justice John Jay had sold the nearby town of Rye to England as one of the conditions for the withdrawal of British troops from the Northwest Territory:

> If Rye to Great Britain was really sold,
> As we by some great men are seriously told,

> Great Britain, not Rye, was ill-treated;
> For if in fulfilling the known maxim of trade,
> Any gold for such a poor purchase was paid,
> Great Britain was confoundedly cheated.[29]

William Plumer added to his impression of Hall Jackson's personality a touch of realism that rings true largely because it is almost the only clue provided by Jackson's memoirists that is less than effusively complimentary: "He was a frank, honest, benevolent man; he spoke freely the language of his heart, & his openness, tho not always admirable, seldom gave offence."[30] It must have been Jackson's openness that had so offended Benjamin Church at the siege of Boston.

Hall Jackson's friends and patients probably cared little for his devotion to reason, science, or poetry, and it was they who awarded him his social standing. Their chief concern would have been with his bedside manner and professional expertise, as far as they could assess it. Jonathan Sewall, the local versifier, probably summarized the feelings of Jackson's neighbors about him in the epitaph for Jackson's headstone in the North Cemetery in Portsmouth, where he lies next to his father, his father-in-law, and his wife:

> To heal disease, to calm the widow's sigh,
> And wipe the tear from poverty's swol'n eye
> Was thine! but ah! that skill on others shown,
> Tho' life to them, could not preserve thy own.
> Yet still thou liv'st in many a grateful breast,
> And deeds like thine, enthrone thee with the blest.[31]

Hall Jackson was a minor figure in that astonishing group of men who, collectively, comprised the American, and last, phase of the Renaissance. He was an inquisitive, efficient, and knowledgeable physician in a time and place that required high standards of medical practice, but in which the demands of a whole new way of political thinking overrode, for a time, almost all other considerations. (It should not diminish Hall Jackson and his fellow surgeons of two centuries ago that they were unable to provide as much care, or to alleviate as much suffering, as is possible today. It is not that the standards have changed, but that the technologies and concepts used in achieving those standards have improved.)

Like many of his fellow countrymen, Jackson took up the cause of American independence with enthusiasm and bad luck. And like many of his fellow physicians, he used the arts and skills of both war and medicine in his country's behalf, a mixture more typical of his century than ours.

Because of the demands that the newly emerging country placed on its citizens, it is no paradox, as it might be today, that Jackson felt no less at home with cannons than with cataract-couching instruments. An eighteenth-century American doctor could not afford to abhor the military as his colleagues in more recent centuries have done. In fact, three Secretaries of War in the period 1796–1813 were physicians (none was a very good war minister): William Eustis, later governor of Massachusetts; James McHenry, for whom the fort over which "The Star Spangled Banner" flew was named; and Henry Dearborn, for whom Ft. Dearborn, later renamed Chicago, was named. Perhaps it is no coincidence that Dearborn had studied medicine with Hall Jackson in Portsmouth.[32]

Jackson was experienced with his century's only solution to its principal infectious disease, smallpox, a disease which our own generation now claims to have eradicated.[33] He performed delicate eye operations that were essentially elective procedures, as well as the major life-saving surgery of the day, amputation. By and large, the population from which his patients came was about as healthy, by all available standards of collective health, as would be expected in a medium-sized early American port city when compared with other populations in England and Europe. Jackson could even improvise imaginative attacks on the most serious injuries, in war as well as in civilian hospitals. He kept up with the latest medical literature, and incorporated such new learning as he thought would be most helpful into his day-to-day practice.

Measured in terms of the respect of his colleagues, patients, and friends, and by his earnings, Hall Jackson was a successful practitioner. In the twentieth century, however, he might not have attracted much attention outside his own town, or his state medical society. Had he not run afoul of politicians, within and without his own profession, he might have been better known today than he is, but he would not have achieved the fame of the Philadelphia academicians. Jackson's practice seems to reflect that of his New England colleagues, based on pragmatic and inductive reasoning from clinical observations, rather than on the deductive logic more extensively employed at Philadelphia (although this generalization requires more extensive documentation).

Hall Jackson was clearly the first to import digitalis for introduction into American medicine, and he made several attempts to disseminate knowledge of the new drug throughout the country, but his was not the only route by which it came to America. The natural course of transatlantic medical communication had resumed sufficiently during the postwar period to ensure the drug several portals of entry into contemporary therapeutic usage.

There were no prestigious research centers, and little widespread advertising, to call the profession's attention to digitalis in the final years of the Enlightenment. It is likely that this eighteenth-century wonder drug gained general acceptance principally by verbal communication among physicians and as the result of journal articles, although they were relatively few and did not incorporate the same kinds of critical analysis and review that are now commonplace. The earlier custom of propagandizing the lay public through newspapers seems to have been diminishing, as physicians and apothecaries increasingly assumed roles as professional drug prescribers. However, even intraprofessional communication was largely anecdotal, in the form of reminiscences of remarkable cures, and not yet dependent on tests of statistical significance.

The limited research efforts devoted to digitalis from 1785 to 1820, in

America and abroad, were for the most part clinically oriented. Some investigators did attempt to describe the pharmacology of the drug in terms of its site and mode of action, but new technologies would be needed before the effects of digitalis could be described in greater and more meaningful detail—a job that is not yet complete. Not only was research into the clinical pharmacology of digitalis hampered by incomplete and erroneous notions of normal cardiovascular physiology and its control, but it was sometimes subject to personal biases and conflicts.

The clinical indications for the use of digitalis, too, were confused because physicians of the period lacked sufficiently detailed information about how the body functions in both health and disease. Yet given the limited physiological knowledge of the period, we can conclude only that the drug was prescribed for what then seemed to be appropriate conditions. The work of Withering alone was not at that time sufficient to indicate that digitalis can provide clinical relief only for people with certain kinds of heart disease. Not until we learned what we now know about cardiovascular physiology and pathology could we realize that his work provides ample guides to understanding and applying the drug's therapeutic properties.

The story of how the foxglove came to America is of more than antiquarian interest. It provides us with a glimpse of the machinery of medicine in the young republic. And it provides us with a terse illustration, spread over many years, of the rise and fall and eventual reemergence of a drug under usual conditions of clinical use and exploration. The data collected at the time exemplify the operation of medicine as a science, but always, as still, operating under constraints, scientific as well as nonscientific. It is no coincidence that a medical revolution began at the same time as the world's most important and most lasting political and social revolution, and in the same cultural milieu.

# Notes

Abbreviations of frequently used names and sources:

EAH    Dr. Edward Augustus Holyoke
EI      Essex Institute, Salem, Massachusetts
HJ     Dr. Hall Jackson
MHS   Massachusetts Historical Society, Boston
MTA   Marblehead Town Archives, Abbot Hall, Marblehead, Mass.
NHHS  New Hampshire Historical Society, Concord
NHSL  New Hampshire State Library, Concord
NWA   Dr. Nathaniel Walker Appleton

## 1. 'The Grand Phiz for Enockalation'

1. See, e.g., J. Worth Estes and Paul Dudley White, "William Withering and the Purple Foxglove," *Scientific American*, 212 (June 1965), 110–119; Erwin H. Ackerknecht, "Aspects of the History of Therapeutics," *Bulletin of the History of Medicine*, 36 (1962), 389–419. One of the oddest retellings of the story is found in Kate C. Hurd-Mead, *A History of Women in Medicine*, 1938 (rep. Boston, Milford House, 1973), p. 478. Dr. Hurd-Mead tells us that it was Withering's famous "old woman of Shropshire"—to whom, without documentation, she gives the name "Mrs. Hutton"—who was the "first to discover that foxglove is useful in the treatment of chronic disease of the heart," and that "Mrs. Hutton" had experimented on several notable personages, including a dean at Oxford (all in contrast with Withering's version). Other patent errors in her story which, unlike most of her vignettes throughout the book, is not documented with any reference to the literature, make me wonder about her sources for this crucial episode in the history of medicine. For more on the pharmacologic setting in which Withering worked, and its limitations, see J. Worth Estes, "Making Therapeutic Decisions with Protopharmacologic Evidence," *Transactions and Studies of the College of Physicians of Philadelphia*, in press.

2. Daniel J. Boorstin, *The Americans: The Colonial Experience* (New York, Vintage, 1958), p. 193.

3. Henry F. May, *The Enlightenment in America* (New York, Oxford, 1976), pp. xiv, 94. Benjamin Franklin, *The Autobiography and Other Writings*, ed. L. Jesse Lemisch (New York, Signet, 1961), pp. 206–207.

4. Russell Leigh Jackson, *The Physicians of Essex County* (Salem, Mass., Essex Institute, 1948), pp. 58–61. William Plumer, "Biog-

raphies," unpublished manuscript, Vol. 3, pp. 654–656 (June 26, 1829), NHHS. Russell Leigh Jackson, "Dr. Hall Jackson of Portsmouth," *Annals of Medical History*, new ser., 5 (1933), 103–128. Some of Plumer's material seems to have been copied from Nathaniel Adams' *Annals of Portsmouth* (n. 11, below), but much is original with Plumer. Russell Leigh Jackson's heretofore definitive paper on Hall Jackson provides no references to any statement or quotation in it, although in a note to the article in his book on the *Physicians of Essex County* he mentions manuscript materials in his own possession. I cannot locate them. When I have been able to find the original locations of primary materials obviously used by R. L. Jackson, I have cited them directly; some of his attributions appear to be in error.

Hall Jackson's birthplace in Hampton is still standing, handsomely restored by its former owners, Judge and Mrs. William Wardwell Treat; it is still in private ownership. The deed by which Clement Jackson sold the property to his brother-in-law Anthony Emery in 1754 is recorded in microfilm Vol. 43 of Deeds, New Hampshire State Archives, NHHS.

Careful searches by the librarians and archivists of the London hospitals that were taking house pupils before 1780, including the Middlesex Hospital, have not revealed further documentation of Hall Jackson's stay there. I am most grateful to Dr. C. Helen Brock and the librarians of the London hospitals who searched their notes and files for me.

5. Whitfield J. Bell, "Medical Practice in Colonial America," *Bulletin of the History of Medicine*, 31 (1957), 442–453. Eric H. Christianson, "Individuals in the Healing Arts and the Emergence of a Medical Community in Massachusetts, 1700–1792: a Collective Biography" (Ph.D. diss., University of Southern California, 1976), p. 29. Philip Cash, "An Analysis of the Social, Political and Professional Impact of the Revolution upon the Boston Medical Community (1759–1789)," paper delivered at the 25th International Congress for the History of Medicine, Quebec City, Canada, August 21–28, 1976. Hyman K. Schonfield, Jean F. Heston, and Isidore S. Falk, "Numbers of Physicians Required for Primary Medical Care," *New England Journal of Medicine*, 286 (1972), 571–576. James K. Cooper and Karen Heald, "Is There a Doctor Shortage?", *Journal of the American Medical Association*, 227 (1974), 1410–11. American Medical Association Coordinating Council on Medical Education, "Physician Manpower and Distribution," ibid., 236 (1976), 3049–55. Barbara J. Culliton, "Health Manpower Act: Aid but Not Comfort for Medical Schools," *Science*, 194 (1976), 700–704. *Physicians for the Future* (New York, Josiah Macy, Jr., Foundation, 1976), pp. 5, 63–64.

6. Richard H. Shryock, *Medicine and Society in America 1660–1860* (New York, New York University, 1960), pp. 2–10. William D. Postell, "Medical Education and Medical Schools in Colonial Amer-

ica," *International Medical Record*, 171 (1958), 364–370. Samuel Lewis, "List of the American Graduates in Medicine in the University of Edinburgh from 1705 to 1866, with Their Theses," *New England Historical and Genealogical Register*, 42 (1888), 159–165. J. H. Baas, *Outlines of the History of Medicine*, trans. H. E. Handerson, 1889 (rep. Huntington, N.Y., Krieger, 1971), pp. 805–806.

7.  Genevieve Miller, "Medical Apprenticeship in the American Colonies," *Ciba Symposia*, 8 (1947), 502–510. Postell, "Medical Education"; Baas, *Outlines*, pp. 805–806.

8.  Fielding H. Garrison, *An Introduction to the History of Medicine* (Philadelphia, Saunders, 1929), p. 405.

9.  Maurice Bear Gordon, *Aesculapius Comes to the Colonies* (1949; rep. New York, Argosy-Antiquarian, 1969), pp. 352–353.

10.  Plumer, "Biographies."

11.  *New England Historical and Genealogical Register*, 97 (1943), 7–9. *New Hampshire Gazette* (Portsmouth), August 25, 1774. Nathaniel Adams, *Annals of Portsmouth* (Portsmouth, published by the author, 1825), p. 315. Although this last work is not documented with footnotes or other forms of citation, the author assures us that he has had access to appropriate documents and to Belknap's *History of New Hampshire* (n. 107, below). At any rate Adams, who lived from 1756 to 1829, witnessed many of the events he describes and probably knew Hall Jackson personally.

  Dr. and Mrs. Jackson had three children: Theodore (1766–1784), died of consumption; Samuel Dalling (1767–1768); and Mary Elizabeth (1769–1808), who married Dr. Joshua Gee Symme of Andover, Mass. Mary Elizabeth's one child, Elizabeth Gee Symme, born about 1800, died an infant. Hall Jackson does have collateral descendants through his sister Sarah (1747–1806), who married Dr. Stephen Little, R.N. (1745–1800). Hall and Sarah Jackson also had four sisters and two brothers, all of whom died without issue.

12.  *New Hampshire Gazette* (Portsmouth), February 26, 1768.

13.  Ibid., March 4, 1768.

14.  David Ramsay, *A Review of the Improvements, Progress and State of Medicine in the XVIIIth Century* (Charleston, S.C., W. P. Young, 1801), p. 5.

15.  HJ, "Meteorological Register...," unpublished manuscript journal, 2 vols., dated consecutively December 1774–June 1795, in the collection of Mr. Joseph W. P. Frost, Eliot, Maine. This manuscript will be discussed in some detail in Chapter 3.

16.  HJ to J[osiah] Bartlett, September 1791, copy, folder 31, Levi Bartlett Papers, Boston Medical Library.

17.  HJ to Mr. Rogers, Boston, September 1, 1791, NHHS, MSS folder 17B-7.

18.  Ruth van Heyningen, "What Happens to the Human Lens in Cataract," *Scientific American*, 222 (December 1975), pp. 70–81. Celsus, *De Medicina*, trans. W. G. Spencer, 3 vols. (Cambridge,

Harvard University, 1935), Vol. 3, pp. 347–352. An excellent diagrammatic representation of couching will be found facing p. 350 of Celsus. Current methods of cataract extraction are reviewed in Norman S. Jaffe, "Cataract Surgery—a Modern Attitude toward a Technologic Explosion," *New England Journal of Medicine*, 299 (1978), 235–237.

19. Burton Chance, "Exposure and Fixation of the Eye in the Early Days of Cataract Extraction," *Archives of Ophthalmology*, 36 (1946), 484–497.

20. Celsus, *De Medicina*, pp. 351–352. The word "couch" is derived from the French *coucher*, "to lay down," which is what is done to the diseased lens when it is dislocated from the ligamentous moorings that normally hold it suspended in the eye.

21. Burton Chance, *Ophthalmology* (New York, Hafner, 1962), pp. 49–51. Arnold Sorsby, *A Short History of Ophthalmology* (New York, Staples, 1948), pp. 46–51.

22. Plumer, "Biographies."

23. Gordon, *Aesculapius*, p. 130. That one of HJ's pupils, Jabez Dow, referred to the operation as "Couching or Depressing Cataract" leads me to believe that HJ did not perform complete lens extraction (Jabez Dow Papers, MS, "Surgery & Local Diseases not Strictly Surgical" July 19, 1813), p. 9, Boston Medical Library.

24. *New Hampshire Gazette* (Portsmouth), October 5, 1770.

25. Ibid., December 6, 1771.

26. HJ, "Register."

27. Plumer, "Biographies." Garrison, *Introduction*, pp. 144, 152. Robert B. Austin, *Early American Medical Imprints, 1668–1820* (Washington, D.C., U.S. Department of Health, Education, and Welfare, 1961), p. 110.

28. *New Hampshire Gazette* (Portsmouth), February 17, 1775.

29. HJ to Jeremy Belknap, December 19, 1789, Belknap Collection, MHS. This theme will be more fully explored in Chapter 3.

30. Ibid.

31. Dale C. Smith, "Quinine and Fever: The Development of the Effective Dosage," *Journal of the History of Medicine and Allied Sciences*, 31 (1976), 343–367.

32. HJ to Jeremy Belknap, December 19, 1789.

33. H. O. J. Collier, "Aspirin," *Scientific American*, 209 (November 1963), 97–108.

34. HJ to Jeremy Belknap, December 19, 1789. Jabez Dow, "Manuscript No. 1, Ointments," Jabez Dow Papers, pp. 22–23, Boston Medical Library. For a detailed discussion of drugs used in New Hampshire and Boston at the same time, see J. Worth Estes, "Therapeutic Practice in Colonial New England," in Philip Cash, Eric Christianson, and J. Worth Estes, eds., *Medicine in Massachusetts, 1630–1830* (Boston, Colonial Society of Massachusetts, in press).

35. Ernest Caulfield, "Some Common Diseases of Colonial Children,"

*Publications of the Colonial Society of Massachusetts,* 35 (1942), 4–65. Timothy Alden, *A Collection of American Epitaphs and Inscriptions,* 2 vols. (New York, 1814), pp. 134–135. [HJ], *Observations and Remarks on the Putrid Malignant Sore Throat...* (Portsmouth, John Melcher, 1786). Jackson's authorship is verified by the inscription in the copy in the American Antiquarian Society, Worcester, Mass.

36. Dr. David L. Morril to Dr. Levi Bartlett, December 23, 1793, Levi Bartlett Collection, Richmond [Virginia] Academy of Medicine. Gordon, *Aesculapius,* p. 129.

37. HJ, *Sore Throat,* p. 3.

38. Garrison, *Introduction,* p. 307.

39. HJ, *Sore Throat,* pp. 5–6.

40. Ibid., p. 6.

41. Ibid., p. 12. For the drug classes mentioned by HJ, see Estes, "Therapeutic Practice."

42. Ibid., pp. 14–15.

43. HJ, "Register."

44. HJ to Dr. Levi Bartlett, August 21, 1788, in Levi Bartlett Collection, Richmond (Virginia) Academy of Medicine.

45. Ibid.

46. Cotton Mather, *The Angel of Bethesda* (MSS, 1724; first published Barre, Mass., American Antiquarian Society and Barre Publishers, 1972), p. 94. A good anecdotal overview of the Boston smallpox experience in 1721–22 is given in Ola Elizabeth Winslow, *A Destroying Angel: the Conquest of Smallpox in Colonial Boston* (Boston, Houghton Mifflin, 1974). A more statistically detailed presentation is in John B. Blake, *Public Health in the Town of Boston* (n. 54, below).

47. Mather, *Angel,* p. 94. William H. McNeill, in *Plagues and Peoples* (New York, Anchor/Doubleday, 1976), pp. 117–119, argues that smallpox may have been known in the ancient Mediterranean world, although it reached severe epidemic proportions in modern Europe only in the late middle ages.

48. Mather, *Angel,* p. 97.

49. Ibid., pp. 113–114.

50. Ibid., p. 115. The word "inoculation" was derived by analogy with the horticultural practice of grafting—that is, "in-eyeing." For instance, in 1767 Thomas Jefferson "inoculated common cherry buds into stocks of large kind at Monticello." Fawn M. Brodie, *Thomas Jefferson: An Intimate History* (New York, Bantam, 1975), p. 74. Mather used the word "transplantation" in the same way.

51. Zabdiel Boylston, *An Historical Account of the Small-Pox Inoculated in New England* (London, S. Chandler, 1726), p. 40.

52. Preserved Smith, *The Enlightenment 1687–1776* (New York, Collier, 1962), pp. 113–115. John Blake, "Smallpox Inoculation in Colonial Boston," *Journal of the History of Medicine,* 8 (1953), 284–300.

53. Adams, *Annals*, p. 207.
54. John B. Blake, *Public Health in the Town of Boston 1630–1822* (Cambridge, Harvard University, 1959), pp. 89–96. Josiah Bartlett, "A Dissertation on the Progress of Medical Sciences in the Commonwealth of Massachusetts," *Medical Communications and Dissertations of the Massachusetts Medical Society*, 2 (1813), 235–270. *Boston Post-Boy & Advertiser*, February 27, 1764. Lyman H. Butterfield, ed., *Adams Family Correspondence*, 4 vols. (Cambridge, Harvard University Press, 1963), Vol. 1, pp. 28–43.
55. *Boston News-Letter*, March 29, 1764. *Boston Gazette*, May 28, 1764. HJ to Robert Hooper, Jr., June 27, 1787, MTA.
56. Blake, "Smallpox Inoculation."
57. *Oxford English Dictionary*, s.v. "Percent."
58. Boylston, *Account of the Small-Pox*, pp. 40–41.
59. Blake, *Public Health*, pp. 92–96.
60. Reginald Fitz, "The Treatment for Inoculated Small-Pox in 1764 and How It Actually Felt," *Annals of Medical History*, Ser. 3, Vol. 4 (1942), 110–113. For an even more detailed account, by a perceptive adult, see *Adams Family Correspondence* (n. 54, above).
61. *Portsmouth Town Records*, microfilm Vol. 2, pp. 283–284, NHSL. HJ, "Register."
62. Adams, *Annals*, pp. 33–34.
63. Ibid., pp. 274–275.
64. HJ, "List of Persons Inoculated at Henzell's Island 1782," unpublished manuscript in collection of Frederick S. Gray, M.D., Portsmouth, N.H., now in the Portsmouth Athenaeum.
65. Jabez Dow, "Observations on the small Pox made at Shapley's Island Hospital during my pupillage," unpublished manuscript in Jabez Dow Papers, Boston Medical Library, 9 pages. About ten or fifteen years later Dow compiled a more professionally oriented series of notes on the subject, gleaned more from standard texts than from personal experience (see his "Pathology 1" manuscript in the same collection). For more details on the drugs administered to the smallpox inoculation patients, see Estes, "Therapeutic Practice." To Dow the word "virus" meant a poisonous material, not a submicroscopic pathogen.
66. *Portsmouth Town Records*, microfilm Vol. 3, n.p., entry for March 25, 1797, NHSL.
67. George Athan Billias, *General John Glover and His Marblehead Mariners* (New York, Henry Holt, 1960), pp. 35–38. Ashley Bowen, "Smallpox Journal," manuscript journal in Marblehead Historical Society, Jeremiah Lee House, item 7569. I am greatly indebted to Philip Chadwick Foster Smith, Curator of Maritime History at the Peabody Museum, Salem, Mass., for the opportunity to study his exact transcriptions of Bowen's journals. They have since been published, with modern spelling and punctuation, as Philip Chadwick Foster Smith, ed., *The Journals of Ashley Bowen (1728–1813) of Marblehead*, 2 vols. (Salem, Mass., Peabody

Museum, 1973). Although the quotations used here are from the journal (save for the poem), the citations to them are to the published journals, Vol. 2.

68. Billias, *Glover*, pp. 38–39. Bowen, *Journals*, pp. 362–370. I have been unable to find any other trace of Doctoress Hawes.
69. Bowen, pp. 328–329, plate XXVI, facing p. 364.
70. Ibid., pp. 361–362.
71. Ibid., pp. 343–344, 351–353. "The 24 day of July" was the date on which Mrs. Bowen came down with smallpox.
72. *Essex Gazette* (Salem, Mass.), October 19–26, 1773.
73. HJ to the Selectmen of the Town of Portsmouth, December 7, 1773, Portsmouth Miscellaneous Town Papers, NHHS.
74. Bowen, *Journals*, p. 361.
75. *Essex Gazette* (Salem, Mass.), October 26 to November 2, 1773.
76. Ibid., October 19–26, 1773.
77. Ibid., October 26 to November 2, 1773. C. W. Dixon, *Smallpox* (London, J. and A. Churchill, 1962), p. 243.
78. British Patent Office, *Abridgements of Specifications Relating to Medicine, Surgery, and Dentistry . . . A.D. 1620–1866*, 2nd ed. (London, Office of the Commissioners for Patents for Inventions, 1872), p. 25. Lester S. King, *The Medical World of the Eighteenth Century* (Chicago, University of Chicago Press, 1958), p. 322. Alan Harwood, "The Hot-Cold Theory of Disease," *Journal of the American Medical Association*, 216 (1971), 1153–58. For more on the Sutton family and their inoculation methods, see David van Zwanenberg, "The Suttons and the Business of Inoculation," *Medical History*, 22 (1978), 71–82.
79. Blake, *Public Health*, pp. 129–130.
80. *Essex Gazette* (Salem, Mass.), October 26 to November 2, 1773.
81. Ibid.
82. Ibid., November 16–23, 1773.
83. "A Forgotten Horror," *Essex Institute Historical Collections*, 35 (1899), 304.
84. *Essex Gazette* (Salem, Mass.), January 11–18, 1774.
85. Bowen, *Journals*, p. 383.
86. Ibid., p. 382.
87. Ibid., p. 383.
88. *Essex Gazette* (Salem, Mass.), January 25 to February 1, 1774. Although the *Gazette* reported that the hospital had 70 beds, Bowen says only 40 (above, n. 69).
89. Bowen, *Journals*, p. 383.
90. Ibid., p. 386.
91. Ibid., p. 388.
92. Billias, *Glover*, pp. 42–48. Pauline Maier, *From Resistance to Revolution* (New York, Vintage, 1974), provides corroborating background information.
93. HJ to Robert Hooper, Jr., June 27, 1787. HJ to Selectmen of Marblehead, February 23, 1788, MTA.

94. Bowen, *Journals*, p. 517. HJ, "List of Persons Inoculated in 1777 (at Marblehead, Mass., by Dr. Hall Jackson)," unpublished manuscript dated December 9, 1793, MTA. HJ to Selectmen of Marblehead, November 22, 1787, MTA. For inflation rates in 1777, see Chapter 2, n. 64.

95. HJ to Selectmen of Marblehead, December 9, 1793, MTA.

96. Peter Force, ed., *American Archives*, Ser. 4, Vol. 4 (Washington, D.C., M. St. Clair Charles and Peter Force, 1843), p. 153.

97. *Portsmouth Town Records*, microfilm Vols. 6, 17, passim, NHSL.

98. Drafts, "His Majesty's Fort William & Mary to Hall Jackson," May 26, 1773, and "Doctor Hall Jackson to Stephen Little," 14 November 1770, both in New Hampshire State Archives, NHSL; Estes, "Therapeutic Practice," n. 34.

99. Baas, *Outlines*, p. 822. Gordon, *Aesculapius*, pp. 129–131.

100. Toby Gelfand, "The Hospice of the Paris College of Surgery (1774–1793)," *Bulletin of the History of Medicine*, 47 (1973), 375–393. Charles G. Child, III, "Surgical Intervention," *Scientific American*, 229 (September 1973), 91–98.

101. Joanne Lynn, "The Health Care System of Pittsfield, New Hampshire" (M.D. thesis, Boston University School of Medicine, 1974), passim.

102. Steven J. Erlanger, *The Colonial Worker in Boston, 1775* (Boston, U.S. Department of Labor New England Regional Office Report 75-2, 1975). Jackson Turner Main, *The Social Structure of Revolutionary America* (Princeton, Princeton University Press, 1965), pp. 116–118.

103. Robert O. Blood, "The Governor's Address," *New England Journal of Medicine*, 226 (1942), 294–297. Stoughton's Elixir was widely advertised—and, presumably, bought—in England: P. S. Brown, "Medicines Advertised in Eighteenth-Century Bath Newspapers," *Medical History*, 20 (1976), 152–168.

104. British Patent Office, *Specifications*, p. 2 (above, n. 78).

105. Item 6386, Probate Records, Rockingham County Register of Probate, Exeter, N.H. Timothy Dwight, *Travels in New England and New York*, 4 vols. (1821–1822; rev. Cambridge, Harvard University Press, 1969), Vol. 3, p. 276. *Early New Hampshire Deeds*, microfilm, NHHS, Vol. 77, p. 248; Vol. 80, p. 336; Vol. 89, pp. 475, 537; Vol. 90, p. 264; Vol. 98, p. 481. Jackson's house stood on the northwest corner of what are now Washington and Court streets in Portsmouth until 1954, when it was razed to make way for a small parking lot, exactly the size of the house foundations, for an automatic laundry just outside the precincts of the Strawbery Banke preservation area. The lowest step of the front-door stoop and faint traces of the foundations are all that are now visible.

106. This volume, in the Portsmouth Athenaeum, was brought to my attention by Joseph W. Hammond of North Hampton, N.H. Gerarde says that foxglove is of "no use" but cites the "Ancients" as his authority.

107. HJ to Jeremy Belknap. Jeremy Belknap, *The History of New Hampshire*, 2nd rev. ed., 3 vols. (Boston, Bradford and Read, 1813), Vol. 3, pp. 73–94. The Latin scientific names given here are Belknap's; some have been changed over the past two centuries.
108. *New Hampshire Medical Society Records 1791–1854* (Concord, N.H., Rumford, 1911), pp. 24–25.
109. Henry R. Viets, *A Brief History of Medicine in Massachusetts* (Boston, Houghton Mifflin, 1930), p. 85.
110. Dr. David L. Morril to Dr. Levi Bartlett (n. 36, above).


## 2. 'A Disagreeable and Dangerous Employment'

1. Nathaniel Adams, *Annals of Portsmouth* (Portsmouth, published by the author, 1825), p. 251.
2. Clifford K. Shipton, *Sibley's Harvard Graduates*, Vol. 14 (Boston, Massachusetts Historical Society, 1968), pp. 177–182.
3. Adams, *Annals*, p. 316.
4. HJ to the Selectmen of the Town of Portsmouth, December 7, 1773, Portsmouth Miscellaneous Town Papers, NHHS. "General Gains" is probably George Gains, a Portsmouth merchant and privateer who was on the town's Committee of Safety with HJ.
5. *Portsmouth Town Records*, NHSL, Vol. 2, pp. 407–408, 414; Vol. 3, p. 72.
6. A. L. Elwyn, ed., *Letters by Josiah Bartlett, William Whipple, and Others* (Philadelphia, Henry B. Ashmead, 1889), p. 15.
7. Howard H. Peckham, *The Toll of Independence: Engagements and Battle Casualties of the American Revolution* (Chicago, University of Chicago, 1974), p. 3. Russell Leigh Jackson, "Dr. Hall Jackson of Portsmouth," *Annals of Medical History*, new ser., 5 (1933), 103–128. However, see above, n. 4 to Chapter 1, on the reliability of R. L. Jackson's evidence. Shipton, *Harvard Graduates*.
8. William Plumer, "Biographies," unpublished manuscript, Vol. 3, pp. 654–656 (June 26, 1829), in NHHS.
9. See, for instance, Jere R. Daniell, *Experiment in Republicanism* (Cambridge, Harvard University, 1970).
10. Petition, HJ and others, to Theodore Atkinson, April 7, 1775, regarding military training, New Hampshire State Archives, Military Records, NHSL. Elwyn, *Letters*, pp. 15–16.
11. Ibid., pp. 16–17. Peckham, *Toll*, p. 4, see n. 7. Portsmouth delegates to the New Hampshire Congress, H. Wentworth, chairman, to the Congress, November 13, 1775, NHHS. HJ to the Hon[bl] President, Counsil, & Representatives of the Colony of New Hampshire, March 19, 1776, NHHS.
12. Richard Frothingham, *History of the Siege of Boston*, 4th ed. (Boston, Little, Brown, 1873), pp. 180–181.
13. Allen C. Wooden, "The Wounds and Weapons of the Revolutionary War from 1775 to 1783," *Delaware Medical Journal*, 44 (1972),

59–65. Pictures and further details of the weapons can conveniently be found in, e.g., H. L. Peterson, *The Book of the Continental Soldier* (Harrisburg, Pa., Stackpole, 1968).

14. John Harris, "Battle of Bunker Hill," special section, *Boston Globe*, June 8, 1975, pp. 23, 28. Frederick Mackenzie, *Diary . . . 1775– 1781*, 2 vols. (Cambridge, Harvard University Press, 1930), Vol. 1, p. 23. Frothingham, *Siege*, pp. 175–206.

15. Louis C. Duncan, *Medical Men in the American Revolution 1775– 1783*, Army Medical Bulletin, No. 25 (Carlisle Barracks, Pa., Medical Field Service School, 1931), p. 375. Howard Lewis Applegate, "The Need for Further Study in the Medical History of the American Revolutionary Army," *Military Medicine*, 126 (1961), 616– 618. Peckham, *Toll*, pp. 130, 133.

16. Henry B. Carrington, *Battle Maps and Charts of the American Revolution*, 1881 (rev. rep. ed., New York, Arno, 1974), passim. Peckham, *Toll*, passim.

17. Elwyn, *Letters*, pp. 17–18. Lawrence Shaw Mayo, *John Langdon of New Hampshire*, 1937 (rep. Port Washington, N.Y., Kennikat, 1970), is the standard biography. See pp. 17–18 for Langdon's courtship of the lady who became Mrs. Jackson.

18. Charles P. Whittemore, "John Sullivan: Luckless Irishman," in George Athan Billias, ed., *George Washington's Generals* (New York, William Morrow, 1964), pp. 137–162. Frank C. Mevers, "Josiah Bartlett: Dedicated Physician, Sterling Patriot," in George E. Gifford, Jr., ed., *Physician Signers of the Declaration of Independence* (New York, Science History Publications, 1976), pp. 99–121. Elwyn, *Letters*, pp. 22–23.

19. Philip Cash, *Medical Men at the Siege of Boston, April, 1775– April, 1776: Problems of the Massachusetts and Continental Armies* (Philadelphia, American Philosophical Society, 1973), pp. 69, 71, 131–133. Charles H. Lesser, ed., *The Sinews of Independence: Monthly Strength Reports of the Continental Army* (Chicago, University of Chicago, 1976), pp. 4–5. All facets of the health care of the troops besieging Boston in 1775–76, and its historical development, are explored in detail in Cash's authoritative study. The most succinct description of the Continental Army hospital system, as it finally evolved, is found in Howard Lewis Applegate, "The American Revolutionary War Hospital Department," *Military Medicine*, 126 (1961), 296–306.

20. James Tilton, *Economical Observations on Military Hospitals* (Wilmington, Del., J. Wilson, 1813), p. 13. See also Morris H. Saffron, "The Tilton Affair," *Journal of the American Medical Association*, 236 (1976), 67–72, for a good description of Tilton's attempts to compromise between the army's needs for both general and regimental hospital services.

21. Quoted in Duncan, *Medical Men*, pp. 120–121.

22. Ibid., p. 129.

23. Tilton, *Economical Observations*, p. 33.

24. C. M. B. Gilman, "Military Surgery in the American Revolution," *Journal of the Medical Society of New Jersey*, 57 (1960), 491–496.
25. Benjamin Rush, *Medical Inquiries and Observations*, rev. ed., 4 vols. (Philadelphia, J. Conrad, 1805), Vol. 1, pp. 269–275.
26. Ibid., p. 273. See Lesser, *Sinews of Independence*, p. xxx, cited in n. 19 above, for at least tentative confirmation of Rush's observation.
27. Ibid., p. 276.
28. *Pennsylvania Packet* (Philadelphia), April 22, 1777. Carl Binger, *Revolutionary Doctor: Benjamin Rush, 1746–1813* (New York, Norton, 1966), p. 119.
29. Elwyn, *Letters*, pp. 23–25.
30. James Thacher, *A Military Journal During the American Revolutionary War* (Boston, Richardson and Lord, 1823), p. 552. Richard Brocklesby, *Oeconomical and Medical Observations . . . Tending to the Improvement of Military Hospitals* (London, T. Beckel and P. A. de Hondt, 1764), p. 48. John Jones, *Plain Concise Practical Remarks on the Treatment of Wounds and Fractures* (New York, John Holt, 1775).
31. Otis G. Hammond, ed., *Letters and Papers of Major-General John Sullivan*, 3 vols. (Concord, New Hampshire Historical Society, 1930), Vol. 1, pp. 84–87.
32. Ibid., pp. 87–88. Cash, *Medical Men at Siege*, p. 137. Allen French, *General Gage's Informers*, 1932 (rep. New York, Greenwood, 1968), pp. 179–182.
33. Elwyn, *Letters*, pp. 24–25.
34. Ibid., pp. 27–28.
35. Ibid., pp. 28–29.
36. Russell Leigh Jackson, "Dr. Stephen Little, R. N.," *Essex Institute Historical Collections* (July 1941), pp. 262–266. Russell Leigh Jackson, *The Physicians of Essex County* (Salem, Mass., Essex Institute, 1948), pp. 72–75.
37. Elwyn, *Letters*, p. 30. The British wounded at Bunker Hill also had to do with salted meat, "which even the healthy often could not stomach," because there was no meat for making broth: R. Arthur Bowler, *Logistics and the Failure of the British Army in America 1775–1783* (Princeton, Princeton University Press, 1975), pp. 158–159.
38. Cash (n. 19 above) has provided a recent assessment of Church's work as Director General, and summarized his treason (*Medical Men at Siege*, pp. 117–128). I have explored the quarrel between HJ and Church in "'A Disagreeable and Dangerous Employment': Medical Letters from the Siege of Boston," *Journal of the History of Medicine and Allied Sciences*, 31 (1976), 271–291, and sketched Church's career in "Treason and Other Medical Problems at the Siege of Boston," *Forum on Medicine* (April 1978), pp. 20 ff. The most extensive documentation of Church's career is found in William Frederick Norwood, "The Enigma of Dr. Benjamin Church: A

High-Level Scandal in the American Colonial Army Medical Service," *Medical Arts and Sciences*, 10 (1956), 71–93. Other accounts, all of which differ in some respects as to their documentations, are found in John Blakeless, *Turncoats, Traitors, and Heroes* (Philadelphia, J. P. Lippincott, 1959), pp. 10–28, 88; Carl van Doren, *Secret History of the American Revolution*, 1941 (rep. New York, Popular Library, 1969), pp. 18–23; and French, *Gage's Informers*, pp. 147–201 (above, n. 32). Church's extensive non-medical writings are listed in John Langdon Sibley and Clifford K. Shipton, *Sibley's Harvard Graduates*, Vol. 13 (Boston, Massachusetts Historical Society, 1952), pp. 380–398. The decoded translation of Church's treasonable letter, dated May 10, 1775, is in Vol. 3 of the Artemas Ward Papers at the MHS and was printed in *New England Historical and Genealogical Register*, 11 (1857), 123–124. Church's own defense appears in Francis R. Packard, *History of Medicine in the United States*, 2 vols. (New York, Paul B. Hoeber, 1931), Vol. 2, pp. 1191–1200.

39. Elwyn, *Letters*, pp. 34–36.
40. Cash, *Medical Men at Siege*, pp. 129–138. Duncan, *Medical Men*, p. 62. Brooke Hindle, *The Pursuit of Science in Revolutionary America, 1735–1789* (Chapel Hill, N.C., University of North Carolina, 1956), p. 235. Applegate, "Hospital Department," p. 300.
41. Ezra Stiles, *The Literary Diary*, ed. Franklin Bowditch Dexter, 2 vols. (New York, Scribner's, 1901), Vol. 1, pp. 618–620; Vol. 2, pp. 117–118, 161. Whitfield J. Bell, Jr., *John Morgan: Continental Doctor* (Philadelphia, University of Pennsylvania, 1965), pp. 179–188. *Pennsylvania Packet* (Philadelphia), June 24, 1779.
42. Peter Force, ed., *American Archives*, Ser. 5, Vol. 1 (Washington, D.C., M. St. Clair Charles and Peter Force, 1843), p. 1266. See also Tables 3–5 in this Chapter.
43. Ibid. George B. Griffenhagen, *Drug Supplies in the American Revolution*, Paper 16, Contributions from the Museum of History and Technology, United States National Museum Bulletin, 225 (Washington, D.C., Smithsonian Institution, 1961), pp. 110–113.
44. HJ to John Langdon, November 3, 1775, Harvard University, Houghton Library, bMS Sparks 49.2(69).
45. Maurice Bear Gordon, *Aesculapius Comes to the Colonies*, 1940 (rep. New York, Argosy-Antiquarian, 1969), p. 110. Jackson, "Dr. Hall Jackson."
46. Ibid. Shipton, *Harvard Graduates* (see above, n. 2).
47. HJ to [John Langdon?], May 13, 1777, Harvard, Houghton Library, Autograph File. For Thornton, see J. Worth Estes, "Honest Dr. Thornton: The Path to Rebellion," in George E. Gifford, Jr., ed., *Physician Signers of the Declaration of Independence* (New York, Science History Publications, 1976), pp. 70–98.
48. HJ to [Langdon?], May 13, 1777.
49. For details of the continuing saga of the difficulties with and among

the army's chief medical officers throughout the war, which do not concern us here, see, for instance, references cited in n. 38 above. Bell, *John Morgan*, pp. 178–239. Binger, *Benjamin Rush*, pp. 119–145.

50. Isaac W. Hammond, ed., *New Hampshire State Papers: Rolls and Documents Relating to Soldiers in the Revolutionary War* (Manchester, John B. Clarke, 1889), Vol. 17, p. 4. Force, *Archives*, pp. 151–154. HJ to the New Hampshire Congress (n.d. but about October 31, 1775), NHHS.

51. "Records of the Committee of Safety," *Collections of the New Hampshire Historical Society*, 7 (1863), 1–340. Nathaniel Bouton, et al., eds., *Documents and Records Relating to New Hampshire*, 40 vols. (Concord and Manchester, 1867–1941), Vol. 14, p. 367; Vol. 15, p. 428. Draft, "The State of New Hampshire to Hall Jackson," 1776, NHSL. Joseph Pierson, order to pay Hall Jackson, December 13, 1776, NHSL. Receipt, "State of New Hampshire to Hall Jackson," December 13, 1776, NHSL. HJ to Nicholas Gilman, March 30, 1780, NHSL. HJ to the Honorable Counsil and Representatives of the State of New Hampshire, October 30, 1778, NHSL. Minute of the Committee for Considering the [illegible] of Doct. Hall Jackson, 1784, signed by John Langdon, NHSL, House of Representatives Records. HJ to the Hon[bl] President and Members of the New Hampshire Congress (n.d. but about 31 October 1775), NHHS. HJ to unknown addressee, October 27, 1775, NHHS. HJ to the Hon[bl] President, Counsil & Representatives of the Colony of New Hampshire, March 19, 1776, NHHS; HJ to the Hon[ble] Congress for the Colony of New Hampshire, November 13, 1775, NHHS.

52. Surgeon's Certificate, signed by HJ, September 15, 1777, Boston Public Library, call no. Ch.C.1.154 (Print Room). Certificate, signed by HJ, February 9, 1786, Pennsylvania Historical Society. Certificate, signed by HJ, February 12, 1780, at Portsmouth, in New Hampshire State Archives, NHSL.

53. Printed circular, February 28, 1792, Keith Collection, MHS.

54. George Athan Billias, *General John Glover and His Marblehead Mariners* (New York, Holt, 1960), pp. 185–188.

55. HJ to John Langdon, November 3, 1775. Packard (*Medicine in United States*, pp. 582–583) states that Dr. Shippen sent Hall Jackson to Bethlehem, Pennsylvania, after the Battle of Brandywine, on September 19, 1777, but I can find no corroborating evidence. In fact there is no evidence that HJ was ever in Pennsylvania.

56. Hammond, *Sullivan Papers*, Vol. 1, p. 309.

57. Charles L. Parsons, *The Capture of Fort William and Mary* (New Castle, N.H., The William and Mary Committee of the New Hampshire American Revolution Bicentennial Commission, 1974). HJ to Matthew Thornton, received October 12, 1775, NHHS. HJ to Phillips White, March 6, 1776, NHHS.

58. HJ to Phillips White, ibid.

59. HJ to the Provincial Congress, November 10, 1777, NHHS. HJ to the Hon^bl President, Counsil & Representatives of the Colony of New Hampshire, March 19, 1776, NHHS. HJ to the Hon^bl the Counsil and Representatives of the Colony of New Hampshire, March 6, 1776.

60. HJ to John Langdon, November 3, 1775.

61. HJ to Elbridge Gerry, April 22, 1777, Gerry Collection, MHS. M. Weare, Josiah Bartlett, E. Thompson, Justices of the Peace, to the Keeper of the Publick Gaol in Exeter, April 18, 1777, in collection of Mr. Joseph W. P. Frost, Eliot, Me.

62. Jackson, "Dr. Hall Jackson" (n. 7 above). Hammond, *State Papers*, Vol. 14, p. 367; Vol. 15, p. 428. S. C. Worthen, "Colonel Pierse Long's Regiment, *Granite Monthly*, 57 (1925), 262–266.

63. HJ to the New Hampshire Congress, November 10, 1777, NHHS.

64. HJ to Elbridge Gerry, September 20, 1778, Gerry Collection, MHS. Billias, *Glover*, p. 176. Peckham, *Toll*, p. 54. In the front of his ledger (now in the American Antiquarian Society, Worcester, Mass.), Dr. Moses Mossman of Sudbury, Mass. (1742–1817) tipped in a "Scale of Depreciation—in Dollars" from 1776 through 1780. From his table we can calculate that money was depreciating at a rate of 2.1 percent per month from January through July 1777; at 17.0 percent per month from July through November 1777; at 3.3 percent per month from November 1777 through November 1778; and at 8.3 percent per month from November 1778 through May 1780 (the overall rate for the entire period was 6.8 percent depreciation per month). Thus Jackson was in Providence during the period of the fastest monetary depreciation of the war in New England.

65. Duncan, *Medical Men*, p. 379. Isobel Stevenson, "Physicians as Soldiers in the Revolutionary Armies," *Ciba Symposia*, 2 (1940), 508–511. Isobel Stevenson, "Political Activities of Revolutionary Physicians," ibid., 512–519. Applegate, "Hospital Department," p. 300.

66. Josiah Bartlett, "A Dissertation on the Progress of Medical Sciences in the Commonwealth of Massachusetts," *Medical Communications and Dissertations of Massachusetts Medical Society*, 2 (1813), 235–270.

67. Hindle, *Pursuit of Science*, pp. 236–240. Howard Lewis Applegate, "Effects of the American Revolution on American Medicine," *Military Medicine*, 126 (1961), 551–553. HJ to Gentlemen [of a Committee to employ physicians for New Hampshire militia], May 29, 1775, New Hampshire State Archives, NHSL.

68. Lesser, *Sinews of Independence*, pp. 2–17. Peckham, *Toll*, pp. 3–14. French, *Gage's Informers*, p. 176.

69. Lesser, *Sinews of Independence*, pp. 2–17. J. Worth Estes, "A Disagreeable and Dangerous Employment" (above, n. 38).

70. Cash, *Medical Men at Siege*, pp. 160–163.

71. Thomas Dickson Reide, *View of the Diseases of the Army...* (London, J. Johnson, 1793), passim.
72. Bowler, *Logistics and British Army*, pp. 53–54, 107, 212–238.
73. Harold Murdock, *Bunker Hill: Notes and Queries* (Boston, Houghton Mifflin, 1927), p. 77. Allen French, *The First Year of the American Revolution* (Boston, Houghton Mifflin, 1934), p. 342.
74. Computed from data given by Lesser (n. 19) and Peckham (n. 7).
75. Howard Lewis Applegate, "Remedial Medicine in the American Revolutionary Army," *Military Medicine*, 126 (1961), 450–453. Cash in *Medical Men at Siege* has shown that preventive medicine was the primary factor in maintaining the health of the patriot troops surrounding Boston.

## 3. Portsmouth: 'As Healthy a Place as Any in America'

1. Timothy Dwight, *Travels in New England and New York*, 4 vols., 1821–22 (rev. ed. Cambridge, Harvard University Press, 1969), Vol. 1, pp. 56–63.
2. Ibid., pp. 311–312.
3. Ibid., p. 311.
4. Ibid., pp. 312–313. Jeremy Belknap, *The History of New Hampshire*, 2nd ed., 3 vols. (Boston, Bradford and Read, 1813), Vol. 3, pp. 162–163.
5. *Heads of Families at the First Census of the United States Taken in the Year 1790: New Hampshire* (Washington, D.C., Government Printing Office, 1907). *Population Schedules of the Second Census of the United States 1800*, microcopy 2, Roll 20, "New Hampshire" (Washington, D.C., National Archives, 1960). *Census of the United States for 1810* (Washington, D.C. 1813). *Census of the United States for 1820: Book I* (Washington, D.C., Gales and Seaton, 1821). U.S. Bureau of the Census, *Historical Statistics of the United States, Colonial Times to 1970*, 2 vols. (Washington, D.C., Government Printing Office, 1975).
6. HJ to Jeremy Belknap, January 7, 1790, Belknap Collection, MHS. The correct total is, of course, 4046. For the writing of Belknap's book and its likeness to those of Dwight and Brissot, see Jere R. Daniell, "Jeremy Belknap and the *History of New Hampshire*," in Lawrence H. Leder, ed., *The Colonial Legacy*, Vol. 3 (New York, Harper and Row, 1973), pp. 241–264.
7. Dwight, *Travels*, Vol. 1, p. 313.
8. Belknap, *History*, Vol. 3, pp. 198–199. Jackson Turner Main, *The Social Structure of Revolutionary America* (Princeton, N.J., Princeton University Press, 1965), pp. 37–38.
9. Marquis de Chastellux, *Travels in North-America in the Years 1780–81–82* (New York, 1828), pp. 313–314, 414.
10. J. P. Brissot de Warville, *New Travels in the United States of*

*America, 1788,* trans. Mara Soceanu Vamos and Durand Echeverria (Cambridge, Harvard University Press, 1964), pp. 366–369. Belknap, *History,* Vol. 3, p. 174.

11. Oliver W. Holmes, "Facts and Traditions Reflecting the Existence of Indigenous Intermittent Fever in New England," *Boylston Prize Dissertations for the Years 1836 and 1837* (Boston, Charles C. Little and James Brown, 1838), p. 117. Percy Stocks, "Measurement of the Public Health," *British Medical Bulletin,* 7 (1951), 312–316.

12. R. Kargon, "John Graunt, Francis Bacon, and the Royal Society: The Reception of Statistics," *Journal of the History of Medicine,* 18 (1963), 337–348. Thomas Robert Malthus, *Population: The First Essay,* 1798 (rep. Ann Arbor, University of Michigan, 1959).

13. Richard H. Shryock, "Eighteenth Century Medicine in America," *American Antiquarian Society Proceedings,* 59 (1949), 275–292.

14. David Ramsay, *A Review of the Improvements, Progress and State of Medicine in the XVIIIth Century* (Charleston, S.C., W. P. Young, 1801), pp. 17–20. See also, e.g., Richard H. Shryock, *The Development of Modern Medicine* (New York, Alfred A. Knopf, 1947).

15. Major Greenwood, *Medical Statistics from Graunt to Farr* (Cambridge, The University Press, 1948), p. 31. Maris A. Vinovskis, "The 1789 Life Table of Edward Wigglesworth," *Journal of Economic History,* 31 (1971), 570–590. Maris A. Vinovskis, "Mortality Rates and Trends in Massachusetts Before 1860," ibid., 32 (1972), 184–213.

16. Lemuel Shattuck, *The Vital Statistics of Boston* (Philadelphia, Lea and Blanchard, 1841), p. xxxii.

17. Census Bureau, *Historical Statistics,* Vol. 1, p. 49.

18. Brissot, *New Travels,* p. 292 (above, n. 10).

19. Census Bureau, *Historical Statistics,* Vol. 2, p. 42. Robert V. Wells, *The Population of the British Colonies in America Before 1776* (Princeton, N.J., Princeton University Press, 1975), pp. 299–300, 313.

20. Brissot, *New Travels,* p. 285.

21. Census Bureau, *Historical Statistics,* Vol. 1, p. 19.

22. Brissot, *New Travels,* pp. 287–290.

23. A. J. Jaffe and W. I. Lourie, Jr., "An Abridged Life Table for the White Population of the United States in 1830," *Human Biology,* 14 (1942), 352–371. Malthus, *Population.*

24. Malthus, *Population,* pp. 38–41.

25. Robert Willan, *Reports on the Diseases in London, Particularly during the Years 1769, 97, 98, 99, and 1800* (London, R. Phillips, 1801). *Dictionary of National Biography,* s.v. "Robert Willan." See Tables 3–5 for similar data in a military population.

26. Jeremiah 8:21–22, 46:11.

27. Brissot, *New Travels,* p. 279. Dwight, *Travels,* Vol. 1, pp. 59–60.

28. Willan, *Reports on Diseases,* pp. 320–323.

29. John Warren, "Remarks on Angina Pectoris," 1812, *New England Journal of Medicine,* 266 (1962), 1–7. C. Sidney Burwell, "A Com-

mentary on Professor John Warren's Paper, 'Remarks on Angina Pectoris'," ibid., 7–9.

30. Francisco Guerra, *American Medical Bibliography, 1639–1783* (New York, Lathrop C. Harper, 1962), pp. 441–447, 469–485, 518–552, 591–594, 618, 641, 658–659, 674. Daniel Adams, ed., *Medical and Agricultural Register*, 1 (1808), 227. A. Matthews, "Notes on Early Autopsies and Anatomical Lectures," *Publications of the Colonial Society of Massachusetts*, 19 (1918), 272–290.

31. Charles S. Hirsch, Norman B. Rushforth, Amasa B. Ford, and Lester Adelson, "Homicide and Suicide in a Metropolitan County. I. Long-Term trends," *Journal of the American Medical Association*, 223 (1973), 900–905. A. Millar, ed., *A Collection of the Yearly Bills of Mortality for 1657 to 1758* . . . (London, A. Millar, 1759), passim. For a valuable treatment of accidental deaths in contemporary London, see Thomas Rogers Forbes, *Crowner's Quest* (Philadelphia, American Philosophical Society, 1978).

32. John Duffy, *Epidemics in Colonial America* (Baton Rouge, Louisiana State University, 1953). Ernest Caulfield, "Early Measles Epidemics in America," *Yale Journal of Biology and Medicine*, 15 (1943), 531–556. Ernest Caulfield, "Some Common Diseases of Colonial Children," *Publications of the Colonial Society of Massachusetts*, 35 (1942), 4–65. John B. Blake, *Public Health in the Town of Boston 1630–1822* (Cambridge, Harvard University Press, 1959). Ernest Caulfield, "A History of the Terrible Epidemic, Vulgarly Called the Throat Distemper, As It Occurred in His Majesty's New England Colonies Between 1735 and 1740," *Yale Journal of Biology and Medicine*, 11 (1939), 219–272.

33. Ibid.

34. Noah Webster, *A Brief History of Epidemic and Pestilential Diseases*, 2 vols. (Hartford, Conn., Hudson & Goodwin, 1799), Vol. 1, p. 264. Edward Augustus Holyoke, "An Account of the Weather and of the Epidemics at Salem, in the County of Essex, for the Year 1786...," *Massachusetts Medical Society Communications*, 1 (1790), 17–40. Brissot, *New Travels*, p. 277.

35. Ibid., p. 290. Blake, *Public Health*, p. 256. For similar seasonal fluctuations in disease that were observed in contemporary New York, see Saul Jarcho, "Cadwallader Colden as a Student of Infectious Disease," *Bulletin of the History of Medicine*, 29 (1955), 99–115.

36. Adams, *Register*, pp. 143–144.

37. A. E. Bender, *Dictionary of Nutrition and Food Technology*, 3rd ed. (London, Archon, 1968); United States National Center for Health Statistics, *Dietary Intake Findings, United States, 1971–1974* (Vital and Health Statistics, Series 11, data from the National Health Survey, No. 202) (DHEW publication [HRA] 77–1647) (Hyattsville, Md., U.S. Department of Health, Education, and Welfare, 1977), pp. 37–39.

38. Shryock, "Eighteenth Century Medicine" (above, n. 13).

39. Ernest Caulfield, "Infant Feeding in Colonial America," *Journal of Pediatrics*, 41 (1952), 673–687.
40. Adams, *Register*, p. 144.
41. HJ, "Meteorological Register," manuscript journal in 2 vols., dated December 1774 to June 1795, collection of Mr. Joseph W. P. Frost, Eliot, Maine.
42. HJ Estate inventory (above, n. 105 of Chapter 1).
43. Everett Mendelsohn, "John Lining and His Contributions to Early American Science," *Isis*, 51 (1960), 278–292. Michael Mendillo and John Keady, "Watching the Aurora from Colonial America," *Transactions of the American Geophysical Union*, 57 (1976), 485–491. Webster, *Epidemic Diseases* (above, n. 34). D. F. Proctor, "The Nose, Ambient Air, and Airway Mucosa: A Pathway in Physiology," *Bulletin of the History of Medicine*, 48 (1974), 352–376.
44. J. Worth Estes, "Genetic Counselling," *Medical Times*, 98, No. 4 (September 1970), 92–106.
45. Ibid.
46. Ambroise Paré, *The Workes*, trans. T. Johnson, 1634 (rep. Pound Ridge, N.Y., Milford House, 1968), pp. 301–303.
47. Brissot, *New Travels*, pp. 283–294. William Barton, "Observations of the Probabilities of the Duration of Human Life, and the Progress of Population, in the United States of America," *Transactions of the American Philosophical Society*, 3 (1793), 25–62. J. Meyer, *Of Insurances on Lives and Life Annuities* (New York, D. and G. Bruce, 1811), pp. 39–43, 78–79. For an example of how mortality statistics were actually used in computing annuities, see W[eyman] L[ee], *An Essay to Ascertain the Value of Leases and Annuities for Years and Lives*...(London, S. Birt, D. Browne, and J. Shackburgh, 1737).
48. Malthus, *Population*, pp. 25–35. Main, *Social Structure*, p. 37. Leonard Hayflick, "The Cell Biology of Human Aging," *New England Journal of Medicine*, 295 (1976), 1302–1308.
49. Brissot, *New Travels*, pp. 279–280. Malthus, while unwilling to conclude that women's "intellectual faculties are inferior," did speculate that "from their different education, there are not so many women as men, who are excited to vigorous mental exertion." Malthus, *Population*, p. 83 (above, n. 12).
50. Edward A. Wigglesworth, "A Table Shewing the Probability of the Duration, the Decrement, and the Expectation of Life, in the States of Massachusetts and New Hampshire," *Memoirs of the American Academy of Arts and Sciences*, Vol. 2, Part II (1804), 62–70. Greenwood, *Medical Statistics* (above, n. 15). See also Vinovskis, "Mortality Rates" (above, n. 15).
51. Brissot, *New Travels*, p. 284.
52. Belknap, *History*, pp. 171–174 (above, n. 4). Belknap's remark about Americans' vigor and robustness has been supported by modern genetic research; see C. O. Carter, *Human Heredity* (Harmondsworth, England, Penguin Books, 1962), p. 102.

53. J. Potter, "The Growth of Population in America, 1700–1860," in D. V. Glass and D. E. C. Eversley, eds., *Population in History* (Chicago, Aldine, 1965), pp. 644–646. James H. Cassedy, *Demography in Early America: Beginnings of the Statistical Mind* (Cambridge, Harvard University Press, 1969), pp. 149–151. William L. Langer, "Checks on Population Growth: 1750–1850," *Scientific American*, 226 (February 1972), 92–99.

54. Dwight, *Travels*, Vol. 1, pp. 63–65 (above, n. 1). Belknap, *History*, Vol. 3, pp. 188–190. Brissot, *New Travels*, p. 291. Robert B. Austin, *Early American Medical Imprints 1668–1820* (Washington, D.C., U.S. Department of Health, Education, and Welfare, 1961), p. 60. W. B. Walker, "Luigi Cornaro, a Renaissance Writer on Personal Hygiene," *Bulletin of the History of Medicine*, 28 (1954), 525–534. See also, for examples of current popular interest in longevity, articles by Alexander Leaf in *National Geographic Magazine*, 143 (1973), 93–118, and in *Scientific American*, 229 (September 1973), 44–52.

55. Cassedy, *Demography*, pp. 210–213. John C. Greene, "Science and the Public in the Age of Jefferson," *Isis*, 49 (1958), 13–25.

56. Brissot, *New Travels*, p. 286.

57. Dwight, *Travels*, Vol. 2, p. 212.

## 4. 'A Weakness and Laxity of the Fibers'

1. Timothy Dwight, *Travels in New England and New York*, 4 vols., 1821–22 (rev. rep. ed. Cambridge, Harvard University Press, 1969). Jeremy Belknap, *The History of New Hampshire*, 2nd ed., 3 vols. (Boston, Bradford and Read, 1813). James Boswell, *The Life of Samuel Johnson LL.D.*, 1791 (rep. New York, Modern Library, 1951), p. 1042.

2. *American Weekly Mercury* (Philadelphia), September 13, 1736; *New Hampshire Gazette and Historical Chronicle* (Portsmouth), July 5, 1765.

3. HJ to William Plumer, February 20, 1786, Plumer Letters, Vol. 1, NHSL. J. Worth Estes, "An 18th Century Clinicopathological Correlation," *Bulletin of the New York Academy of Medicine*, 52 (1976), 617–626.

   For the moment, this exercise in clinicopathological correlation must remain a mystery on two counts. For the first, we wonder just why Jackson sent the account of his post-mortem findings to William Plumer (1759–1850), a lawyer and future United States senator, in Epping, N.H. Plumer may have had some professional need to know, as an attorney, or he may have been soliciting data for the biographical notes he was compiling (e.g., his notes on Jackson, cited above in n. 4, Chapter 1). The other mystery concerns the modern diagnostic equivalent of General Whipple's cardiac disease. Several interpretations of the autopsy protocol have been suggested to me. Dr. Richard Van Praagh suggests that this is the first known case of overriding tricuspid valve with right atrial to left ventricular communication, and tricuspid stenosis. However, overriding tricuspid valve is a very rare and not well understood congenital heart defect. The true underlying problem may have been that the right ventricle was unusually small rather than that the valve was actually misplaced during a fault in embryological development. Dr. Helen B. Taussig and her colleagues, on the other hand, feel that there is no evidence that an overriding tricuspid valve was present, but that the unequivocal right atrial to left ventricular shunt was accompanied by extraordinary tricuspid stenosis and ossification. Although there is no evidence that cyanosis was present, as would have been expected in a patient with that kind of shunting, there must have been some oxygen deficit in the arterial blood, because very little blood was circulated through the lungs. Dr. Taussig is amazed at "the way the General was able to carry on." At any rate, the dynamics of so-called "criss-cross atrioventricular relationships" are not well understood even today. It is clear, however, that Whipple died as the result of tricuspid stenosis, probable ante-mortem mural thrombosis of the right atrium, atrial fibrillation, and consequent congestive heart failure with hydrothorax, coupled with insufficient oxygenation of the peripheral tissues and, perhaps, myocardial infarction as the terminal event. (Richard Van Praagh, M.D., to Alexander S. Nadas, M.D., November 8, 1971; Helen B. Taussig, M.D., to J. Worth Estes, M.D., November 6, 1971, December 7, 1971, and June 12, 1972—all in the author's possession.) Regardless of the exact diagnosis, Jackson's detailed and knowledgeable description of General Whipple's illness, and his explanation based on the autopsy findings, show that Jackson had a remarkably keen comprehension of cardiovascular physiology and its pathology.

4.  Nathaniel Adams, *Annals of Portsmouth* (Portsmouth, published by the author, 1825), pp. 283–284.

5.  Cotton Mather, *The Angel of Bethesda*, 1724 (first published Barre, Mass., American Antiquarian Society and Barre Publishers, 1972), p. 28. When he dedicated his great work to Charles I, Harvey established the precedent of regarding the heart as the absolutely essential central organ of the body (William Harvey, *Exercitatio Anatomica de Motu Cordis*, Chauncey D. Leake, trans., Springfield, Ill., Charles C. Thomas, 1928, p. 3).

6.  Ralph Major, *A History of Medicine*, 2 vols. (Springfield, Ill., Charles C. Thomas, 1954), pp. 182–206. Celsus, *De Medicina*, trans. W. G. Spencer, 3 vols. (Cambridge, Harvard University Press, 1935), Vol. 1, p. 313.

7.  Ambroise Paré, *The Workes*, trans. T. Johnson, 1634 (rep. Pound Ridge, N.Y., Milford House, 1968), p. 299. Cantharides, or powdered "Spanish fly," was used as a skin irritant to draw off diseased body fluids; its use as a putative aphrodisiac was a later development in its mythology.

8.  Jerome J. Bylebyl, "The Growth of Harvey's *De Motu Cordis*," *Bulletin of the History of Medicine*, 47 (1973), 427–470. Bylebyl presents a very clear and succinct description of Galen's cardio-vascular concepts, as well as of the evolution of Harvey's thinking about them. Harvey's own illness and death prevented him from translating his discovery to practical uses at the bedside, although he had intended to do so, according to one near-contemporary biographer (John Freind, *History of Physick from the Time of Galen to the Beginning of the XVI Century*, 4th ed., 2 vols., London, M. Cooper, 1750, pp. 237–238).

9.  Audrey B. Davis, "Some Implications of the Circulation Theory for Disease Theory and Treatment in the Seventeenth Century," *Journal of the History of Medicine and Allied Sciences*, 26 (1971), 28–39. Thomas Willis, *The London Practice of Physick*, 1692 (rep. Boston, Milford House, 1973), pp. 527–533. Lester S. King, "Medical Theory and Practice at the Beginning of the 18th Century," *Bulletin of the History of Medicine*, 46 (1972), 1–15. Lester S. King, *The Growth of Medical Thought* (Chicago, University of Chicago Press, 1963), pp. 133–135. For modern concepts of fever and its causes, see Elisha Atkins and Phyllis Bodel, "Clinical fever: Its history, manifestations and pathogenesis," *Federation Proceedings*, 38 (1979), 57–63.

10.  Willis, *London Practice*, pp. 133–137.

11.  Kenneth Dewhurst, *John Locke (1632–1704): Physician and Philosopher: A Medical Biography* (London, Wellcome Historical Medical Library, 1963), pp. 128, 146–147, 169–170, 194, 283.

12.  K. J. Franklin, trans., *De Corde (1669) by Richard Lower. Early Science in Oxford*, ed. R. T. Gunther, Vol. 9 (Oxford, for the subscribers, 1932), pp. 117–118.

13.  Richard H. Shryock, *Medicine and Society in America 1660–1860* (New York, New York University, 1960), p. 66. Lester S. King, *The Medical World of the Eighteenth Century* (Chicago, University of Chicago, 1958), p. 77.

14.  King, pp. 126–127. E. Ashworth Underwood, "The History of the Quantitative Approach in Medicine," *British Medical Bulletin*, 7 (1951), 265–274.

15.  King, *Medical World*, pp. 125–129. William Withering, *An Account of the Foxglove* (Birmingham, M. Swinney, 1785), pp. xiv–xv.

16.  Saul Jarcho, trans. and ed., *Practical Observations on Dropsy of the Chest. Transactions of the American Philosophical Society*, new ser., 61, Part 3 (1971), 3–46.

17.  Ibid., pp. 14–22.

18.  Ibid., pp. 25–28.

19.  Ibid., pp. 25–28.

20.  Ibid., pp. 35–44.

21.  John Floyer, *The Physician's Pulse-Watch* (London, Sam. Smith and Benj. Walford, 1707), pp. 3, 16–19. Underwood, "Quantitative Approach."

22. Underwood. Floyer, *Pulse-Watch*, pp. 40, 46.
23. [Giovanni Maria Lancisi], *De Subitaneis Mortibus*, trans. and ed. Paul Dudley White and Alfred V. Boursy (New York, St. John's University, 1971), pp. 115–130, 133–139, 147. Patrick A. McKee, William P. Castelli, Patricia M. McNamara, and William B. Kennel, "The Natural History of Congestive Heart Failure: the Framingham Heart Study," *New England Journal of Medicine*, 285 (1971), 1441–1446.
24. Giovanni Maria Lancisi, *De [Motu Cordis et] Aneurysmatibus*, trans. Wilmer Cave Wright (New York, Macmillan, 1952).
25. Raymond Vieussens, *Traité Nouveau de la Structure et des Causes du Mouvement Naturel du Coeur* (Toulouse, Jean Guillemette, 1715), pp. 105–106. The portion cited is translated and quoted in Paul Dudley White, *Heart Disease*, 4th ed. (New York, Macmillan, 1951), p. 675.
26. Bernardo Ramazzini, *Diseases of Workers (De Morbis Artificium)*, trans. W. C. Wright (New York, Hafner, 1964), pp. 131, 151, 231, 243, 253, 267, 281–285, 343, 449.
27. Mather, *Angel of Bethesda*, pp. 125–129. Mather named his book for the angel who stirred up the water in the pool of Bethesda near the sheep gate in Jerusalem; whoever stepped into the water next after the angel was healed of his disease (John 5:2–4).
28. Paul Dudley White, "Heart Failure," *Bulletin of the New York Academy of Medicine*, 18 (1942), 18–35.
29. Stephen Hales, *Statical Essays: Containing Haemastaticks...*, 1733 (rep. New York, Hafner, 1964), pp. 113–118.
30. Ibid. See also n. 5, Chapter 5.
31. Donald Monro, *An Essay on the Dropsy* (London, D. Wilson and T. Durham, 1755), pp. 8–10.
32. Ibid., pp. 8–10, 25.
33. John Baptist Morgagni, *The Seats and Causes of Diseases*, trans. B. Alexander, 3 vols. (London, A. Millar, T. Cadell, and Johnson and Payne, 1769), Vol. 1, pp. 378–379; Vol. 2, pp. 280–361.
34. Leopold Auenbrugger, *Inventum Novum ex Percussione Thoracis Humani*, trans. John Forbes, 1761 (rep. C. N. B. Camac, *Classics of Medicine and Surgery*, New York, Dover, 1959), pp. 142–143.
35. William Heberden, *Commentaries on the History and Cure of Diseases*, 1782 (rep. New York, Hafner, 1962), pp. 216–224.
36. Samuel Clossey, *The Existing Works*, 1763 et seq. (rep. New York, Hafner, 1967), p. 28. David C. Humphrey, "The King's College Medical School and its Professionalization in Pre-Revolutionary New York," *Bulletin of the History of Medicine*, 49 (1975), 206–234.
37. Clossey, *Works*, pp. 47, 54.
38. Ibid., pp. 50–55.
39. Ibid., p. 90.
40. Ibid., pp. 111–113.
41. William Cullen, *First Lines of the Practice of Physic*, 3 vols. (Edin-

burgh, Bell and Bradfute, and William Creech, 1791), Vol. 3, pp. 262–267.

42. Shryock, *Medicine and Society in America*, pp. 64–67; see n. 13. King, *Medical World*, pp. 147–149; see n. 13. Benjamin Rush, *Medical Inquiries and Observations* (Philadelphia, T. Dobson, 1789).

43. George W. Corner, ed., *The Autobiography of Benjamin Rush*, 2 vols. (Princeton, Princeton University, 1948), Vol. 2, pp. 361–366. I have not included John Brown's ideas here because his influence seems to have been small. They are outlined well in W. R. Trotter, "John Brown, and the Nonspecific Component of Disease," *Perspectives in Biology and Medicine*, 21 (Winter, 1978), 258–264. The expiration of humoral concepts of disease is summarized in Robert J. Miciotto, "Carl Rokitansky: A Reassessment of the Hematohumoral Theory of Disease," *Bulletin of the History of Medicine*, 52 (1978), 183–199.

44. Jean-Nicholas Corvisart, *An Essay on the Organic Diseases and Lesions of the Heart and Great Vessels*, trans. Jacob Gates (Boston, Bradford and Read, 1812), pp. 278, 313–314, 323–324.

45. Allan Burns, *Observations on Some of the Most Frequent and Important Diseases of the Heart* (Edinburgh, Thomas Bryce; John Murray; J. Callow, 1809), p. 164. Joseph Hodgson, *A Treatise on the Diseases of the Arteries and Veins* . . . (London, Thomas Underwood, 1815), pp. 28–30. James Hope, *A Treatise on the Diseases of the Heart and Great Vessels*, 2nd ed. (London, W. Kidd, 1835), pp. 196, 205.

46. Robert James, *A Medicinal Dictionary*, 3 vols. (London, Osborne, 1745), Vol. 2, p. 3, s.v. "Hydrops."

47. Ibid.

48. For a skeletal treatment of the immediate effects of digitalis, see J. Worth Estes and Paul Dudley White, "William Withering and the Purple Foxglove," *Scientific American*, 212 (1965), 110–119. The development of thinking about the action of digitalis after Withering is tersely summarized in Sir John MacMichael, "The History of Ideas on Digitalis Action," in B. H. Marks and A. M. Weissler, eds., *Basic and Clinical Pharmacology of Digitalis* (Springfield, Ill., Charles C. Thomas, 1972), pp. 5–14.

   Recent reviews of current thinking about the physiology and biochemistry of heart failure include Alberto Ramirez and Walter H. Abelmann, "Cardiac Decompensation," *New England Journal of Medicine*, 290 (1974), 499–501; Eugene Morkin and Paul J. LaRaia, "Biochemical Studies on the Regulation of Myocardial Contractility," ibid., 445–451; Glenn A. Langer, "The Intrinsic Control of Myocardial Contraction—Ionic Factors," ibid., 285 (1971), 1065–71; Arnold M. Katz, "Congestive Heart Failure: Role of Altered Myocardial Cellular Control," ibid., 293 (1975), 1184–1191.

   The most recent detailed review of the site and mode of digitalis action is Thomas W. Smith and Edgar Haber, "Digitalis," *New England Journal of Medicine*, 289 (1973), 945–952, 1010–15, 1063–72, 1125–29. The standard text reference is Gordon K. Moe and Alfred E. Farah, "Digitalis and Allied Cardiac Glycosides," in Louis S. Goodman and Alfred Gilman, eds., *The Pharmacological Basis of Therapeutics*, 5th ed. (New York, Macmillan, 1975), pp. 653–682. Subcellular details of digitalis action are explored in "Newer Aspects of Cardiac Glycoside Action," The Digitalis Bicentennial Symposium presented by the American Society for Pharmacology and Experimental Therapeutics at Anaheim, California, April 13, 1976, *Federation Proceedings*, 36 (1977), 2207–46; and Tai Akera, "Membrane Adenosinetriphosphatase: A Digitalis Receptor?," *Science*, 198 (1977), 569–574. Extracardiac sites of digitalis action are discussed in Lynne C. Weaver, Tai Akera, and Theodore M. Brody, "Digoxin Toxicity: Primary Sites of Drug Action on the Sympathetic Nervous System," *Journal of Pharmacology and Experimental Therapeutics*, 197 (1976), 1–9.

For a detailed comprehensive review of current thinking about factors which control the heart and blood flow, see Eugene Braunwald, "Regulation of the Circulation," *New England Journal of Medicine*, 290 (1974), 1124–29.

The disposition of digitalis in the body is reviewed in James E. Doherty, William H. Hall, Marvin L. Murphy, and Owen W. Beard, "New Information Regarding Digitalis Toxicity," *Chest*, 59 (1971), 433–437.

The relationship of basic scientific information about digitalis to its use in the treatment of disease is summarized in David H. Huffman and Daniel L. Azarnoff, "Indications for Digitalis Therapy: A New Look," *Journal of the American Medical Association*, 229 (1974), 1911–14.

Just as this book was going to press a new drug called amrinone, which shares many therapeutic properties with digitalis but has few side effects, was announced. The new drug's mechanisms have not been determined, but so far it appears to facilitate the action of digitalis in patients who otherwise respond poorly to the older drug: Joseph R. Benotti, William Grossman, Eugene Braunwald, Dominick D. Davolos, and Adawia A. Alousi, "Hemodynamic Assessment of Amrinone: A New Inotropic Agent," *New England Journal of Medicine*, 299 (1978), 1373–1377. Lawrence K. Altman, "A New Drug Is Reported to Help Failing Heart Pump More Blood," *New York Times*, December 22, 1978.

## 5. 'The Great Abstractor of Arterial Action'

1. Robert E. Schofield, *The Lunar Society of Birmingham* (Oxford, Clarendon Press, 1963), p. 125. Preserved Smith, *The Enlightenment 1687–1776* (New York, Collier, 1962), p. 118.

2.  George A. Beller, Thomas W. Smith, Walter H. Abelmann, Edgar Haber, and William B. Hood, Jr., "Digitalis Intoxication," *New England Journal of Medicine*, 284 (1971), 989–997.
3.  Edward W. Pelikan, M.D., to J. Worth Estes, May 25, 1964, in the author's collection, and summarized in J. Worth Estes and Paul Dudley White, "William Withering and the Purple Foxglove," *Scientific American*, 212 (1965), 110–119.
4.  William Withering, *An Account of the Foxglove*... (Birmingham, M. Swinney, 1785), pp. 184, 189.
5.  Louis H. Roddis, "William Withering and the Introduction of Digitalis into Medical Practice," *Annals of Medical History*, new ser., 8 (1936), 93–112, 185–201. Maurice S. Jacobs, "The History of Digitalis Therapy," ibid., 492–499. Maurice B. Strauss, ed., *Familiar Medical Quotations* (Boston, Little, Brown, 1968), p. 183. Sarah Hoare, *Memoirs of Samuel Hoare*, ed. F. R. Pryor (London, Headley Brothers, 1911). Harold Feil, "The Story of a Verse on the Foxglove," *Bulletin of the Cleveland Medical Library*, 14 (1966), 12–14. Dr. Feil presents a slightly different version of the same poem prepared by Miss Hoare in 1825:

    > And Digitalis wisely given,
    > Another boon of favoring Heaven
    >   Will Happily display;
    > The rapid pulse it can abate,
    > The hectic flush can moderate,
    > And blest by him, whose will is fate,
    >   May give a happier day.

    Feil also cites evidence that the poem, in either version, was written with the foxglove's supposed ability to cure consumption in the author's mind, chiefly because the word "hectic" was applied to consumption in many medical writings; he thinks that the poem does not refer to the efficacy of digitalis in dropsy. The evidence from the poem itself, however, is slim. Robert Willan defined hectic as characterized by the daily recurrence, usually in the morning, of skin warmth ("the hectic flush"), accompanied by increased heart rate and increased sweating, all of which are compatible with advanced tuberculosis. But sixty years earlier Stephen Hales had specified that hectic fevers occur when "the Pulse is weak and quick, when the Heart is supplied with little Blood," as often happens in congestive heart failure. William Heberden noted in 1782 that "the precise meaning of the word hectic has not been settled" and that it "is always occasioned by some other disease." And Benjamin Rush was confused by it, because it "differs from all the other states of fever, by the want of regularity in its paroxysms," and is associated chiefly with consumption, but also with cases of lues, scrofula, and gout. All of this exemplifies, for an almost trivial instance, the con-fusion, even distress, that can arise among historians of medicine when concepts of disease change, following changes in methods of making observations and/or changes in physiological models. Robert Willan, *Reports on the Diseases in London*...(London, R. Phillips, 1801), p. x. Stephen Hales, *Statical Essays*...(1733; rep. New York, Hafner, 1964), p. 13. William Heberden, *Commentaries on the History and Cure of Diseases* (1802; rep. New York, Hafner, 1962), pp. 186–198. Benjamin Rush, *Medical Inquiries and Observations*, 2d ed., 4 vols. (Philadelphia, J. Conrad Co., 1805), Vol. 3, p. 50.

6.  Charles Darwin, "An Account of the Retrograde Motions of the Absorbent Vessels...," trans. from Latin by Erasmus Darwin, in Charles Darwin, *Experiments Establishing a Criterion Between Mucaginous and Purulent Matter* (Lichfield, J. Jackson et al., 1780). Fulton has demolished Erasmus Darwin's claim of priority with little difficulty, and has demonstrated that the cases of dropsy included in young Charles Darwin's paper were posthumous additions by his father: John F. Fulton, "Charles Darwin (1758–1778) and the History of the Early Use of Digitalis," *Bulletin of the New York Academy of Medicine*, 10 (1934), 496–506; John F. Fulton, "The Place of William Withering in Scientific Medicine," *Journal of the History of Medicine and Allied Sciences*, 8 (1953), 1–15.

7.  Erasmus Darwin, "An Account of the Successful Use of Foxglove in Some Dropsies, and in the Pulmonary Consumption," *Medical Transactions of the Royal College of Physicians of London*, 3 (1785), 255–286. Withering, *Account of the Foxglove*, pp. 11–16 (above, n. 4).

8.  Erasmus Darwin, *Zoonomia, or the Laws of Organic Life*, 2nd American ed., 2 vols. (Boston, Thomas and Andrews, 1803), pp. 256–257. Sir George Baker, "An Appendix to the Preceding Paper," *Medical Transactions of the Royal College of Physicians of London*, 3 (1785), 287–308.

9.  Erasmus Darwin, *The Botanic Garden* (Dublin, Moore, 1793), p. 107. That Darwin's influence, for better or worse, was wide-ranging cannot be disputed, and it must have been augmented by his poetry. For instance, in 1831 Mary Shelley recalled a discussion between Lord Byron and her husband some fifteen years earlier: "Various philosophical doctrines were discussed, and among others the nature of the principle of life, and whether there was any probability of its ever being discovered and communicated. They talked of the experiments of Dr. Darwin...who preserved a piece of vermicelli in a glass case till by some extraordinary means it began to move with voluntary motion. Perhaps a corpse would be reanimated; galvanism had given token of such things: perhaps the component parts of a creature might be manufactured, brought together, and endued with vital warmth." The immediate fruit of this discussion was, of course, Mary Shelley's *Frankenstein* (1816; rep. New York, Lancer, 1968), pp. 10–11.

10. William Jones, "An Account of Two Cases of Insanity...," *Medical Commentaries* (Edinburgh), Decade 2, Vol. 1 (1787), 302–316. Withering, *Account of the Foxglove*, pp. 134–137 (above, n. 4).

11. William Cullen, *A Treatise of the Materia Medica*, 2 vols. (Edinburgh, 1789), Vol. 1, p. 375. William Cullen, *First Lines of the Practice of Physic*, 3 vols. (Edinburgh, 1790), Vol. 3, p. 262. William Heberden, too, considered foxglove to be a "narcotic," that is, a sedative; but because he wrote in 1782, before Withering's book had appeared, and because he seems not to have been in personal contact with Withering (except, perhaps, second-hand), Heberden may have had in mind the age-old use of foxglove leaves in promoting uneventful wound healing or as treatment for the falling sickness. Heberden, *Commentaries*, p. 9 (above, n. 5).

12. John Coakley Lettsom, "Of the Digitalis Purpurea, in Hydropic Diseases," *Memoirs of the Medical Society of London*, 2 (1794), 145–180.

13. Thomas Beddoes, "An Account of the Good Effects of Opium in the Case of a Person Poisoned by Digitalis," *Medical Facts and Observations*, 5 (1794), 17–20. Withering, *Account of the Foxglove*, p. 188.

14. Ibid., pp. xv–xvi.

15. François Salerne, "Observation de Botanique," *Histoires de l'Academie Royale des Sciences* (1748), 120–122.

16. Thomas Beddoes, *Observations on the Medical and Domestic Management of the Consumption* (Troy, N.Y., O. Penniman, 1803), pp. 114–115, 126–130 (one of a number of reprintings).

17. Ibid., pp. 130–132.

18. Ibid., pp. 132–134.

19. William Currie, "Observations of the Digitalis Purpurea, or Fox-Glove," *Memoirs of the Medical Society of London*, 4 (1795), 10–15. This paper was completed on October 26, 1789.

20. John Ferriar, *An Essay on the Medical Properties of the Digitalis Purpurea or Foxglove* (Manchester, Sowler and Russell, 1799), p. 4.

21. Ibid., pp. 5–9.

22. Ibid., p. 13.

23. Ibid., pp. 13–14.

24. Ibid., pp. 34–36.

25. Ibid., pp. 17, 27–28.

26. John Ferriar, *Medical Histories and Reflections*, 1st American ed. (Philadelphia, Thomas Dobson, 1816), pp. 18–30, 212.

27. Robert Kinglake, ["On the Medical Effects of Digitalis"], *Medical and Physical Journal of London*, 3 (1800), 120–126. Eli Rodin Movitt, *Digitalis and Other Cardiotonic Drugs* (New York, Oxford University Press, 1946), p. 6.

28. John Bailey, ["On Digitalis"], *Medical and Physical Journal of London*, 3 (1800), 127–128.

29. Nathan Drake, "On Digitalis," ibid., p. 305. John Sherwen, ["On Digitalis"], ibid., pp. 307–311. Thomas Harrington, ["On Digitalis"], ibid., pp. 202–206. William Carson, "On the Use of Digitalis," ibid., pp. 513–514.

30. John Penkivil, "On Digitalis," ibid., pp. 315–321.

31. George Mossman, "On the Action of Digitalis," ibid., pp. 311–315.

32. James Magennis, "On the Effects of Digitalis," ibid., pp. 128–135. Sir Charles Aldis, *On the Nature and Cure of Glandular Diseases* ...(London, S. Highley, 1832), p. iv. The time course of digitalis' action in reducing the heart rate in Magennis' patient is consistent with more recent data, e.g., those of Paul D. White and R. R. Sattler, "The Effect of Digitalis on the Normal Human Electrocardiogram, with Especial Reference to A-V Conduction," *Journal of Experimental Medicine*, 23 (1916), 613–629; Paul D. White, Gerardo M. Balboni, and Louis E. Viko, "Clinical Observations on the Digitalis-like Action of Squill," *Journal of the American Medical Association*, 75 (1920), 971–976; and below, n. 80. It would be fruitless, even though tempting, to assess these studies, performed some 120 years apart, in terms of the relative potencies of the preparations used by Magennis and White. Besides, Magennis continued to increase his patient's dose, while White and his co-workers used fixed daily doses to achieve, in normal men, a mean reduction of heart rate of 5 beats per minute.

33. Aldis, *Glandular Diseases*, pp. iii–iv, see n. 32; Magennis, "Effects of Digitalis."

34. Ibid.

35. Ibid.

36. Ibid.

37. John Murray, *Elements of Materia Medica and Pharmacy*, 2 vols. (Edinburgh, A. Neill, 1804), Vol. 1, pp. 131, 300.

38. Charles William Quin, *A Treatise on the Dropsy of the Brain...* [*and*] *on the Use and Effect of Digitalis Purpurea in Dropsies* (London, J. Murray and W. Jones, 1790), pp. 91–92. Quin presented to Withering a copy of Quin's 1779 M.D. thesis on digitalis when they met in Edinburgh that year (Withering, *Account of the Foxglove*, pp. 199–200). Quin did not name the author of the paper he heard at the Royal Medical Society.

39. L. Maclean, *An Inquiry into the Nature, Causes, and Cure of Hydrothorax*, 1810 (1st American ed. Hartford, 1814).

40. L. Maclean, ["Remarks on Digitalis Purpurea"], *Medical and Physical Journal of London*, 2 (1799), 113–127.

41. William Hamilton, *Observations on the Preparation, Utility, and Administration of the Digitalis Purpurea, or Foxglove* (London, Longman, Hurst, Rees, and Orme, 1807), p. 15.

42. John Blackall, *Observations on the Nature and Cure of Dropsies*, 3rd ed. (London, Longman, Hurst, Rees, Orme, and Browne, 1818), pp. 300–302, 340. William Withering, *An Account of the Scarlet Fever* (London, T. Cadell, 1799). For Blackall's role in the development of concepts of proteinuria in dropsy, see William Dock, "Proteinuria: The Story of 280 Years of Trials, Errors, and Rectifications," *Bulletin of the New York Academy of Medicine*, 50 (1974), 659–666.

43. Richard H. Shryock, *Medicine and Society in America 1660–1860* (New York, New York University, 1960), p. 138.
44. Ibid., pp. 35–37.
45. Brooke Hindle, *The Pursuit of Science in Revolutionary America, 1735–1789* (Chapel Hill, University of North Carolina, 1956), pp. 186–187, 236–240.
46. "Books and Stationary...for Sale by Charles Pierce, Portsmouth, 1799," and "Catalogue of Books for Sale at Lamson and Odiorne's, Exeter, [N.H.,] 1794," broadsheets in NHHS. Archibald Malloch, *Medical Interchange Between the British Isles and America Before 1801* (London, Royal College of Physicians, 1946), pp. 127–131.
47. Lawrence Farmer, ed., *Doctors' Legacy* (New York, Harper and Bros., 1955), pp. 54–55.
48. John Shaw Billings, "Literature and Institutions," in E. H. Clarke, ed., *A Century of American Medicine* (Philadelphia, Henry C. Lea, 1876), p. 294. See also above, Chapter 3. Study of the Austin List (above, n. 26 of Chapter 1) would probably reveal more publications in each of Billings' categories.
49. J. Worth Estes, "The New Frontier in 1809: A Brief Look at the World and Work of Dr. Ephraim McDowell of Danville, Kentucky," *Boston Medical Quarterly*, 14 (1963), 153–156.
50. Shryock, *Medicine and Society*, pp. 61, 136 (above, n. 43). Benjamin Spector, "Guideposts in the History of American Medicine," *International Record of Medicine*, 171 (1958), 323–330. "American Philosophical Society Minutes, 1743–1838," *Proceedings of the American Philosophical Society*, 22, Pt. 3 (1885), 1–875. L. Jesse Lemisch, ed., *Benjamin Franklin: The Autobiography and Other Writings* (New York, New American Library, 1961), p. 207. John C. Greene, "Science and the Public in the Age of Jefferson," in Brooke Hindle, ed., *Early American Science* (New York, Science History Publications, 1976), pp. 201–213. Dorothy Long, ed., *Medicine in North Carolina* (Raleigh, North Carolina Medical Society, 1972), p. 34. For a recent study of early American medical theses, see Edward C. Atwater, "'Squeezing Mother Nature': Experimental Physiology in the United States before 1870," *Bulletin of the History of Medicine*, 52 (1978), 313–335.
51. Ibid., p. 97. J. Davidson Frame and Francis Narin, "The International Distribution of Biomedical Publications," *Federation Proceedings*, 36 (1977), 1790–1795.
52. George W. Corner, *Two Centuries of Medicine* (Philadelphia, J. B. Lippincott, 1965), p. 52. Rush, *Medical Inquiries*, Vol. 3, p. 234 (above, n. 5).
53. Benjamin Rush, *Medical Inquiries and Observations*, 2nd ed., 2 vols. (Philadelphia, T. Dobson, 1793), Vol. 2, pp. 166, 173. George W. Corner, ed., *The Autobiography of Benjamin Rush* (Princeton, Princeton University Press, 1948), p. 281.
54. James Mease, "On the Digitalis Purpurea," *Medical Repository*, 1 (1797), 145–152.

55. James S. Stringham, "On the Efficacy of the Digitalis Purpurea in Allaying Excessive Action of the Sanguiferous System," ibid., 4 (1801), 108–112.
56. [Editorial], "Digitalis Purpurea," ibid., 312–314.
57. Mahlon Gregg, "On the Salivating Effects of Digitalis Purpurea, or Common Foxglove," *Philadelphia Medical and Physical Journal*, 1 (1804), 80–81. Benjamin Smith Barton, "Editor's Note," ibid., 81–82.
58. Benjamin Smith Barton, *Collections for an Essay Towards a Materia Medica* ... (Philadelphia, Way and Groff, 1798), p. 34. Benjamin Smith Barton, *Elements of Botany*, 3rd ed. (Philadelphia, Robert DeSilver, 1827), p. 79.
59. Isaac Rand, *Observations on Phthisis Pulmonalis* (Boston, The Repertory Office, 1804), pp. 7–8, 13.
60. John Redman Coxe, *The American Dispensatory* (Philadelphia, Carey and Lea, 1806), pp. 270–272.
61. John Collins Warren, "Organic Diseases of the Heart," *Medical Communications and Dissertations of the Massachusetts Medical Society*, 2 (1813), 49–109, p. 87.
62. John Welsh Croskey, *History of Blockley* (Philadelphia, F. A. Davis, 1929), p. 446.
63. John Moore, *An Inaugural Dissertation on Digitalis Purpurea, or Fox-Glove, and Its Use in Some Diseases* (Philadelphia, Way and Groff, 1800), p. 5.
64. Charles D. O'Malley, "A Translation of William Withering's *De Angina Gangraenosa*," *Journal of the History of Medicine*, 8 (1953), 16–45.
65. Moore, *Dissertation on Digitalis*, p. 10.
66. Ibid., pp. 17–18.
67. "Urbanitas," [Correspondence], *Philadelphia Medical Museum*, 4 (1807), 152.
68. Moore, *Dissertation on Digitalis*, pp. 19–20. "Digitalis Purpurea," *Medical Repository*, 1 (1797), 312–314. Moore performed his experiments IV and VII on his "worthy friend and colleague, Dr. Enoch Wilson," who later reported "On the Salivating and Other Effects of the Digitalis Purpurea, in a Case of Dropsy," *Philadelphia Medical and Physical Journal*, 1 (1805), 48–54. Wilson saw his patient in 1801, a year or so after he had participated in Moore's experiments.
69. Information kindly supplied by Mrs. Kathleen Conway, Assistant Executive Secretary, Medical Alumni Society of the University of Pennsylvania.
70. Lewis Burwell, *Observations on the Digitalis Purpurea, or Fox-Glove* (Philadelphia, printed for the author by Hugh Maxwell, 1805), pp. 10, 13, 17.
71. Ibid., pp. 16–18.
72. Information kindly supplied by Mrs. Mary D. McGuire, Director of

Alumni Affairs, College of Physicians and Surgeons, Columbia University.

73. Thomas Edward Steell, *An Inaugural Dissertation on the Use of the Digitalis Purpurea in the Cure of Certain Diseases* (New York, T. and J. Swords, 1811), pp. 7–8.

74. Daniel J. Boorstin, *The Americans: The Colonial Experience* (New York, Vintage, 1958), p. 214. Richard N. Goodwin, "The American Condition," *The New Yorker* (January 21, 1974), 35–60.

75. Steell, *Dissertation on the Use of Digitalis*, pp. 10–12.

76. Ibid., pp. 16–17.

77. Ibid., pp. 20–21.

78. Ibid., pp. 23–25.

79. Ibid., pp. 25–31.

80. Harry Gold, McKeen Cattell, Theodore Greiner, et al., "Clinical Pharmacology of Digoxin," *Journal of Pharmacology and Experimental Therapeutics*, 109 (1953), 47–57.

81. Steell, *Dissertation on the Use of Digitalis*, p. 29.

82. *Medical Repertory*, 15 (1812), 86.

83. William Currie, *An Historical Account of the Climates and Diseases of the United States of America* (Philadelphia, T. Dobson, 1792), pp. 61, 240; see also above, n. 7.

84. Ibid., p. 244.

85. James Ewell, *The Planter's and Mariner's Medical Companion* (Philadelphia, John Bioren, 1807), pp. 144–146.

86. Bryce A. Smith, "Notes on the Materia Medica of Nathan Smith," *Yale Journal of Biology and Medicine*, 11 (1939), 189–205.

87. Solomon Drowne, manuscript note, n.d. [probably 1811–1830], in Drowne Papers, no. A8850, John Hay Library, Brown University, Providence, R.I.

88. Actually, the chain can be traced back to the Hippocratic and Galenic writings. It *could* not be broken until the rise of experimental medicine and pharmacology in the mid-nineteenth century, when the ancient theories and hypotheses could first be tested and, only then, rejected. For details of the chain, see Owsei Temkin, *Galenism: Rise and Decline of a Medical Philosophy* (Ithaca, Cornell University Press, 1973), and Lester S. King, *The Growth of Medical Thought* (Chicago, University of Chicago Press, 1963). As Temkin and King point out, the results of eighteenth-century experiments could only be interpreted in the light of the experimenters' understanding of medicine, as is exemplified by the theses of Moore, Burwell, and Steell. I have begun to study the implications of this dictum for the overall efficacy of general medical therapy in late colonial New England (see Estes, "Therapeutic Practice," cited in n. 34, above, Chapter 1).

## 6. The Purple Foxglove

1. HJ to William Withering, February 9, 1786, collection of Withering letters bequeathed to the Royal Society of Medicine, London, by Sir William Osler. An incomplete draft or copy of this letter is in Vol. 1 of the Plumer Papers, NHSL, pp. 23–26. See, for a discussion of Withering's specific contributions in his 1785 volume, J. Worth Estes and Paul Dudley White, "William Withering and the Purple Foxglove," *Scientific American*, 212 (1965), 110–119.

   Hall Jackson's correspondence with Withering and with Holyoke and Appleton, as outlined below, exemplifies the critical role of the postal service in disseminating information in colonial and early republican America. Not only did letters carry new information, they multiplied the audiences for that which was contained in books, which were seldom printed in editions of more than 300 to 500. William K. Beatty and Virginia L. Beatty, "Sources of Medical Information," *Journal of the American Medical Association*, 236 (1976), 78–82. Hellmut Lehmann-Haupt, *The Book in America*, 2nd ed. (New York, R. R. Bowker, 1952), pp. 33, 40.

2. Russell Leigh Jackson, "Dr. Hall Jackson of Portsmouth," *Annals of Medical History*, new ser., 5 (1933), 103–128. But see also above, n. 4 to Chapter 1; R. L. Jackson wrote that his collateral ancestor spent several years in England, and that he had known Withering and Dr. Erasmus Darwin there; obviously, neither of these assertions is true.

3. *Dictionary of National Biography*, s.v. "Thomas Percival" and "Charles White."

4. British Patent Office, *Abridgements of Specifications Relating to Medicine, Surgery, and Dentistry . . . A. D. 1620–1866* (London, Office of the Commissioners of Patents for Inventions, 1872), pp. 5, 12, 19, 34, 42. For a summary of the medical uses of squill, see "Symposium on Squill," with papers by Saul Jarcho, Jerry Stannard, David L. Cowen, and Chalmers L. Gemmill, *Bulletin of the New York Academy of Medicine*, 50 (1974), 682–750. It will be clear from these papers that digitalis did not *replace* squill, which seems to have been regarded as unpredictable in its efficacy. Squill may provide a good historical example of a drug which, by 1785, had been around for too long to permit further systematic study of its efficacy in the treatment of the disease it had long been presumed to be able to cure (this paradox still finds exemplification today). That squill offers no significant or consistent advantage over digitalis was forcefully demonstrated in Paul D. White, Gerardo M. Balboni, and Louis E. Viko, "Clinical Observations on the Digitalis-like Action of Squill," *Journal of the American Medical Association*, 75 (1920), 971–976.

5. Withering's other published works follow:
   *De Angina Gangraenosa* (Edinburgh, Auld and Smellie, 1766). For

an English translation, see *Journal of the History of Medicine*, 8 (1953), 16–45.

"Experiments upon the Different Kinds of Marle Found in Staffordshire," *Philosophical Transactions of the Royal Society*, 63 (1773), 161.

*A Botanical Arrangement of All the Vegetables Naturally Growing in Great Britain*, 2 vols. (Birmingham, M. Swinney, 1776).

*An Account of the Scarlet Fever* ... (London, T. Cadell, 1779; 2nd ed., Birmingham, M. Swinney, 1793).

"An Analysis of Two Mineral Substances, viz. the Rowley Rag-Stone and the Toad-Stone," ibid., 72 (1782), 327–336.

Trans. of Torbern Bergman, *Outlines of Mineralogy* (Birmingham, Piercy and Jones, 1783).

"Experiments and Observations on the Terra Ponderosa," ibid., 74 (1784), 293–311.

"A Letter on Arsenical Solution," in Thomas Fowler, *Medicinal Reports of the Effects of Arsenic* ... (London: J. Johnson and William Brown, 1786), pp. 113–131.

"A Letter to Joseph Priestley, L.L.D. on the Principle of Acidity, the Decomposition of Water," ibid., 78 (1788), 319–330.

"An Account of Some Extraordinary Effects of Lightning," ibid., 80 (1790), 293–295.

*A Botanical Arrangement of British Plants*, 2nd ed., 3 vols. (Birmingham, M. Swinney, 1787–92).

"A New Method of Preserving Fungi, Ascertained by Chymical Experiment," *Transactions of the Linnean Society*, 2 (1794), 263–266.

"A Letter on Pulmonary Consumption," in Thomas Beddoes, ed., *Letters from Dr. Withering, Dr. Ewart, Dr. Thornton, and Dr. Briggs* ... (Bristol, 1794).

*Analyse Chimica da Aqua das Caldas da Rainha. A Chemical Analysis of the Water of Caldas da Rainha* (Lisbon, Printed by the Academy, 1795).

*An Arrangement of British Plants*, 3rd ed., 3 vols. (Birmingham, M. Swinney, 1796). The 4th edition was edited by William Withering, Jr., and the 14th and last edition was published in 1877.

"Observations on Pneumatic Medicine," *Annals of Medicine*, 1 (1796), 392–393.

"An Account of a Convenient Method of Inhaling the Vapour of Volatile Substances," ibid., 3 (1799), 447–451.

6.  William Withering to HJ, October 27, 1786. Boston Medical Library. This letter had been among the family papers of Mrs. Henry B. Shepard of West Newton, Mass., along with some HJ manuscript letters, all of which descended to her through her great-grandfather, Dr. William Perry of Exeter, N.H. Dr. Perry (1788–1887), who had studied with Drs. James Thacher of Plymouth and John Collins

Warren of Boston, received his M.D. degree from Harvard in 1814 (Isaac A. Watson, *Physicians and Surgeons of America*, Concord, N.H., Republican Free Press Association, 1898). It is not known how the HJ materials came into Dr. Perry's possession, but Mrs. Shepard suggests that they may have been given to him by Dr. William Parker, Jr., of Exeter, whose name was on the wrappers enclosing them. Parker must have known Jackson, for both were among the founding members of the New Hampshire Medical Society.

Following a clue in Francis Packard's *History of Medicine in America*, I had searched for the Withering letter for about ten years but had given up the quest as a lost cause when, in a prototypical serendipitous encounter, Mrs. Shepard brought it to my attention in March 1970 after hearing me lecture on plants of medical importance, during which I had discussed Withering's contribution at some length. I would never have found it otherwise, since it was not in any public collection. Subsequently, Mrs. Shepard very generously gave it to the Boston Medical Library.

The abridgment of Withering's letter that HJ sent to Yale's president Ezra Stiles has been reprinted several times, most recently in Douglas Carroll, "Introduction of Digitalis into North America," *New England Journal of Medicine* 235, (1946), 808–810; that reprinting had been taken directly from *The American Museum* (Philadelphia), 3 (1788), 59–60, to which it had probably been contributed by Stiles. Before the discovery of the original Withering letter, it must have been that abridgment which constituted the evidence used to support modern but undocumented claims (e.g. by Packard) that Jackson was the first to introduce digitalis to America. Dr. Carroll has written to me that Dr. Reginald Fitz had written to him that descendants of Jackson's foxglove seeds still grew at Yale earlier in this century.

7. *Biographical Directory of the American Congress, 1774–1961* (Washington, D.C., U.S. Government Printing Office, 1963), p. 1140. A. G. Brown, Jr., "Virginia's Physician-Generals in the Revolution," *Sons of the Revolution in State of Virginia Quarterly Magazine*, 2 no. 2 (April 1923), 12–22. James Thacher, *American Medical Biography* (Boston, Richardson and Lord; Cottons and Barnard, 1828), p. 344. Jackson Turner Main, *The Social Structure of Revolutionary America* (Princeton, Princeton University Press, 1965), p. 146. T. W. Peck and K. D. Wilkinson, *William Withering of Birmingham* (London, Simpkin Marshall, 1950), p. 41. The last reference, the only detailed biography of Withering, is difficult to use as source material, because it contains no specific citations of the authors' primary sources. Main points out that Walter Jones spent 118 pounds a year during his three years at Edinburgh, about 30 or 40 pounds less than the average amount required to keep up a "tolerable genteel character." His papers are at the Virginia His-

torical Society, Richmond, and the University of Virginia Library, Manuscripts Division, Charlottesville.

8. Manasseh Cutler, *An Account of Some of the Vegetable Productions Naturally Growing in This Part of America* (Boston, American Academy of Arts and Sciences, 1785), pp. 401, 465. William Withering, *A Botanical Arrangment of All the Vegetables Naturally Growing in Great Britain...*, 2 vols. (Birmingham, M. Swinney, 1776), Vol. 1, p. 376. Cutler must have used this first edition (see above, n. 5, for other editions). In the book, published just as he began his ten-year study of the foxglove, Withering had only this to say about the plant's medical properties: "A dram of it taken inwardly excites violent vomiting. It is certainly a very active medicine, and merits more attention than modern practice bestows upon it."

9. *Dictionary of American Biography*, s.v. "Manasseh Cutler."

10. William Parker Cutler and Julia Perkins Cutler, *Life, Journals, and Correspondence of Reverend Manasseh Cutler*, 2 vols. (Cincinnati, R. Clarke & Co., 1888), Vol. 1, p. 43.

11. Ibid., Vol. 2, p. 296.

12. James H. Cassedy, "An Early American Hangover: The Medical Profession and Intemperance 1800–1860," *Bulletin of the History of Medicine*, 50 (1976), 405–413. Daniel J. Boorstin, *The Americans: The Colonial Experience* (New York, Vintage, 1958), p. 238.

13. HJ, "Meteorological Register"; see above, Chapter 3 and n. 41, for a detailed discussion of this manuscript. Robert E. Schofield, *The Lunar Society of Birmingham* (Oxford, Clarendon Press, 1963), pp. 3–4.

14. Thomas Fowler, *Medical Reports of the Effects of Arsenic in the Cure of Agues, Remitting Fevers, and Periodic Headaches* (London, J. Johnson and William Brown, 1786), pp. 113–131. William Withering, *An Account of the Foxglove* (Birmingham, M. Swinney, 1785), pp. 121–122. According to the custom of the day, perhaps a thousand copies of Withering's book were printed. No subsequent editions, save for twentieth-century facsimile or reprint editions, in whole or in part, have been issued. In his letter to Fowler, Withering notes that 75 percent of the 48 patients whom he treated with arsenic were cured of their illness; of those 36 who were cured, 8 percent showed signs of arsenic toxicity.

15. Withering, *Account of the Foxglove*, p. 192.

16. Ibid., pp. 80–81, 144–146.

17. Russell Leigh Jackson, *The Physicians of Essex County* (Salem, Mass., The Essex Institute, 1948), pp. 58–61. Stephen W. Williams, *American Medical Biography* (Greenfield, Mass., L. Merriam and Co., 1845), pp. 251–275. Dr. Holyoke's Scrapbook, EAH Manuscripts, EI.

18. Williams, pp. 18–19.

19. NWA to EAH, October 14, 1786, EAH, EI, Vol. 2, p. 64.

20. HJ to EAH, April 24, 1787, ibid., p. 68.
21. EAH to HJ, May 3, 1787, ibid., p. 69. HJ to EAH, May 24, 1787, ibid., p. 70.
22. NWA to EAH, May 17, 1787, ibid., p. 69.
23. Walter L. Burrage, *A History of the Massachusetts Medical Society* (privately printed, 1923), p. 25.
24. NWA to EAH, October 10, 1787, EAH, EI, Vol. 2, p. 72. NWA to EAH, October 22, 1787, ibid., p. 72. William Jones, "An Account of Two Cases of Insanity, One of Which Was Cured by the Use of the Fox-glove. Also a Case of Hemoptysis, Cured by the Same Remedy," *Medical Commentaries* (Edinburgh), Decade 2, Vol. 1 (1787), 302–316. Withering, *Account of the Foxglove*, pp. 134–137.
25. HJ to EAH, February 27, 1788, EAH, EI, Vol. 2, p. 73.
26. NWA to EAH, n.d. (? spring 1788), ibid., p. 142.
27. NWA to EAH, February 8, 1788, ibid., p. 74. NWA to EAH, March 20, 1788, ibid., p. 74. NWA to EAH, April 18, 1789, ibid., p. 80.
28. HJ to EAH, July 12, 1790, ibid., p. 90.
29. HJ, "Some Cases of the Administration of the Foxglove," manuscript, 8 pages, n.d. (? 1790), ibid., Vol. 1, p. 53. HJ's first draft of this report was among the papers given to the Boston Medical Library by Mrs. Shepard (n. 6 above).
30. Estes and White, "William Withering and the Purple Foxglove."
31. Rev. Matthew Merriam to HJ, February 5, 1789, EAH, EI, Vol. 2, p. 79.
32. HJ to EAH, July 12, 1790, ibid., p. 90.
33. NWA to EAH, January 22, 1791, ibid., p. 92.
34. NWA to EAH, March 11, 1791, ibid., p. 94. NWA to EAH, April 5, 1791, ibid., p. 96.
35. NWA to EAH, April 18, 1791, ibid., p. 96.
36. NWA to EAH, April 26, 1791, ibid., p. 97. Essex South Medical District, *Memoir of Edward Augustus Holyoke, M.D., LL.D.* (Boston, Perkins and Marvin, 1829). Williams, *American Medical Biography*, p. 265.
37. Dr. J. Barker to EAH, May 1, 1799, EAH, EI, Vol. 2, p. 112.
38. Dr. Isaac Rand to EAH, March 1, 1813, ibid., p. 127. Dr. Isaac Rand to EAH, March 15, 1813, ibid., p. 128.
39. Isaac Rand, *Observations on Phthisis Pulmonalis* (Boston, Repertory Office, 1804).
40. James Thacher, *American Medical Biography* (Boston, Richardson and Lord; Cottons and Barnard, 1828), pp. 311–313.
41. James Thacher, *American Medical Practice* (Boston, Ezra Reed, 1817), pp. 554–555.
42. HJ to Ezra Stiles, April 30, 1787, Beinecke Rare Book and Manuscript Library, Yale University. Jackson's draft of this letter is in Vol. 1 of the Plumer Papers in the NHSL. *American Museum* (Philadelphia), 3 (1788), 59–60. Nathaniel Adams, *Annals of Ports-*

*mouth* (Portsmouth, published by the author, 1825), pp. 266–267.

43. Thomas Jefferson, *Notes on the State of Virginia* (1781; rep. New York, Harper and Row, 1964). J. U. Lloyd, "Digitalis. Foxglove," *American Journal of Pharmacy*, 85 (1913), 214–228.

44. Anne Leighton, *Early American Gardens: For Meate or Medicine* (Boston, Houghton Mifflin, 1970). E. G. Swem, *Brothers of the Spade: Correspondence of Peter Collinson, of London, and of John Custis, of Williamsburg, Virginia, 1734–1746* (Barre, Mass., Barre Gazette, 1957), p. 46.

45. Ibid., pp. 48, 53, 58.

46. Adolph B. Benson, ed., *Peter Kalm's Travels in North America: The English Version of 1770* (New York, Dover, 1966), pp. 100, 107.

47. Thomas Short, *Medicina Britannica*, 3rd ed. (Philadelphia, B. Franklin and D. Hall, 1751), p. 108. Helen G. Cruikshank, ed., *John and William Bartram's America* (New York, Anchor, 1961).

48. John Hill, *The British Herbal* (London, 1756), plate 17, no. 15. George S. Rousseau, "The Much-Maligned Doctor: 'Sir' John Hill (1707–1775)," *Journal of the American Medical Association*, 212 (1970), 103–108.

49. William Darlington, *Memorials of John Bartram and Humphrey Marshall* (Philadelphia, Lindsay and Blakiston, 1849), pp. 568–569. John Fothergill in England had written to Humphrey Marshall in 1771, four years before Withering began his studies, to ask if there were any native American plants that could cure dropsy. "We can vomit, purge, sweat, to what degree we please, but have no certain diuretic. This is much wanted in the cure of dropsies and other complaints." Betsy Copping Corner and C. C. Booth, eds., *Chain of Friendship* (Cambridge, Harvard University Press, 1971), p. 327. However, we have no clues as to whether the desired anti-dropsical drug plant was in Dr. Marshall's garden at that time. Even if it had been, it would have been imported, for it was not native to America. Professor Robert Benson Gordon very kindly searched the Marshall herbaria at West Chester State College for me.

50. William P. C. Barton, *Compendium Florae Philadelphicae* (Philadelphia, 1818). John Torrey, *Catalog of Plants Growing Spontaneously Within Thirty Miles of the City of New York* (Albany, 1819). Amos Eaton, *Manual of Botany for North America* (Albany, Webster and Skinners, 1829).

51. Jacob Bigelow, *Florula Bostoniensis*, 3rd ed. (Boston, Charles C. Little; James Brown, 1840). J. Worth Estes, "Concordance of Dr. Waterhouse's *Hortus Siccus*," in Lloyd E. Hawes, *Benjamin Waterhouse, M.D.* (Boston, Countway Library of Medicine, 1974), pp. 18–28.

52. Jacob Bigelow, *A Treatise on the Materia Medica, Intended as a Sequel to the Pharmacopoeia of the United States* (Boston, Charles Ewer, 1822), pp. 162–166.

53. Henry T. Drowne, ed., *Journal . . . by Solomon Drowne, M.D.*

(New York, Charles L. Moreau, 1972). [Solomon Drowne], "Catalogue of Trees, Shrubs, & Herbaceous Plants in my Garden," manuscript, n.d. (probably 1792–94), Drowne Papers, no. D566, John Hay Library, Brown University.

54. HJ to Mr. Avery, October 15, 1791, Boston Medical Library (above, n. 6).
55. William Plumer, "Biographies," manuscript in NHHS, Vol. 3, pp. 654–656, June 26, 1829.

## 7. Patterns and Conclusions

1.  Erwin H. Ackerknecht, "Aspects of the History of Therapeutics," *Bulletin of the History of Medicine*, 36 (1962), 389–419.
2.  Milton G. Bohrod, "Medical Genealogy," *Journal of the History of Medicine*, 24 (1969), 292–293.
3.  William Currie, *A View of the Diseases Most Prevalent in the United States of America at Different Seasons of the Year* (Philadelphia, J. and A. Y. Humphreys, 1811), p. 168.
4.  Ackerknecht, "Therapeutics."
5.  David H. Crombe, "Determination and Correlation of Factors Influencing New Drug Acceptance by Physicians," unpublished manuscript, 1972, in the author's possession.
6.  However, retail drug advertising, directed toward the suffering, flourished during this period. See, for instance, P. S. Brown, "Medicines Advertised in Eighteenth-Century Bath Newspapers," *Medical History*, 20 (1976), 152–168.
7.  [William Brown], *Pharmacopoeia Simplicorum et Efficaciorum in Usum Nosocomii Militaris ad Exercitum Foederatarum Americae Civitatum* (Philadelphia, Styner and Cist, 1778).
8.  *The Pharmacopoeia of the Massachusetts Medical Society* (Boston, E. and J. Larkin, 1808), pp. 14, 97, 183.
9.  *Pharmacopoeia Nosocomii Neo-Eboracensis* (New York, Collins, 1816), pp. 59, 120. *The Pharmacopoeia of the United States of America* (Boston, Wells, 1820), pp. 34, 148, 227.
10. Ernest Jawetz, "Infectious Diseases: Problems of Antimicrobial Therapy," *Annual Review of Medicine*, 5 (1954), 1–26.
11. The precipitous rise and fall and the gradual reemergence of chloramphenicol can be studied in, among other sources, the following: Quentin R. Bartz, "Isolation and Characterization of Chloromycetin," *Journal of Biological Chemistry*, 172 (1948), 445–450; Eugene H. Payne, Jose A. Knaudt, and Sylvio Palacios, "Treatment of Epidemic Typhus with Chloromycetin," *Journal of Tropical Medicine and Hygiene*, 51 (1948), 68–71; J. Worth Estes, *Post Hoc Quantitative Assessment of Drug Side Effects in Man* (M.A. thesis, Boston University, 1963, abstract in *Pharmacologist*, 15, 1973, 189); William R. Best, "Chloramphenicol-Associated Blood Dys-

crasias," *Journal of the American Medical Association*, 201 (1967), 181–188; package insert for chloramphenicol, distributed by Food and Drug Administration, USDHEW, May 7, 1968; "Putting Chloramphenicol into Perspective," *Medical World News* (September 13, 1968), pp. 36–38; Louis S. Goodman and Alfred Gilman, eds., *The Pharmacological Basis of Therapeutics*, 5th ed. (New York, Macmillan, 1975), pp. 1194–98; Henry E. Simmons and Paul B. Stolley, "This Is Medical Progress?," *Journal of the American Medical Association*, 227 (1974) 1023–28; John C. Ballin, Michael H. M. Dykes, Joseph B. Jerome, et al., "In Comment," ibid., 1029–30; Calvin M. Kunin, "In Comment," ibid., 1030–32; Milton M. Howell, "In Comment," ibid., 1032.

12. Jawetz, "Infectious Diseases" (above, n. 10).

13. Sir Charles Aldis, *On the Nature and Cure of Glandular Diseases* (London, S. Highley, 1832), pp. iii–iv.

14. A. L. J. Bayle, *Bibliotheque de Therapeutique* . . . (Paris, J.-B. Bailliere, 1835), Vol. 3, pp. 362–363, 370.

15. Jabez Dow, "Manuscript No. 1, Ointments," Jabez Dow Papers, Boston Medical Library, pp. 19–23.

16. George B. Wood, *A Treatise on Therapeutics and Pharmacology*, 2nd ed. (Philadelphia, J. B. Lippincott, 1860), pp. 118–119. J. A. Myers, "Development of Knowledge of Unity of Tuberculosis and of the Portals of Entry of Tubercle Bacilli," *Journal of the History of Medicine and Allied Sciences*, 29 (1974), 213–228.

17. Franz J. Ingelfinger, "Shattuck Lecture—The General Medical Journal: for Readers or Repositories?," *New England Journal of Medicine*, 296 (1977), 1258–64.

18. Andrew Katsampes, "The Sources of Different Views of the Accumulation of Knowledge about Digitalis," unpublished term paper, Boston University Graduate School, Department of Pharmacology and Experimental Therapeutics, December 17, 1975. Sir John MacMichael, "The History of Ideas on Digitalis Action," in B. H. Marks and A. M. Weissler, eds., *Basic and Clinical Pharmacology of Digitalis* (Springfield, Ill., Charles C. Thomas, 1972), pp. 5–14. Richard H. Orr and Alice A. Leeds, "Biomedical Literature: Volume, Growth, and Other Characteristics," *Federation Proceedings*, 23 (1964), 1310–31.

19. Lester S. King, "Rationalism in Early Eighteenth Century Medicine," *Journal of the History of Medicine*, 18 (1963), 257–271.

20. *The Charter of the New Hampshire Medical Society* (Exeter, N.H., Henry Ranlet, 1792). Nathaniel Adams, *Annals of Portsmouth* (Portsmouth, published by the author, 1825), pp. 315–316. Clifford K. Shipton, *Sibley's Harvard Graduates* (Boston, Massachusetts Historical Society, 1968), Vol. 14, s.v. "Jackson, Hall." *Federal Fire Society of Portsmouth, N. H.* (Portsmouth, published by the Society, 1905), pp. 5–7. *Medical Papers Contributed to the Massachusetts Medical Society*, 1 (Boston, Thomas and Andrews,

1790), p. xiii. HJ to NWA, November 9, 1783, *Massachusetts Medical Society Documents*, Boston Medical Library, Vol. 1, shelf list B MS b 75.1, p. 155.

21. HJ, "Meteorological Register," manuscript journal (see above, n. 41 of Chapter 3). Lawrence Shaw Mayo, *John Langdon of New Hampshire*, 1937 (rep. Port Washington, N.Y., Kennikat, 1970), pp. 216–221. Adams, *Annals*, passim. Broadside, "Procession in Honor of President Washington," October 19, 1789, MHS. J. Worth Estes, "Honest Dr. Thornton: The Path to Rebellion," in George E. Gifford, Jr., ed., *Physician Signers of the Declaration of Independence* (New York, Science History Publications, 1976), pp. 70–98.

22. The portrait of HJ is in the Department of Fine Arts, Amherst College, Amherst, Mass. Miss Margaret C. Toole, former curator of Amherst's collection, has written to me: "The portrait...was bequeathed...by Herbert Lee Pratt of Long Island in 1945. According to a letter from Mr. Russell Leigh Jackson [above, n. 4 of Chapter 1], 'The portrait was painted in Portsmouth, N. H., and was hanging in Dr. Jackson's house at the time of his death when his sister...took it off the wall and carried it to Newbury, Mass.' The painting descended in the family to her daughter Mary Little Pearson, wife of Silas Pearson, Jr.; to her daughter Sarah Jackson Pearson Leigh, wife of Benjamin Leigh, the 3rd; then to her son, Hall Jackson Leigh; and then to his son, Amos Little Leigh, who was the grandfather of Russell Leigh Jackson. Mr. Jackson also stated that the family had had Copley's bill, dated April 2, 1772, for well over a hundred years." Experts on eighteenth-century American portraits are, however, uncertain whether Copley did, in fact, paint the portrait of Jackson. At any rate, it is the only portrait even thought to be of him.

23. Judge W. Parker, Exeter, to HJ, November 29, 1779, MSS file 17B-7, NHHS. HJ to Selectmen of Marblehead, November 22, 1787, MTA.

24. Adams, *Annals*, p. 315. *Oracle of the Day* (Portsmouth), September 30, 1797. *Columbian Centinel* (Boston), (October 7, 1797). Russell P. Stearns, *Science in the British Colonies of America* (Urbana, University of Illinois Press, 1970), p. 274.

25. Adams, *Annals*, p. 316.

26. Timothy Alden, *A Collection of American Epitaphs and Inscriptions* (New York, 1814), Vol. 2, pp. 134–135.

27. David Nichol Smith, ed., *The Oxford Book of Eighteenth Century Verse* (Oxford: Clarendon Press, 1928), p. 391. Henry F. May, *The Enlightenment in America* (New York, Oxford University Press, 1976), p. 18.

28. HJ, "Meteorological Register" (above, n. 41 of Chapter 3); the poem is inscribed on the flyleaves of Vol. 1, and is dated July 1785. I cannot verify that HJ was the author of the poem; it may be one that he had read and liked, so copied it into his journal.

29. *Portsmouth Herald* (April 29, 1976), p. 4.
30. William Plumer, "Biographies," unpublished manuscript, Vol. 3, pp. 654–656 (June 26, 1829), NHHS.
31. Jonathan N. Sewall, *Miscellaneous Poems* (Portsmouth, William Treadwell, 1801). The last line of the poem on the gravestone in Portsmouth's North Cemetery has become buried by the turf around the stone.
32. Louis C. Duncan, *Medical Men in the American Revolution 1775–1783*, Army Medical Bulletin 25 (Carlisle Barracks, Pa., Medical Field Service School, 1931), pp. 105–106. Maurice Bear Gordon, *Aesculapius Comes to the Colonies*, 1940 (rep. New York, Argosy-Antiquarian, 1969), pp. 140–141.
33. Donald A. Henderson, "The Eradication of Smallpox," *Scientific American*, 235 (October 1976), 25–33.

# Index

Asterisks (*) indicate pages with patients known to have been treated by Dr. Hall Jackson. The title Dr. is used to indicate physicians, including surgeons who in England preferred to use the traditional honorific Mr.

Library of Congress Cataloging in Publication Data

Estes, J　Worth, 1934–
　Hall Jackson and the purple foxglove.

　Includes bibliographical references and index.
　　1. Jackson, Hall, 1739–1797. 2. Physicians—
New Hampshire—Portsmouth—Biography. 3. Digitalis—
History—18th century. 4. Withering, William,
1741–1799. 5. Edema—History—18th century.
6. Congestive heart failure—History—18th century.
7. Portsmouth, N.H.—Statistics, Medical. 8. Medicine—United States—History—18th century. I. Title.
R154.J27E83　610'.92'4 [B]　79–63083
ISBN 0-87451-173-9

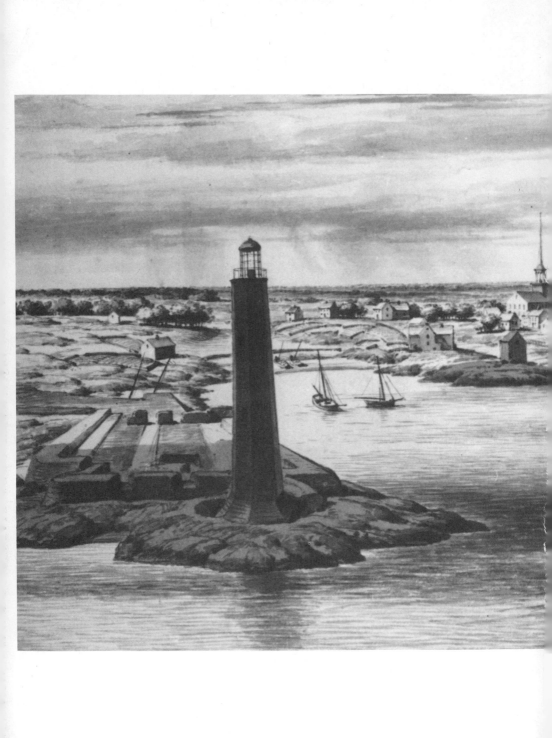